New Perspectives in Health: Gut Microbiota

New Perspectives in Health: Gut Microbiota

Editors

Diana María Cardona Mena
Pablo Roman

MDPI • Basel • Beijing • Wuhan • Barcelona • Belgrade • Manchester • Tokyo • Cluj • Tianjin

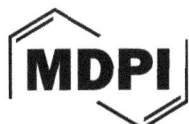

Editors
Diana María Cardona Mena
Department of Nursing,
Physiotherapy and Medicine,
Health Research
Center (CEINSA),
University of Almeria,
04120 Almeria, Spain

Pablo Roman
Department of Nursing,
Physiotherapy and Medicine,
Health Research
Center (CEINSA),
University of Almeria,
04120 Almeria, Spain

Editorial Office
MDPI
St. Alban-Anlage 66
4052 Basel, Switzerland

This is a reprint of articles from the Special Issue published online in the open access journal *International Journal of Environmental Research and Public Health* (ISSN 1660-4601) (available at: https://www.mdpi.com/journal/ijerph/special_issues/health_microbiota).

For citation purposes, cite each article independently as indicated on the article page online and as indicated below:

LastName, A.A.; LastName, B.B.; LastName, C.C. Article Title. *Journal Name* **Year**, *Volume Number*, Page Range.

ISBN 978-3-0365-5279-8 (Hbk)
ISBN 978-3-0365-5280-4 (PDF)

© 2022 by the authors. Articles in this book are Open Access and distributed under the Creative Commons Attribution (CC BY) license, which allows users to download, copy and build upon published articles, as long as the author and publisher are properly credited, which ensures maximum dissemination and a wider impact of our publications.

The book as a whole is distributed by MDPI under the terms and conditions of the Creative Commons license CC BY-NC-ND.

Contents

Diana Cardona and Pablo Roman
New Perspectives in Health: Gut Microbiota
Reprinted from: *Int. J. Environ. Res. Public Health* **2022**, *19*, 5828, doi:10.3390/ijerph19105828 . . . 1

Diana Cardona, Pablo Roman, Fernando Cañadas and Nuria Sánchez-Labraca
The Effect of Multiprobiotics on Memory and Attention in Fibromyalgia: A Pilot Randomized Controlled Trial
Reprinted from: *Int. J. Environ. Res. Public Health* **2021**, *18*, 3543, doi:10.3390/ijerph18073543 . . . 5

Oscar Lorenzo, Marta Crespo-Yanguas, Tianyu Hang, Jairo Lumpuy-Castillo, Artur M. Hernández, Carolina Llavero, MLuisa García-Alonso and Jaime Ruiz-Tovar
Addition of Probiotics to Anti-Obesity Therapy by Percutaneous Electrical Stimulation of Dermatome T6. A Pilot Study
Reprinted from: *Int. J. Environ. Res. Public Health* **2020**, *17*, 7239, doi:10.3390/ijerph17197239 . . . 17

Miguel Rodriguez-Arrastia, Adrian Martinez-Ortigosa, Lola Rueda-Ruzafa, Ana Folch Ayora and Carmen Ropero-Padilla
Probiotic Supplements on Oncology Patients' Treatment-Related Side Effects: A Systematic Review of Randomized Controlled Trials
Reprinted from: *Int. J. Environ. Res. Public Health* **2021**, *18*, 4265, doi:10.3390/ijerph18084265 . . . 31

Lidia Stasiak-Różańska, Anna Berthold-Pluta, Antoni Stanisław Pluta, Krzysztof Dasiewicz and Monika Garbowska
Effect of Simulated Gastrointestinal Tract Conditions on Survivability of Probiotic Bacteria Present in Commercial Preparations
Reprinted from: *Int. J. Environ. Res. Public Health* **2021**, *18*, 1108, doi:10.3390/ijerph18031108 . . . 47

Lucía Guadamuro, M. Andrea Azcárate-Peril, Rafael Tojo, Baltasar Mayo and Susana Delgado
Impact of Dietary Isoflavone Supplementation on the Fecal Microbiota and Its Metabolites in Postmenopausal Women
Reprinted from: *Int. J. Environ. Res. Public Health* **2021**, *18*, 7939, doi:10.3390/ijerph18157939 . . . 65

Felipe Papa Pellizoni, Aline Zazeri Leite, Nathália de Campos Rodrigues, Marcelo Jordão Ubaiz, Marina Ignácio Gonzaga, Nauyta Naomi Campos Takaoka, Vânia Sammartino Mariano, Wellington Pine Omori, Daniel Guariz Pinheiro, Euclides Matheucci Junior, Eleni Gomes and Gislane Lelis Vilela de Oliveira
Detection of Dysbiosis and Increased Intestinal Permeability in Brazilian Patients with Relapsing–Remitting Multiple Sclerosis
Reprinted from: *Int. J. Environ. Res. Public Health* **2021**, *18*, 4621, doi:10.3390/ijerph18094621 . . . 77

Emanuele Rinninella, Marco Cintoni, Pauline Raoul, Vincenzina Mora, Antonio Gasbarrini and Maria Cristina Mele
Impact of Food Additive Titanium Dioxide on Gut Microbiota Composition, Microbiota-Associated Functions, and Gut Barrier: A Systematic Review of In Vivo Animal Studies
Reprinted from: *Int. J. Environ. Res. Public Health* **2021**, *18*, 2008, doi:10.3390/ijerph18042008 . . . 95

Keith Bernard Woodford
Casomorphins and Gliadorphins Have Diverse Systemic Effects Spanning Gut, Brain and Internal Organs
Reprinted from: *Int. J. Environ. Res. Public Health* **2021**, *18*, 7911, doi:10.3390/ijerph18157911 . . . 113

Laura Sanchis-Artero, Juan Francisco Martínez-Blanch, Sergio Manresa-Vera, Ernesto Cortés-Castell, Josefa Rodriguez-Morales and Xavier Cortés-Rizo
Evaluation of Changes in Gut Microbiota in Patients with Crohn's Disease after Anti-Tnfα Treatment: Prospective Multicenter Observational Study
Reprinted from: *Int. J. Environ. Res. Public Health* **2020**, *17*, 5120, doi:10.3390/ijerph17145120 . . . **133**

Jordie A. J. Fischer and Crystal D. Karakochuk
Feasibility of an At-Home Adult Stool Specimen Collection Method in Rural Cambodia
Reprinted from: *Int. J. Environ. Res. Public Health* **2021**, *18*, 12430, doi:10.3390/ijerph182312430 . **147**

Lola Rueda Ruzafa, José Luis Cedillo and Arik J. Hone
Nicotinic Acetylcholine Receptor Involvement in Inflammatory Bowel Disease and Interactions with Gut Microbiota
Reprinted from: *Int. J. Environ. Res. Public Health* **2021**, *18*, 1189, doi:10.3390/ijerph18031189 . . . **155**

Maria Maddalena Sirufo, Francesca De Pietro, Alessandra Catalogna, Lia Ginaldi and Massimo De Martinis
The Microbiota-Bone-Allergy Interplay
Reprinted from: *Int. J. Environ. Res. Public Health* **2022**, *19*, 282, doi:10.3390/ijerph19010282 . . . **175**

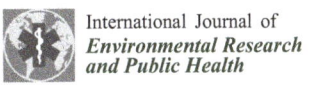

Editorial

New Perspectives in Health: Gut Microbiota

Diana Cardona [1,2,*] and Pablo Roman [1,2]

1. Department of Nursing, Physiotherapy and Medicine, University of Almeria, 04120 Almeria, Spain; pablo.roman@ual.es
2. Health Research Center (CEINSA), University of Almeria, 04120 Almeria, Spain
* Correspondence: dcardona@ual.es; Tel.: +34-950-214580

The gut microbiota has an important role in different physiological functions, exerting effects from energy metabolism to psychiatric well-being. Several factors alter the gut microbiota, indeed altering the quality of health. The gut microbiota dysbiosis has been related to an increased susceptibility to intestinal, cardiovascular and nervous pathologies. This Special Issue focusing on "New perspectives in Health: Gut Microbiota" aims to cover recent and novel advancements, as well as future trends in the field of gut microbiota and health, given that more research is required to elucidate the role of microbiota, its outcomes in health, diseases and the pathways which are involved.

Topics addressed in this Special Issue include the influence of gut microbiota in several health diseases such as cancer, fibromyalgia or multiple sclerosis, as well as the development of new methods to analyze fecal samples or to detect probiotic bacteria, including different types of manuscripts such as clinical trials, reviews or observational studies. Twelve papers were published, covering different aspects of gut microbiota and health.

Two papers are clinical trials focused on the modulatory effects of probiotics in gut microbiota. The first one proved that a multispecies probiotic is effective to produce an improvement in attention in fibromyalgia [1]. The second one showed that combined strategy of a hypocaloric diet, percutaneous electrical stimulation and probiotics administration promoted a positive influence on anti-obesogenic gut bacteria by increasing muconutritive (*Akkermansia muciniphila*) and immunomodulatory (*Bifidobacterium* spp.) microbiota and Bacteroidetes phylum (*Prevotella* spp.) and reducing the ratio of *Firmicutes/Bacteroidetes* ratio [2]. On the topic of probiotics, a published systematic review in this Special Issue has shown that some probiotic strains (*Lactobacillus acidophilus, L. casei, Bifidobacterium longum,* or *L. rhamnosus*, among others) are an effective therapeutic strategy in some common treatment-related side effects in adult oncology patients [3]. In this context, it is important to elucidate which probiotic species has the best capability for withstand, thus, one study of this Special Issue compares five strains of probiotic (*Bifidobacterium* BB-12, *Lactobacillus rhamnosus* GG, *L. casei, L. acidophilus, L. plantarum*) and concludes that the *L. plantarum* strain had the best capability for growth [4].

Diet is an important modulator of gut microbiota so there are several papers in the Special Issue about this topic. One of them showed gut microbial and fatty acids changes after the ingestion of isoflavones, contributing to the understanding of the modulation of the gut microorganisms. Specifically, after isoflavone supplementation, the abundance of the genera *Slackia* significantly increased and the fecal microbial communities of menopausal women equol producers were more like no producers [5]. In fact, diet also plays an important role in multiple sclerosis, in which dysbiosis has been detected in relapsing–remitting patients receiving disease-modifying therapies. This gut microbiota alteration could be involved in increased intestinal permeability and affect clinical response and disease progression [6]. Related to the diet, the systematic review published about the effects of Titanium dioxide (TiO_2) revealed that TiO_2 alters the composition and the activity of intestinal bacteria. In addition, this food additive used in pastries, sweets and sauces, promoting an inflammatory environment in the gut and immune responses in animals with colitis or obesity [7]. In the same line, casomorphins from dairy and gliadorphin peptides from cereals produce intestinal inflammation and permeability, as well altered gut microbiota via opioid receptors, point to the importance to the vigilance to food-derived opioids [8].

One study protocol was also published in this Special Issue. This prospective study with 44 patients with Crohn's disease with anti-TNFα treatment will provide additional evidence regarding potential non-invasive tools such as microbiota-based biomarkers to improve clinical management of these patients [9]. In this context, the development of new techniques of stool recollection such us a low-cost at-home stool collection kit for rural or low-resource settings are relevant [10].

Two review papers complete this Special Issue. The first one reviewed the relationship between nicotine receptors and gut microbiota, showing that the control of gut inflammation through $\alpha 7$ and $\alpha 9$ nAChRs, the vagus nerve, and the cholinergic anti-inflammatory pathway is fundamental [11]. The second one points to the relevance of gut microbiota in both osteoporosis (OP) and food allergy (FA). The disbyosis observed in these diseases causes the development of an important inflammatory substrate in the intestine, which leads to FA and the loss of estrogen typical of primary OP [12].

Overall, these 12 contributions published in this Special Issue further strengthen the essential function of gut microbiota in health and in various diseases. However, there are still many fundamental questions that remain unanswered, promising a great future for this field. Therefore, more research is necessary, and a second edition about this topic is proposed. Finally, the Guest Editors would like to sincerely thank all the authors for their valuable contributions.

Funding: This research received no external funding.

Institutional Review Board Statement: Not applicable.

Informed Consent Statement: Not applicable.

Conflicts of Interest: The authors declare no conflict of interest.

References

1. Cardona, D.; Roman, P.; Cañadas, F.; Sánchez-Labraca, N. The Effect of Multiprobiotics on Memory and Attention in Fibromyalgia: A Pilot Randomized Controlled Trial. *Int. J. Environ. Res. Public Health* **2021**, *18*, 3543. [CrossRef] [PubMed]
2. Lorenzo, O.; Crespo-Yanguas, M.; Hang, T.; Lumpuy-Castillo, J.; Hernández, A.M.; Llavero, C.; García-Alonso, M.L.; Ruiz-Tovar, J. Addition of Probiotics to Anti-Obesity Therapy by Percutaneous Electrical Stimulation of Dermatome T6. A Pilot Study. *Int. J. Environ. Res. Public Health* **2020**, *17*, 7239. [CrossRef] [PubMed]
3. Rodriguez-Arrastia, M.; Martinez-Ortigosa, A.; Rueda-Ruzafa, L.; Ayora, A.F.; Ropero-Padilla, C. Probiotic Supplements on Oncology Patients' Treatment-Related Side Effects: A Systematic Review of Randomized Controlled Trials. *Int. J. Environ. Res. Public Health* **2021**, *18*, 4265. [CrossRef] [PubMed]
4. Stasiak-Różańska, L.; Berthold-Pluta, A.; Pluta, A.S.; Dasiewicz, K.; Garbowska, M. Effect of Simulated Gastrointestinal Tract Conditions on Survivability of Probiotic Bacteria Present in Commercial Preparations. *Int. J. Environ. Res. Public Health* **2021**, *18*, 1108. [CrossRef] [PubMed]
5. Guadamuro, L.; Azcárate-Peril, M.A.; Tojo, R.; Mayo, B.; Delgado, S. Impact of Dietary Isoflavone Supplementation on the Fecal Microbiota and Its Metabolites in Postmenopausal Women. *Int. J. Environ. Res. Public Health* **2021**, *18*, 7939. [CrossRef] [PubMed]
6. Pellizoni, F.P.; Leite, A.Z.; de Campos Rodrigues, N.; Ubaiz, M.J.; Gonzaga, M.I.; Takaoka, N.N.C.; Mariano, V.S.; Omori, W.P.; Pinheiro, D.G.; Matheucci Junior, E.; et al. Detection of Dysbiosis and Increased Intestinal Permeability in Brazilian Patients with Relapsing-Remitting Multiple Sclerosis. *Int. J. Environ. Res. Public Health* **2021**, *18*, 4621. [CrossRef] [PubMed]
7. Rinninella, E.; Cintoni, M.; Raoul, P.; Mora, V.; Gasbarrini, A.; Mele, M.C. Impact of Food Additive Titanium Dioxide on Gut Microbiota Composition, Microbiota-Associated Functions, and Gut Barrier: A Systematic Review of In Vivo Animal Studies. *Int. J. Environ. Res. Public Health* **2021**, *18*, 2008. [CrossRef] [PubMed]
8. Woodford, K.B. Casomorphins and Gliadorphins Have Diverse Systemic Effects Spanning Gut, Brain and Internal Organs. *Int. J. Environ. Res. Public Health* **2021**, *18*, 7911. [CrossRef] [PubMed]
9. Sanchis-Artero, L.; Martínez-Blanch, J.F.; Manresa-Vera, S.; Cortés-Castell, E.; Rodriguez-Morales, J.; Cortés-Rizo, X. Evaluation of Changes in Gut Microbiota in Patients with Crohn's Disease after Anti-Tnfα Treatment: Prospective Multicenter Observational Study. *Int. J. Environ. Res. Public Health* **2020**, *17*, 5120. [CrossRef] [PubMed]

10. Fischer, J.A.J.; Karakochuk, C.D. Feasibility of an At-Home Adult Stool Specimen Collection Method in Rural Cambodia. *Int. J. Environ. Res. Public Health* **2021**, *18*, 12430. [CrossRef] [PubMed]
11. Ruzafa, L.R.; Cedillo, J.L.; Hone, A.J. Nicotinic Acetylcholine Receptor Involvement in Inflammatory Bowel Disease and Interactions with Gut Microbiota. *Int. J. Environ. Res. Public Health* **2021**, *18*, 1189. [CrossRef] [PubMed]
12. Sirufo, M.M.; De Pietro, F.; Catalogna, A.; Ginaldi, L.; De Martinis, M. The Microbiota-Bone-Allergy Interplay. *Int. J. Environ. Res. Public Health* **2021**, *19*, 282. [CrossRef] [PubMed]

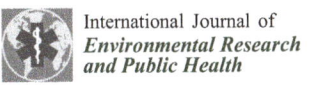

International Journal of
Environmental Research and Public Health

Article

The Effect of Multiprobiotics on Memory and Attention in Fibromyalgia: A Pilot Randomized Controlled Trial

Diana Cardona [1], Pablo Roman [1,*], Fernando Cañadas [2] and Nuria Sánchez-Labraca [1]

[1] Department of Nursing, Physiotherapy and Medicine, Health Research Center (CEINSA), University of Almeria, 04120 Almeria, Spain; dcardona@ual.es (D.C.); msl397@ual.es (N.S.-L.)
[2] Department of Psychology, University of Almeria, 04120 Almeria, Spain; jcanadas@ual.es
* Correspondence: pablo.roman@ual.es; Tel.: +34-950214563

Citation: Cardona, D.; Roman, P.; Cañadas, F.; Sánchez-Labraca, N. The Effect of Multiprobiotics on Memory and Attention in Fibromyalgia: A Pilot Randomized Controlled Trial. *Int. J. Environ. Res. Public Health* **2021**, *18*, 3543. https://doi.org/10.3390/ijerph18073543

Academic Editor: María José Benito

Received: 22 February 2021
Accepted: 23 March 2021
Published: 29 March 2021

Publisher's Note: MDPI stays neutral with regard to jurisdictional claims in published maps and institutional affiliations.

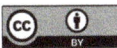

Copyright: © 2021 by the authors. Licensee MDPI, Basel, Switzerland. This article is an open access article distributed under the terms and conditions of the Creative Commons Attribution (CC BY) license (https://creativecommons.org/licenses/by/4.0/).

Abstract: Fibromyalgia syndrome (FMS) is a chronic, generalized and diffuse pain disorder accompanied by cognitive deficits such as forgetfulness, concentration difficulties, loss of vocabulary and mental slowness, among others. In recent years, FMS has been associated with altered intestinal microbiota, suggesting that modulating gut microbiota (for example, through probiotics) could be an effective therapeutic treatment. Thus, the aim of the present study was to continue exploring the role of probiotics in cognitive processes in patients with FMS. A pilot randomized controlled trial was conducted in 31 patients diagnosed with FMS to compare the effects of a multispecies probiotic versus a placebo on cognitive variables (memory and attention) after eight weeks. Results showed that treatment with a multispecies probiotic produced an improvement in attention by reducing errors on an attention task, but it had no effect on memory. More specifically, a tendency to reduce errors of omission (Go trials) during the Go/No-Go Task was observed after treatment. These findings, along with our previous results in impulsivity, underline the relevance of using probiotics as a therapeutic option in FMS, although more research with a larger sample size is required.

Keywords: probiotics; memory; attention; microbiota; gut–brain axis; gastrointestinal microbiome; fibromyalgia

1. Introduction

Fibromyalgia syndrome (FMS) is a chronic, generalized and diffuse pain disorder accompanied by symptoms such as morning stiffness, fatigue, depression and sleeping disorders [1]. Another prevalent complaint is cognitive deficits such as forgetfulness, concentration difficulties, loss of vocabulary and mental slowness, among others [2,3]. Some previous research found that FMS patients show poor performance in some executive functions [4], such as concentration, working memory deficits [5] and reduced ability to inhibit irrelevant information [6], as well as low cognitive flexibility and poor decision-making [4]. Likewise, in these patients, there is also less brain activation in the cortical structures of the inhibition network (specifically in the areas involved in response selection/motor preparation) and the attention network [7].

Recently, FMS has been associated with altered intestinal microbiota [8], as well as with chronic widespread musculoskeletal pain, a symptom of FMS which has shown reduced diversity in the microbiome, particularly of *Coproccocus*, indicating the involvement of the gut microbiota [9]. The gut microbiota plays an important role in different physiological functions, exerting effects from energy metabolism to psychiatric well-being [10]. Research has documented lower levels of *Bifidobacterium* and higher levels of *Enterococcus* spp. in these patients [11]. Furthermore, it has been stated that the higher the aerobic enterococcal count, the worse the neurological and cognitive deficits, such as nervousness, memory loss, forgetfulness and confusion [12]. This is related to the gut–brain axis pathway, which is a bidirectional communication network between the brain and the gut microbiota that occurs via three different pathways: neural, endocrine and immune [13]. It is worth mentioning that neural communication takes place through the vagus nerve and the enteric nervous system (ENS), while endocrine communication occurs via the production of hormones such as cortisol, and immune system communication takes place via the modulation of cytokines [14,15]. In this context, bacterial products activate the ENS [16] and stimulate primary afferent nerves, as well as bacterial metabolites that cause behavioral changes [17]. For these reasons, the gut–brain axis, which allows gut bacteria to affect the central nervous system (for example, with probiotic administration), has been used as a treatment option for a variety of health and mental disorders [18].

Probiotics are defined as live microorganisms which, when administered in adequate amounts, confer a health benefit on the host [19]. Probiotics have been shown to specifically catalyze oligosaccharides, increasing short-chain fatty acid (SCFA) production [20]. SCFAs are metabolic byproducts of the anaerobic fermentation of dietary carbohydrates and some amino acids, and they play a variety of roles in health maintenance, not only in the intestine as an energy source that improves transit, but also in the immune system [21]. Fibromyalgia (FM) patients have an altered composition of SCFAs, and *Parabacteroides merdae* increases neurotransmitters in FMS patients, which could explain the cognitive dysfunction [22].

In fact, FMS and irritable bowel syndrome (IBS) are common co-occurring disorders [23] for which modulation of the gut microbiota is a treatment strategy [24]. Moreover, FMS is frequently associated with other immuno-rheumatic diseases, such as chronic fatigue syndrome [25], which appears to improve after probiotics administration [26], or rheumatoid arthritis, in which probiotics also improve symptoms [27]. However, even though the gut microbiota may play a role in FMS, according to a recent systematic review, the data are insufficient [28], and more research is required to obtain conclusive answers in relation to the effectiveness of dietary interventions [29].

According to all of the above, changes in gut microbiota could be involved in FMS, so modulating the gut microbiota is a therapeutic treatment that needs to be explored. Therefore, we carried out a pilot study on the effect of multispecies probiotics on the cognitive and emotional symptoms of FMS [30]. In the first part of this study, we showed the beneficial effects of probiotics on impulsivity [31]. In this context, the current study aims to continue exploring the role of probiotics in cognitive processes in patients with FMS, specifically the effects of a multispecies probiotic on attention and memory function in FMS patients. Given the role of gut microbiota in central nervous system functions, we expect that oral intake of probiotics will have beneficial effects on memory and attention in FM.

2. Materials and Methods

2.1. Study Design and Participants

This study is part of a large, double-blinded study and a parallel group design that was registered with ClinicalTrial.gov (NCT02642289) and approved by the Human Research Ethics Committee of the University of Almeria (Spain). The study protocol and recruitment procedure have been previously described [30]. Fibromyalgia patients were recruited from the Almeria Fibromyalgia Association (AFIAL—Spain) or from El Ejido Fibromyalgia Association (AFIEL—Spain) and were diagnosed at least 1 year before entering the study according to the criteria of the American College of Rheumatology [1,32]. Exclusion criteria involved: (1) use of antibiotics and nutritional supplements, (2) allergies, (3) current participation in other psychological or medical studies, (4) being pregnant or breastfeeding, (5) severe intestinal disease and (6) meeting the criteria for psychiatric disorders other than depression and/or anxiety. More information about the participants' characteristics can be found in the first part of the study [31].

2.2. Procedure

Participants were randomly assigned to the following groups: experimental (ERGYPHILUS Plus (Laboratorios NUTERGIA S.L., San Sebastián, Spain)), which contained *Lactobacillus rhamnosus GG*, *L. paracasei*, *L. acidophilus* and *Bifidobacterium bifidus* (revivification of 6 million germs per capsule, 4 capsules per day, $n = 16$), or placebo ($n = 15$). The placebo capsules were composed of cellulose and provided by Complementos Fitonutricionales S.L. (Spain). The evaluation was performed both before the treatment (baseline) and after 8 weeks of treatment (post-intervention). More information about the procedure can be found in the first part of the study [31]. The duration of treatment was selected according to similar, previous research [33,34].

The selected probiotic species have been used previously to improve functions related to the gut–brain axis [33,35,36] and are therefore expected to be capable of attenuating the cognitive and emotional changes caused by FMS.

2.3. Outcome Measures

2.3.1. Demographic Measures

All participants provided the following demographic and clinical information: gender, age, FM diagnosis onset, years of formal education and body mass index (BMI). The BMI index was calculated by dividing the weight by the square of the height.

2.3.2. Cognitive Task

All cognitive tasks, except that of digits, were processed using the computer program E-Prime® version 2.0 (Psychology Software Tools, Pittsburgh, PA, USA).

Memory Tasks: Working Memory

Digit Task

The Digit Span Task is a subtest belonging to the Wechsler Scale of Intelligence for Adults—WAIS [37], which measures the verbal component of working memory. It consists of two parts: digits in direct order and digits in reverse order. In both, the experimenter reads aloud a series of numbers (specifically, 7 pairs of sequences consisting of between 1 and 9 numbers that are incrementally increased) that the participant must repeat in the same order (direct condition) or in reverse order (reverse condition). The test ends when both attempts at a certain level fail.

Corsi Task

This task evaluates the spatial component of working memory. The task consists of two blocks: direct and inverse condition, respectively. Each trial begins with the appearance of a pattern of nine white squares on a gray background. These are colored red in a rapid sequence of two, three... up to nine squares in the direct condition, and eight in the reverse. After the sequence, the nine-square pattern appears again, and the participant must touch the squares that have changed color with the mouse in the same order (direct condition) in which this happened or in reverse order (reverse condition). Span (or capacity) memory was calculated based on the longest sequence that each participant recalled correctly, directly and inversely, in at least one of the two sequences. Reaction Times (RTs) of the sequences correctly reproduced in forward and reverse order were also calculated.

Attention Tasks

Go/No-Go Task

The Go/No-Go Task is a classical paradigm to investigate inhibition control [38]. The stimulus in this task was a rectangle presented in different corners of the screen. When the rectangle was presented in the upper left, upper right and lower right corners of the computer screen, these are known as Go trials, and when all the rectangles are presented in the lower left corner, these are No-Go trials. The participants were required to press the space bar for Go trials and not to press the space bar for No-Go trials. The error rate on the Go conditions, or errors of omission trials, and the percentage of errors in the No-Go conditions, or errors of commission, were analyzed. In addition, RTs obtained in Go trials by participants were taken into account by both groups.

Stroop Task with Negative Priming (NP)

This task was employed to evaluate inhibitory mechanisms and also interference effects in the NP condition [39]. Each trial started with the presentation of a fixation point (a cross) located in the center of the screen. Immediately afterwards, a word written in a determinate color appeared (for example, the word BLUE written in red ink). Participants had to press, as quickly as possible, the key that corresponded to the color of the ink in which the word was written (red), regardless of the word's meaning. There were four possible colors (red, green, blue and yellow), and each was assigned to a key on the keyboard. Congruent trials were those in which the color of the word coincided with the color in which it was presented. Incongruent trials were those in which the color word did not coincide with the color in which it was displayed. Trials were also coded according to the congruency of the previous trial (N-1) in order to evaluate the NP effect for each trial. The measures of the RTs obtained by participants in congruent and incongruent trials were compared to calculate the Stroop effect. The negative priming effect was also calculated by comparing the measures of the RTs obtained by participants in control trials vs. incongruent trials.

2.4. Statistical Analyses

Statistical analyses and graphics were performed using SPSS v19.0 (SPSS, Inc., Chicago, IL, USA) and GraphPad Prism v7.0 (GraphPad Software, La Jolla, CA, USA), respectively. All alpha levels were set at $p < 0.05$. As this was a pilot study, no power analysis was performed to predetermine sample size.

First, a descriptive analysis was performed, and the normal distribution of variables was verified by the Kolmogorov–Smirnov test. Baseline demographics were compared between both groups using χ^2 tests for categorical data and Student's *t*-tests for continuous data. For the cognitive task, the mean scores (total and/or partial) were subjected to a repeated-measures analysis of variance (ANOVA). In addition, the Student's *t*-test was employed to compare means between groups.

Due to technical problems, some data were missing. The exact number of participants is indicated in each task.

3. Results

3.1. Participant Characteristics

A total of 31 patients diagnosed with FMS were allocated to the probiotic or placebo group (Figure 1). Sociodemographic variables are shown in Table 1, which describe the sample that participated in the study. No statistically significant differences in any of the variables between either group ($p > 0.05$) were observed.

Table 1. Sociodemographic characteristics of study population.

	PROBIOTIC ($n = 16$)	PLACEBO ($n = 15$)
Gender (%)		
Men	6.25	13.33
Women	93.75	86.67
Age	55.00 ± 8.37	50.27 ± 7.86
Years of diagnosis	8.56 ± 5.90	8.47 ± 5.80
Formal education (years)	12.75 ± 0.95	12.27 ± 1.29
BMI (kg/m^2)	29.40 ± 1.64	30.23 ± 1.63

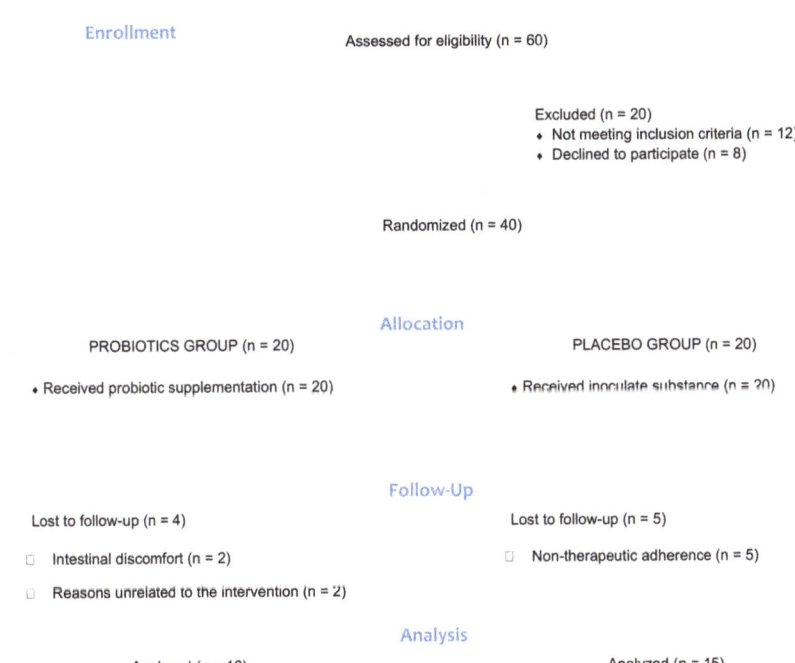

Figure 1. Flow diagram of the progress through the phases of the pilot parallel randomized trial of two groups.

3.2. Performance on Cognitive Task

3.2.1. Memory Task

Digit Task

For each participant, the memory span (or capacity) score was calculated based on the longest sequence that was correctly remembered, forward and reverse (see Table 2), adding the corresponding score to all sequences answered correctly (two points were awarded when the two attempts of the sequence were reproduced correctly and one point when only one of them was remembered). These data were analyzed using an analysis of variance with one inter-subject manipulated factor, group (placebo, probiotic), and two within-subject manipulated factors, order (forward and reverse) and treatment (pre-, post-). No effect or interaction was statistically significant ($p > 0.05$).

Table 2. Span of memory expressed by mean and standard error.

	PLACEBO ($n = 15$)		PROBIOTIC ($n = 16$)	
	PRE-	POST-	PRE-	POST-
Forward	8.42 (0.48)	8.78 (0.48)	8.06 (0.54)	8.31 (0.59)
Reverse	5.35 (0.26)	5.50 (0.47)	5.56 (0.60)	5.62 (0.56)

Corsi Task

Span (or capacity) memory was calculated based on the longest sequence that each participant recalled correctly, directly and inversely, in at least one of the two sequences (Table 3). The average median RTs of the sequences correctly reproduced in forward and reverse order was also calculated (Table 4). These data were analyzed using analysis of variance with one factor manipulated between subjects, group (placebo, probiotic), and two factors manipulated within subjects, order (forward and reverse) and treatment (pre-, post-). No effect or interaction was statistically significant ($p > 0.05$).

Table 3. Span of memory expressed by mean and standard error.

	PLACEBO ($n = 12$)		PROBIOTIC ($n = 13$)	
	PRE-	POST-	PRE-	POST-
Forward	4.92 (337)	5.08 (37)	5.00 (311)	5.39 (288)
Reverse	4.50 (324)	4.83 (299)	5.08 (356)	4.92 (356)

Table 4. The average median of Reaction Times (RTs) expressed by mean and standard error.

	PLACEBO ($n = 12$)		PROBIOTIC ($n = 13$)	
	PRE-	POST-	PRE-	POST-
Forward	4602 (378)	4600 (474)	3823 (362)	3839 (454)
Reverse	3998 (316)	4520 (417)	3911 (303)	3615 (399)

3.2.2. Attention Task

Go/No-Go Task

In this task, we analyzed the error rate for the Go conditions, or errors of omission trials, the percentage of errors in the No-Go conditions, or errors of commission, and the average of the medians of the RTs obtained in the Go trials (Table 5) by participants in both groups. These data were analyzed using analysis of variance with one factor manipulated between subjects, group (placebo, probiotic), and one factor manipulated within subjects, treatment (pre-, post-). The ANOVA of errors of omission showed a marginal effect of the interaction group x treatment ($F1, 24 = 3.62$; $p = 0.069$). Furthermore, a marginal effect of group ($F1, 24 = 3.56$; $p = 0.071$) was observed post-treatment in the Go condition (Figure 2). No other effect or interaction was statistically significant ($p > 0.05$).

Table 5. The average median of RTs expressed by mean and standard error.

	PLACEBO ($n = 12$)		PROBIOTIC ($n = 14$)	
	PRE-	POST-	PRE-	POST-
Go trials	400 (47.3)	378 (35.7)	344 (43.8)	365 (33.1)

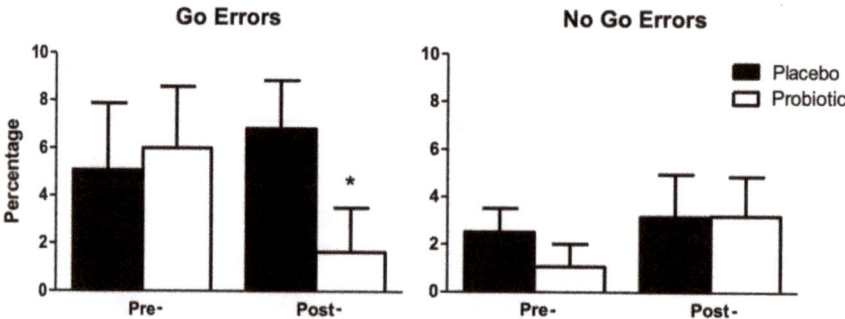

Figure 2. Percentage of omission errors (Go Errors) and of commission (No Go Errors) committed by participants in both groups depending on the treatment. Error bars represent the standard error of the mean. * marginal effect of the interaction group x treatment.

Stroop Task

In this task, the measures of the median RTs obtained by participants in congruent and incongruent trials were compared to calculate Stroop effects. These data were analyzed using analysis of variance with two factors manipulated between subjects, group (placebo, probiotic) and condition (congruent, incongruent), and one factor manipulated within subjects, treatment (pre-, post-). The results only showed a significant effect of condition ($p < 0.01$); no other significant effects were observed ($p > 0.05$). The negative priming effect was also calculated by comparing the measures of the median RTs obtained by participants in control trials vs. incongruent trials. No effect or interaction was statistically significant ($p > 0.05$) (Table 6).

Table 6. The average median of RTs and errors expressed by mean and standard error.

	PLACEBO (*n* = 11)		PROBIOTIC (*n* = 12)	
	PRE-	POST-	PRE-	POST-
RTs				
Congruent	1013 (60)	998 (59)	987 (58)	979 (57)
Incongruent	1094 (69)	1044 (61)	1075 (66)	1065 (58)
Control	1076 (68)	1036 (57)	1061 (66)	1045 (55)
Ignored	1051 (72)	1023 (69)	1052 (69)	1050 (66)
Errors				
Congruent	0.6 (0.4)	0.5 (0.2)	0.5 (0.4)	0.7 (0.2)
Incongruent	3.1 (2.8)	2.3 (0.9)	4.7 (2.7)	1.6 (0.8)
Control	2.5 (1.6)	2.5 (0.9)	4.8 (2.5)	0.7 (0.9)
Ignored	3.4 (2.5)	1.4 (0.5)	4.4 (2.4)	0.7 (0.5)

4. Discussion

The purpose of the present study was to continue exploring the beneficial effects of treatment with a multispecies probiotic in patients diagnosed with FMS. For this, a group of patients with a mean time of 8 and a half years since diagnosis and a mean age of 52 years were treated for 8 weeks with a multispecies probiotic or with a placebo substance and evaluated immediately for its effects on attention and memory.

To our knowledge, the only study evaluating the role of probiotics in cognition in FMS patients is our previous study, which showed a reduction in impulsivity after treatment [31]. In the current research, we found no significant differences in memory after treatment. Although no other studies have used probiotics to improve memory in FMS, a recent systematic review and meta-analysis of preclinical and clinical studies indicates that probiotics could be a useful strategy to improve dementia and cognitive decline [35] in both healthy [36] and elderly populations [40]. Similarly, a probiotic-treated Alzheimer's experimental model demonstrated an improvement in learning [41] and memory [42]. In clinical studies of elderly people with mild cognitive impairment, an improvement in cognitive function (memory and attention) and an increase in brain-derived neurotrophic factor (BDNF) were reported after treatment with *Lactobacillus plantarum C29*-fermented soybean (DW2009) for 12 weeks [43]. Similar data were collected after the administration of *Bifidobacterium* A1 for 12 weeks in older adults with memory deficits, although the data are not conclusive and further research is required in this regard [44]. According to these studies, one possible explanation for the lack of positive results in our study could be the short length of treatment; studies demonstrating memory benefits were of significantly longer duration.

Regarding the attentional tasks, no differences in the Stroop effect or the negative priming effect (Stroop Task with Negative Priming) were observed among the participants after the treatment, implying that the probiotic treatment used did not affect the inhibitory mechanisms of attention. However, patients with FMS treated with the probiotic showed a tendency towards reduced errors of omission (Go trials) during the Go/No-Go Task and the group that received the placebo presented a number of errors that was slightly higher than those registered in the pre-treatment phase. This type of error occurs when there is an absence of response to a relevant stimulus, and it is assumed that it reflects symptoms of inattention [45]. Therefore, FMS patients treated and not treated with the probiotic showed similar levels of inhibitory motor control and similar ability to inhibit information irrelevant to the task objective, but they differed in their ability to maintain attention for an extended period with the objective of responding to specific stimuli. This difference could be attributed to the effect that probiotics produced in these patients, which improved their ability to maintain attention, as evidenced by the results obtained in the Go/No-Go Task in the post-treatment phase.

Despite studies finding that the effects of probiotics on attention are reduced, similar results have been observed in other populations. In this regard, after 8 weeks of treatment with *Lactobacillus plantarum* 299v, patients with major depression showed an improvement in attention and work speed on the attention and perceptivity test, but no significant effects on the Stroop test [46]. Similarly, *Lactobacillus plantarum* DR7 treatment for 12 weeks improved basic attention and memory in healthy adults, as measured by the computerized CogState Brief Battery [47].

A recent systematic review and meta-analysis showed a positive effect of probiotics on cognition in both humans and animals [48]. Human studies showed an improvement in attention and memory in patients with Alzheimer's, in the healthy elderly individuals or those with depression. The only FMS study included in this analysis was the first part of our current research [31]. Most included studies used *Lactobacillus* and *Bifidobacterium* probiotic strains, but it is worth noting that the meta-analysis found that using just one probiotic was more effective than using a combination. In the same manner, the 12-week treatment was more effective than the 8-week treatment, implying that our findings on FM cognition could be significant after additional weeks of treatment.

The putative mechanisms of action of probiotics in cognitive function, as suggested by Lv and collaborators [48], are related to neuroinflammation. In this regard, the decline in cognitive function associated with aging is related to changes in brain immunoregulation, including decreases in IL-4 [49]. Several studies suggest a decrease in the diversity of microbiota with cognition and inflammatory markers [50], in which changes in the intestinal metagenome appear to be associated with cognitive function and brain iron deposition [51]. In this context, factors associated with aging, such as oxidative stress and inflammation, are related to the intestinal microbiota [52], which influences the different sequences of cognitive impairment [53], and probiotic treatment could reverse this cognitive impairment via cytokine systems.

Interestingly, elevations of proinflammatory chemokines/cytokines could negatively impact symptoms of FMS. Proinflammatory cytokines have been shown to have an important modulatory role in pain transmission and perception. It is not surprising that high levels of them have been found, specifically of interleukins 1, 2, 6 and 8, in patients with FMS [54]. Therefore, probiotic administration could be an effective approach to treat cognitive deficits in FMS, as can be seen in our results. In other words, a multispecies probiotic treatment can improve some cognitive functions in FMS patients, such as impulse control, sustained attention and the ability to maintain attentional control in a context of change. The clinical relevance of microbiota modulation in FMS patients should be considered as an adjuvant treatment.

However, these results must be taken with caution, given that this study had several limitations. First of all, we had a limited number of subjects, since this was a pilot randomized controlled trial. Secondly, the nutritional habits of the participants should have been registered because they could influence or interfere with the results—for example, the effect of the consumption of other fermented foods. Finally, measuring the gut microbiota would have given us more information about probiotic modulation. In this manner, future studies should be designed with a large sample size while keeping these limitations in mind.

5. Conclusions

Treatment of FMS patients with a multispecies probiotic for 8 weeks resulted in a tendency towards fewer errors in attention to relevant stimuli, particularly in a task that required inhibitory control at the motor level. However, this treatment had no effect on memory, specifically on working memory. These findings, along with those of our previous research on impulsivity, point to the importance of using probiotics as a therapeutic option in FMS. Nonetheless, more research is needed given the potential role of probiotics in FMS, especially since dysbiosis has been reported in FMS patients. In future studies, authors should consider exploring the effect of a specific probiotic strain on the treatment of cognitive impairment.

Author Contributions: D.C., N.S.-L., F.C. and P.R. designed research, conducted research, analyzed data and performed statistical analysis; D.C. and P.R. wrote the initial manuscript; N.S.-L. and F.C. critically reviewed the manuscript. All authors have read and agreed to the published version of the manuscript.

Funding: This research received no external funding.

Institutional Review Board Statement: The study was conducted according to the guidelines of the Declaration of Helsinki and approved by the Institutional Review Board of Universidad de Almeria (UAL/1-270415).

Informed Consent Statement: Informed consent was obtained from all subjects involved in the study.

Data Availability Statement: The data presented in this study are available on request from the corresponding author. The data are not publicly available due to ethical considerations.

Acknowledgments: We would like to thank the staff of the Almeria Fibromyalgia Association (AFIAL—Spain) and the El Ejido Fibromyalgia Association (AFIEL—Spain) for their assistance throughout the development of this study. In addition, we wish to thank Nutergia and Complementos Fitonutricionales for providing the probiotics and placebo free of charge.

Conflicts of Interest: The authors declare no conflict of interest.

References

1. Wolfe, F.; Smythe, H.A.; Yunus, M.B.; Bennett, R.M.; Bombardier, C.; Goldenberg, D.L.; Tugwell, P.; Campbell, S.M.; Abeles, M.; Clark, P. The American College of Rheumatology 1990 Criteria for the Classification of Fibromyalgia. Report of the Multicenter Criteria Committee. *Arthritis Rheum.* **1990**, *33*, 160–172. [CrossRef]
2. Glass, J.M. Fibromyalgia and cognition. *J. Clin. Psychiatry* **2008**, *69* (Suppl. 2), 20–24.
3. Glass, J.M. Review of Cognitive Dysfunction in Fibromyalgia: A Convergence on Working Memory and Attentional Control Impairments. *Rheum. Dis. Clin. N. Am.* **2009**, *35*, 299–311. [CrossRef]
4. Verdejo-García, A.; López-Torrecillas, F.; Calandre, E.P.; Delgado-Rodríguez, A.; Bechara, A. Executive function and decision-making in women with fibromyalgia. *Arch. Clin. Neuropsychol.* **2009**, *24*, 113–122. [CrossRef]
5. Park, D.C.; Glass, J.M.; Minear, M.; Crofford, L.J. Cognitive Function in Fibromyalgia Patients. *Arthritis Rheum.* **2001**, *44*, 2125–2133. [CrossRef]
6. Leavitt, F.; Katz, R.S. Normalizing memory recall in fibromyalgia with rehearsal: A distraction-counteracting effect. *Arthritis Care Res.* **2009**, *61*, 740–744. [CrossRef] [PubMed]
7. Glass, J.M.; Williams, D.A.; Fernandez-Sanchez, M.L.; Kairys, A.; Barjola, P.; Heitzeg, M.M.; Clauw, D.J.; Schmidt-Wilcke, T. Executive function in chronic pain patients and healthy controls: Different cortical activation during response inhibition in fibromyalgia. *J. Pain* **2011**, *12*, 1219–1229. [CrossRef] [PubMed]
8. Minerbi, A.; Gonzalez, E.; Brereton, N.J.B.; Anjarkouchian, A.; Dewar, K.; Fitzcharles, M.A.; Chevalier, S.; Shir, Y. Altered microbiome composition in individuals with fibromyalgia. *Pain* **2019**, *160*, 2589–2602. [CrossRef]
9. Freidin, M.B.; Stalteri, M.A.; Wells, P.M.; Lachance, G.; Baleanu, A.-F.; Bowyer, R.C.E.; Kurilshikov, A.; Zhernakova, A.; Steves, C.J.; Williams, F.M.K. An association between chronic widespread pain and the gut microbiome. *Rheumatology* **2020**. [CrossRef]
10. Moloney, R.D.; Johnson, A.C.; O'Mahony, S.M.; Dinan, T.G.; Greenwood-Van Meerveld, B.; Cryan, J.F. Stress and the Microbiota-Gut-Brain Axis in Visceral PaRelevance to Irritable Bowel Syndrome. *CNS Neurosci. Ther.* **2016**, *22*, 102–117. [CrossRef] [PubMed]
11. Logan, A.C.; Katzman, M. Major depressive disorder: Probiotics may be an adjuvant therapy. *Med. Hypotheses* **2005**, *64*, 533–538. [CrossRef]
12. Butt, H.; Dunstan, R.; McGregor, N.; Roberts, T. Bacterial colonosis in patients with persistent fatigue. In Proceedings of the AHMF International Clinical and Scientific Conference, Sydney, Australia, 1–2 December 2001.
13. Mayer, E.A.; Tillisch, K.; Gupta, A.; Mayer, E.E.A.; Rhee, S.; Pothoulakis, C.; Mayer, E.E.A.; Cryan, J.; Dinan, T.; Mayer, E.E.A.; et al. Gut/brain axis and the microbiota. *J. Clin. Investig.* **2015**, *125*, 926–938. [CrossRef]
14. Bercik, P.; Collins, S.M. The effects of inflammation, infection and antibiotics on the microbiota-gut-brain axis. *Adv. Exp. Med. Biol.* **2014**, *817*, 279–289.

15. De Palma, G.; Collins, S.M.; Bercik, P.; Verdu, E.F. The microbiota-gut-brain axis in gastrointestinal disorders: Stressed bugs, stressed brain or both? *J. Physiol.* **2014**, *592*, 2989–2997. [CrossRef] [PubMed]
16. Al-Nedawi, K.; Mian, M.F.; Hossain, N.; Karimi, K.; Mao, Y.-K.; Forsythe, P.; Min, K.K.; Stanisz, A.M.; Kunze, W.A.; Bienenstock, J. Gut commensal microvesicles reproduce parent bacterial signals to host immune and enteric nervous systems. *FASEB J.* **2015**, *29*, 684–695. [CrossRef] [PubMed]
17. Chichlowski, M.; Rudolph, C. Visceral pain and gastrointestinal microbiome. *J. Neurogastroenterol. Motil.* **2015**, *21*, 172–181. [CrossRef] [PubMed]
18. Dinan, T.G.; Stanton, C.; Cryan, J.F. Psychobiotics: A novel class of psychotropic. *Biol. Psychiatry* **2013**, *74*, 720–726. [CrossRef] [PubMed]
19. WHO. *Report of the Joint FAO/WHO Expert Consultation on Evaluation of Health and Nutritional Properties of Probiotics in Food Including Powder Milk with Live Lactic Acid Bacteria, Córdoba, Argentina, 1–4 October 2001*; Food and Agriculture Organization of the United Nations: Quebec City, QC, Canada, 2001; 30p.
20. Hardy, H.; Harris, J.; Lyon, E.; Beal, J.; Foey, A.D. Probiotics, prebiotics and immunomodulation of gut mucosal defences: Homeostasis and immunopathology. *Nutrients* **2013**, *5*, 1869–1912. [CrossRef]
21. Wichmann, A.; Allahyar, A.; Greiner, T.U.; Plovier, H.; Lundén, G.Ö.; Larsson, T.; Drucker, D.J.; Delzenne, N.M.; Cani, P.D.; Bäckhed, F. Microbial Modulation of Energy Availability in the Colon Regulates Intestinal Transit. *Cell Host Microbe* **2013**, *14*, 582–590. [CrossRef]
22. Minerbi, A.; Fitzcharles, M.A. Gut microbiome: Pertinence in fibromyalgia. *Clin. Exp. Rheumatol.* **2020**, *38*, 99–104.
23. Rodrigo, L.; Blanco, I.; Bobes, J.; De Serres, F.J. Effect of one year of a gluten-free diet on the clinical evolution of irritable bowel syndrome plus fibromyalgia in patients with associated lymphocytic enteritis: A case-control study. *Arthritis Res. Ther.* **2014**, *16*, 1–11.
24. Pusceddu, M.M.; Murray, K.; Gareau, M.G. Targeting the Microbiota, From Irritable Bowel Syndrome to Mood Disorders: Focus on Probiotics and Prebiotics. *Curr. Pathobiol. Rep.* **2018**, *6*, 1–13. [CrossRef] [PubMed]
25. Penfold, S.; Denis, E.S.; Mazhar, M.N. The association between borderline personality disorder, fibromyalgia and chronic fatigue syndrome: Systematic review. *BJPsych Open* **2016**, *2*, 275–279. [CrossRef] [PubMed]
26. Roman, P.; Carrillo-Trabalón, F.; Sánchez-Labraca, N.; Cañadas, F.; Estévez, A.F.; Cardona, D. Are probiotic treatments useful on fibromyalgia syndrome or chronic fatigue syndrome patients? A systematic review. *Benef. Microbes* **2018**, *9*, 603–611. [CrossRef]
27. Nelson, J.; Sjöblom, H.; Gjertsson, I.; Ulven, S.M.; Lindqvist, H.M.; Bärebring, L. Do Interventions with Diet or Dietary Supplements Reduce the Disease Activity Score in Rheumatoid Arthritis? A Systematic Review of Randomized Controlled Trials. *Nutrients* **2020**, *12*, 2991. [CrossRef] [PubMed]
28. Erdrich, S.; Hawrelak, J.A.; Myers, S.P.; Harnett, J.E. Determining the association between fibromyalgia, the gut microbiome and its biomarkers: A systematic review. *BMC Musculoskelet. Disord.* **2020**, *21*, 1–12. [CrossRef]
29. Pagliai, G.; Giangrandi, I.; Dinu, M.; Sofi, F.; Colombini, B. Nutritional interventions in the management of fibromyalgia syndrome. *Nutrients* **2020**, *12*, 2525. [CrossRef]
30. Roman, P.; Estévez, Á.F.; Sánchez-Labraca, N.; Cañadas, F.; Miras, A.; Cardona Mena, D. Probióticos en fibromialgia: Diseño de un estudio piloto doble ciego y randomizado. *Nutr. Hosp.* **2017**, *34*, 1246–1251.
31. Roman, P.; Estévez, A.F.; Miras, A.; Sánchez-Labraca, N.; Cañadas, F.; Vivas, A.B.; Cardona, D. A Pilot Randomized Controlled Trial to Explore Cognitive and Emotional Effects of Probiotics in Fibromyalgia. *Sci. Rep.* **2018**, *8*, 1–9. [CrossRef]
32. Wolfe, F.; Clauw, D.J.; Fitzcharles, M.-A.; Goldenberg, D.L.; Katz, R.S.; Mease, P.; Russell, A.S.; Russell, I.J.; Winfield, J.B.; Yunus, M.B. The American College of Rheumatology preliminary diagnostic criteria for fibromyalgia and measurement of symptom severity. *Arthritis Care Res.* **2010**, *62*, 600–610. [CrossRef]
33. Kato-Kataoka, A.; Nishida, K.; Takada, M.; Suda, K.; Kawai, M.; Shimizu, K.; Kushiro, A.; Hoshi, R.; Watanabe, O.; Igarashi, T.; et al. Fermented milk containing *Lactobacillus casei* strain Shirota prevents the onset of physical symptoms in medical students under academic examination stress. *Benef. Microbes* **2016**, *7*, 153–156. [CrossRef] [PubMed]
34. Kelly, J.R.; Allen, A.P.; Temko, A.; Hutch, W.; Kennedy, P.J.; Farid, N.; Murphy, E.; Boylan, G.; Bienenstock, J.; Cryan, J.F.; et al. Lost in translation? The potential psychobiotic Lactobacillus rhamnosus (JB-1) fails to modulate stress or cognitive performance in healthy male subjects. *Brain. Behav. Immun.* **2017**, *61*, 50–59. [CrossRef] [PubMed]
35. Ruiz-Gonzalez, C.; Roman, P.; Rueda-Ruzafa, L.; Rodriguez-Arrastia, M.; Cardona, D. Effects of probiotics supplementation on dementia and cognitive impairment: A systematic review and meta-analysis of preclinical and clinical studies. *Prog. Neuro-Psychopharmacol. Biol. Psychiatry* **2020**, 110189. [CrossRef] [PubMed]
36. Benton, D.; Williams, C.; Brown, A. Impact of consuming a milk drink containing a probiotic on mood and cognition. *Eur. J. Clin. Nutr.* **2007**, *61*, 355–361. [CrossRef]
37. Ibor, J. Escala de Inteligencia de Wechsler para Adultos III. *Schizophr. Res.* **2005**, 147–156.
38. Casey, B.J.; Trainor, R.J.; Orendi, J.L.; Schubert, A.B.; Nystrom, L.E.; Giedd, J.N.; Castellanos, F.X.; Haxby, J.V.; Noll, D.C.; Cohen, J.D.; et al. A developmental functional MRI study of prefrontal activation during performance of a Go-No-Go task. *J. Cogn. Neurosci.* **1997**, *9*, 835–847. [CrossRef] [PubMed]
39. Mayas, J.; Fuentes, L.J.; Ballesteros, S. Stroop interference and negative priming (NP) suppression in normal aging. *Arch. Gerontol. Geriatr.* **2012**, *54*, 333–338. [CrossRef]

40. Inoue, T.; Kobayashi, Y.; Mori, N.; Sakagawa, M.; Xiao, J.Z.; Moritani, T.; Sakane, N.; Nagai, N. Effect of combined bifidobacteria supplementation and resistance training on cognitive function, body composition and bowel habits of healthy elderly subjects. *Benef. Microbes* **2018**, *9*, 843–853. [CrossRef]
41. Rezaeiasl, Z.; Salami, M.; Sepehri, G. The effects of probiotic Lactobacillus and Bifidobacterium strains on memory and learning behavior, long-term potentiation (LTP), and some biochemical parameters in β-amyloid-induced rat's model of Alzheimer's disease. *Prev. Nutr. Food Sci.* **2019**, *24*, 265–273. [CrossRef]
42. Rezaei Asl, Z.; Sepehri, G.; Salami, M. Probiotic treatment improves the impaired spatial cognitive performance and restores synaptic plasticity in an animal model of Alzheimer's disease. *Behav. Brain Res.* **2019**, *376*, 112183. [CrossRef]
43. Hwang, Y.H.; Park, S.; Paik, J.W.; Chae, S.W.; Kim, D.H.; Jeong, D.G.; Ha, E.; Kim, M.; Hong, G.; Park, S.H.; et al. Efficacy and safety of lactobacillus plantarum C29-fermented soybean (DW2009) in individuals with mild cognitive impairment: A 12-week, multi-center, randomized, double-blind, placebo-controlled clinical trial. *Nutrients* **2019**, *11*, 305. [CrossRef]
44. Kobayashi, Y.; Kuhara, T.; Oki, M.; Xiao, J.Z. Effects of bifidobacterium breve a1 on the cognitive function of older adults with memory complaints: A randomised, double-blind, placebo-controlled trial. *Benef. Microbes* **2019**, *10*, 511–520. [CrossRef]
45. Barkley, R.A. Behavioral inhibition, sustained attention, and executive functions: Constructing a unifying theory of ADHD. *Psychol. Bull.* **1997**, *121*, 65–94. [CrossRef]
46. Rudzki, L.; Ostrowska, L.; Pawlak, D.; Małus, A.; Pawlak, K.; Waszkiewicz, N.; Szulc, A. Probiotic Lactobacillus Plantarum 299v decreases kynurenine concentration and improves cognitive functions in patients with major depression: A double-blind, randomized, placebo controlled study. *Psychoneuroendocrinology* **2019**, *100*, 213–222. [CrossRef]
47. Chong, H.X.; Yusoff, N.A.A.; Hor, Y.Y.; Lew, L.C.; Jaafar, M.H.; Choi, S.B.; Yusoff, M.S.B.; Wahid, N.; Abdullah, M.F.I.L.; Zakaria, N.; et al. Lactobacillus plantarum DR7 alleviates stress and anxiety in adults: A randomised, double-blind, placebo-controlled study. *Benef. Microbes* **2019**, *10*, 355–373. [CrossRef]
48. Lv, T.; Ye, M.; Luo, F.; Hu, B.; Wang, A.; Chen, J.; Yan, J.; He, Z.; Chen, F.; Qian, C.; et al. Probiotics treatment improves cognitive impairment in patients and animals: A systematic review and meta-analysis. *Neurosci. Biobehav. Rev.* **2021**, *120*, 159–172. [CrossRef]
49. Frank, M.G.; Fonken, L.K.; Watkins, L.R.; Maier, S.F.; Lowry, C.A. Could Probiotics Be Used to Mitigate Neuroinflammation? *ACS Chem. Neurosci.* **2019**, *10*, 13–15. [CrossRef] [PubMed]
50. Claesson, M.J.; Cusack, S.; O'Sullivan, O.; Greene-Diniz, R.; De Weerd, H.; Flannery, E.; Marchesi, J.R.; Falush, D.; Dinan, T.; Fitzgerald, G.; et al. Composition, variability, and temporal stability of the intestinal microbiota of the elderly. *Proc. Natl. Acad. Sci. USA* **2011**, *108*, 4586–4591. [CrossRef]
51. Blasco, G.; Moreno-Navarrete, J.M.; Rivero, M.; Pérez-Brocal, V.; Garre-Olmo, J.; Puig, J.; Daunis-i-Estadella, P.; Biarnés, C.; Gich, J.; Fernández-Aranda, F.; et al. The gut metagenome changes in parallel to waist circumference, brain iron deposition, and cognitive function. *J. Clin. Endocrinol. Metab.* **2017**, *102*, 2962–2973. [CrossRef] [PubMed]
52. Heyck, M.; Ibarra, A. Microbiota and memory: A symbiotic therapy to counter cognitive decline? *Brain Circ.* **2019**, *5*, 124. [PubMed]
53. Brüssow, H. Microbiota and healthy ageing: Observational and nutritional intervention studies. *Microb. Biotechnol.* **2013**, *6*, 326–334. [CrossRef] [PubMed]
54. Theoharides, T.C.; Tsilioni, I.; Bawazeer, M. Mast Cells, Neuroinflammation and Pain in Fibromyalgia Syndrome. *Front. Cell. Neurosci.* **2019**, *13*, 353. [CrossRef] [PubMed]

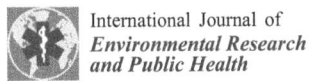

Article

Addition of Probiotics to Anti-Obesity Therapy by Percutaneous Electrical Stimulation of Dermatome T6. A Pilot Study

Oscar Lorenzo [1,2,*], Marta Crespo-Yanguas [1], Tianyu Hang [1], Jairo Lumpuy-Castillo [1], Artur M. Hernández [3], Carolina Llavero [4], MLuisa García-Alonso [1] and Jaime Ruiz-Tovar [4,5]

[1] Laboratory of Diabetes and Vascular Pathology, Instituto de Investigaciones Sanitarias-Fundación Jiménez Díaz, Universidad Autónoma, 28040 Madrid, Spain; marta.crespo@fjd.es (M.C.-Y.); taniahang9318@gmail.com (T.H.); jairo.lumpuy@estudiante.uam.es (J.L.-C.); mga@eaac.es (M.G.-A.)
[2] Spanish Biomedical Research Centre on Diabetes and Associated Metabolic Disorders (CIBERDEM) Network, 28040 Madrid, Spain
[3] Department of Sport Sciences, Universidad Europea de Madrid, 28670 Villaviciosa de Odón-Madrid, Spain; ahernandez@urj.es
[4] Obesity Unit, Clinica Garcilaso, 28010 Madrid, Spain; cllavero@urj.es (C.L.); jruiztovar@gmail.com (J.R.-T.)
[5] Department of Health Sciences, Universidad Rey Juan Carlos, 28933 Mostoles-Madrid, Spain
* Correspondence: olorenzo@fjd.es; Tel.: +34-915-504-800 (ext. 2818)

Received: 7 September 2020; Accepted: 29 September 2020; Published: 3 October 2020

Abstract: Obesity is becoming a pandemic and percutaneous electrical stimulation (PENS) of dermatome T6 has been demonstrated to reduce stomach motility and appetite, allowing greater weight loss than isolated hypocaloric diets. However, modulation of intestinal microbiota could improve this effect and control cardiovascular risk factors. Our objective was to test whether addition of probiotics could improve weight loss and cardiovascular risk factors in obese subjects after PENS and a hypocaloric diet. A pilot prospective study was performed in patients ($n = 20$) with a body mass index (BMI) > 30 kg/m^2. Half of them underwent ten weeks of PENS in conjunction with a hypocaloric diet (PENS-Diet), and the other half was treated with a PENS-Diet plus multistrain probiotics (*L. plantarum LP115*, *B. brevis B3*, and *L. acidophilus LA14*) administration. Fecal samples were obtained before and after interventions. The weight loss and changes in blood pressure, glycemic and lipid profile, and in gut microbiota were investigated. Weight loss was significantly higher (16.2 vs. 11.1 kg, $p = 0.022$), whereas glycated hemoglobin and triglycerides were lower (−0.46 vs. −0.05%, $p = 0.032$, and −47.0 vs. −8.5 mg/dL, $p = 0.002$, respectively) in patients receiving PENS-Diet + probiotics compared with those with a PENS-Diet. Moreover, an enrichment of anti-obesogenic bacteria, including *Bifidobacterium spp*, *Akkermansia spp*, *Prevotella spp*, and the attenuation of the Firmicutes/Bacteroidetes ratio were noted in fecal samples after probiotics administration. In obese patients, the addition of probiotics to a PENS intervention under a hypocaloric diet could further improve weight loss and glycemic and lipid profile in parallel to the amelioration of gut dysbiosis.

Keywords: obesity; percutaneous electrical stimulation; dermatome T6; microbiota

1. Introduction

About a third of the population in developed countries is obese in some degree [1]. The WHO has proposed the classification of normal weight to be when the body mass index (BMI) ranges between 18.5 and 24.9 kg/m^2, overweight (BMI 25–29.9 kg/m^2), class I obesity (BMI 30–34.9 kg/m^2), class II obesity (BMI 35–39.9 kg/m^2), and class III obesity (BMI ≥ 40 kg/m^2) [2]. Obesity itself is a health risk factor that influences the development and progression of various metabolic and cardiovascular diseases, such as dyslipidemia, type-2 diabetes mellitus (T2D), hypertension, and ischemic heart disease, thereby worsening the quality of life of patients and survival [3]. This non-communicable disease is also associated with low-grade, chronic systemic inflammation by dysregulation of adipokines and pro-inflammatory mediators (i.e., cytokines, chemokine), and subsequent alterations in the immune cell composition and distribution [4]. Obesity is a multifactorial disease and thus, therapeutic approaches should be diverse [5]. In this sense, dietary treatments associated with body exercise are primary anti-obesity approaches. Other strategies, such as behavior therapy, have been also considered [6]. However, long-term strategies with hypocaloric diets and physical exercise are not frequently attained, and psychological comorbidities may be chronic in these patients. In consequence, alternative procedures should be explored. In this regard, by percutaneous electrical neurostimulation (PENS) of the sensory nerve terminals located in dermatome T6, the gastric wall can be stimulated to produce distention in the fasting state, and to block contractions in the postprandial phase [7]. As a result, stomach emptying is slowed and early satiety is promoted. Moreover, the associated modulation of neuronal activities influences on appetite reduction [8]. Indeed, we previously demonstrated that PENS achieved a significantly greater weight loss than an isolated hypocaloric diet in patients with BMI > 30 kg/m^2, and this effect could be due, at least in part, to ghrelin inhibition [9,10].

Importantly, pathogenesis of obesity has been linked with alterations in gut microorganisms. The intestinal microbiota is composed of tens of trillions of microorganisms, including at least 1000 different species of known bacteria, placed in the gut lumen or adhered to the mucus layer [11]. The five dominant bacterial phyla in the human gut are Firmicutes, Bacteroidetes, Actinobacteria, Proteobacteria, and Verrumicrobia [12]. The immunomodulatory bacteria are of great importance for local and systemic immunity, whereas the muconutritive microbiota are responsible of mucus layer formation, and the proteolytic bacteria have key metabolic functions in protein digestion [13]. Among other functions, microbiota participates in the metabolism of proteins, plant polyphenols, bile acids, and vitamins, and in the assimilation of non-absorbable carbohydrates by conversion into monosaccharides and short chain fatty acids (SCFA) and gases. However, though the intestinal microbiota is highly diverse in "healthy" individuals, those exhibiting adiposity, insulin resistance and/or dyslipidemia are characterized by low bacterial diversity [14]. Furthermore, obesity is associated with substantial changes in the composition and metabolic functions of bacteria, making an "obese microbiota", which involves a greater extraction of nutrients from the diet [15]. Bacteroidetes prevalence is generally lower in obese people, in contrast with that of Firmicutes. However, the complexity of how the gut microbiome modulates obesity can be more than a simple disproportion between these commensal phyla [16,17]. In this line, different probiotics have demonstrated that they can balance microbiota bacteria and subsequently reduce body weight and metabolic and cardiovascular factors [18]. Thus, the aim of this study was to investigate the effect of probiotics on anti-obesity actions of PENS in conjunction with a hypocaloric diet.

2. Methodology

2.1. Subjects of Study

A pilot prospective study (NCT03872245) was completed in the Obesity Unit of Garcilaso Clinic (Madrid, Spain). The inclusion criteria were adult patients with a body mass index (BMI) > 30 kg/m^2, with previous failure in dietary treatment. The exclusion criteria were (i) untreated endocrine diseases causing obesity, (ii) portable electric devices, (iii) diagnosis of previous cardiovascular events (acute myocardial infarction or coronary syndrome, heart failure) or cancer, and (iv) earlier treatment with hormone, prebiotics, probiotics, or nutritional supplements. In a previous study, we had observed that PENS of dermatome T6 (PENS) associated with the hypocaloric (1200 Kcal) diet produced a significantly greater weight loss (BMI = −5.1 kg/m^2) than only PENS (BMI = −1.4 kg/m^2) or the isolated hypocaloric diet (BMI = −2.0 kg/m^2) [9]. Moreover, data from the literature have shown that single or multistrain probiotics alone produced minimal changes in body weight (BMI = −0.36 and −0.15 kg/m^2, respectively) and in glycemic/lipidemic factors [19]. Therefore, we have now treated obese subjects, who previously were unsuccessfully treated only with the hypocaloric diet, with PENS with or without probiotics under the same diet in order to observe the potential differences in weight loss, associated cardiovascular factors (i.e., blood pressure, glycemia, and lipidemia), and microbiota. Thus, patients ($n = 20$) were randomized into two groups for anti-obesity interventions; PENS in conjunction with a hypocaloric diet ($n = 10$) (PENS-Diet), and the same strategy plus an administration of probiotics ($n = 10$) (PENS-Diet + probiotics). We followed a simple randomization using a random number table. All patients signed an informed consent for inclusion in the study and the use of clinical data for this research project. The Ethical Committee of Clinical Research (Medicine, Esthetic and longevity Foundation) approved this investigation (ref.: Garcilas-19-3; Feb 2019). The work was carried out in accordance with The Code of Ethics of the World Medical Association (Declaration of Helsinki). All participants finished the study.

2.2. Percutaneous Electrical Stimulation (PENS)

The PENS of dermatome T6 was performed as previously described [10] by using the Urgent PC 200 Neuromodulation System® (Uroplasty, Minnetonka, MN, USA). Patients were placed in a supine position without anesthesia, and PENS was delivered by a needle electrode inserted in the left upper quadrant along the medio-clavicular line, at two centimeters below the ribcage, at a 90° angle towards the abdominal wall, and at 0.5–1 cm of depth. Successful insertion was confirmed by the feeling of electric movement at least 5 cm beyond the dermatome territory. The PENS was undertaken at a frequency of 20 Hz at the highest amplify (0–20 mA) without causing any pain. The participants underwent one 30-min session every week for ten consecutive weeks.

2.3. Hypocaloric Diet, Exercise, and Probiotics Administration

A 1200 Kcal/day diet was uniformly prescribed during PENS interventions in both groups of patients, as we previously published. The diet followed a Mediterranean style (carbohydrates 51%, proteins 23% and fat 26%) with a high intake of fruit and vegetables, a moderate intake of meats, and olive oil as the main source of fat [20]. Briefly, patients were recommended to take skimmed milk (200 mL) or natural yogurt and bread (200 g) as breakfast, 100 g of fruit (e.g., apple, pear) mid-morning, and 200 g of vegetables (e.g., spinach, lettuce, cauliflower) or pasta soup, fish (120 g) or chicken (100 g), and fruit (100 g), at lunch and dinner. Olive oil (30 cc) could be also taken as a complement, and skimmed milk (200 mL) with coffee or tea as a snack. A record of food intake was applied along the study. The intake of alcohol and nutritional supplements was not allowed during the study. Moreover, patients received instructions for regular exercise practice (1 h of brisk walking/day), following a counselling protocol against obesity in patients under 50 years [21]. Brisk walking consisted of a moderate-intensity exercise of walking to a minimum speed of 100 steps per minute (about 4.8 km/h). Since obese patients have many difficulties in adhering to nutritional advice and exercise recommendations, we did a weekly follow-up of food intake and exercise practice. Our dietician phoned all the patients to remind them of the need to stick to these recommendations. The dietician wrote down the daily intake of food and the time/speed of brisk walking. At the end of the study (10 weeks), the dietician confirmed a full adherence rate to the Mediterranean diet and daily exercise. In a previous work, we described a 98% and 94% diet compliance in patients undergoing PENS or PENS-Diet interventions, respectively [9]. The reduction of appetite induced by PENS and the short length of the study could facilitate this high adherence. Some patients additionally received two tablets per day of probiotics Adomelle® (4th generation technology, Bromatech, Italy) during the ten weeks of treatment. The composition of Adomelle® was *Lactobacillus plantarum LP115* ($<1 \times 10^9$ colony forming units; CFU), *Bifidobacterium brevis B3* ($<1 \times 10^9$ CFU), and *Lactobacillus acidophilus LA14* (1×10^9 CFU). The probiotics were given after meals with drinking water and did not alter the food intake. Participants were also compliant with probiotics intake.

2.4. Variables

2.4.1. Anthropometric Variables

Anthropometric parameters at baseline and after interventions included the body mass index (BMI, as the body weight in kg/m^2), weight loss (WL, as ([Initial BMI]—[Post-intervention BMI])), percent of total weight loss (%TWL, as ([Initial Weight]—[Post-intervention Weight])/([Initial Weight])) × 100, and the percentage excess BMI loss (%EBMIL, as (ΔBMI/[Initial BMI–25]) × 100). We evaluated systolic and diastolic blood pressures by using automatic tensiometer device (Omron M2-HEM-7121-E, Kyoto, Japan). Blood samples were centrifuged for 20 min at 2.500 g and the obtained plasma was tested for glucose and lipid determinations. The fasting glucose and glycated hemoglobin (A1C), and the lipid profile (triglycerides, total cholesterol, LDL-cholesterol, and HDL-cholesterol) were quantified by standard methods (ADVIA 2400 Chemistry System, Siemens, Germany) in the Analytical department of Hospital Fundación Jiménez Díaz. All variables were measured before and after interventions.

2.4.2. Analysis of Microbiota

Fecal samples were obtained in OMNIgene-GUT tubes (Abyntek, Spain) at the beginning and after treatments, and stored at −80 °C. Patients did a self-collection at home, following the manufacturer's instructions. They took fecal samples free from urine or toilet water with a spatula, and transferred them into provided tubes (with homogenizer and stabilizing liquid). Samples were kept for one week at room temperature and delivered to the dietician, who froze them (−80 °C) until use. The OMNIgene-GUT kit provides a valid method to keep RNA at room temperature [22]. After two months, total RNA was extracted from feces (~50 mg) by dissolving in Trizol reagent (Thermo Fisher). RNA concentration and purity were assessed by the 260/280 nm-ratio using the Nanodrop spectrophotometer (Nirko). Equal amounts of RNA were reverse-transcribed to obtain the cDNA for quantitative-PCR (qPCR), as previously described [23]. The gene expression assays were labelled with Fam fluorophore, whereas the housekeeping gene was labelled by VIC fluorophore. Amplification conditions were: 2′ at 50 °C, 10″ at 95 °C and 40 cycles of 15″ at 95 °C and 1′ at 60 °C (AB7500 fast y Quant Studio 5; Thermo Fisher). All samples were prepared in triplicate to obtain their threshold cycle (Ct). If deviation for each triplicate were higher than 0.3 cycles, Ct was not considered. The relative expression for each gene was achieved following the model $R = 2^{-\Delta\Delta Ct}$. The primer setup was designed to target the ribosomal RNA genes (16S) of the major bacterial groups present in the mammalian intestinal microbiota, including the Firmicutes, Bacteroidetes, Proteobacteria, Fusobacteria, Actinobacteria, and Verrucomicrobia phyla [24]. To gain an insight into the bacterial composition, we used specific primers for bacterial species (Table 2). The specificity of primers was checked in silico with the "probe match" facility of the Ribosomal Database Project (http://rdp.cme.msu.edu/), and further validated on the BLAST search (NCBI) [25]. The primers were purchased from Thermo Scientific, and stored at −20 °C. The reference ranges for intestinal bacteria were calculated as an average of number of gene copies (NGC) from fecal samples of a control population of volunteer patients (Supplementary Materials Figure S1). These subjects (Spanish; 50% females; 45.0 ± 5.0 years-old; $n = 100$) were non-obese; normoglycemic and normolipidemic; and free from known cardiovascular, malignant, and digestive or intestinal diseases. Thus, characteristics of this control group could be compared with those of the study group.

2.5. Statistics

Quantitative variables were summarized as mean values and standard deviation, or by median and interquartile range, depending on the symmetry of the data distribution. Variables with normal distribution were expressed as mean values and standard deviation, whereas those variables with non-normal distribution were shown as median and interquartile ranges. Normality of quantitative variables was analyzed by the Shapiro Wilk test. Variables with normal distribution were compared using Student's t test for independent and paired samples, while variables with non-normal distribution were compared using the Mann–Whitney U test for independent samples, and a Wilcoxon Signed Rank test for relate samples. Associations between variables were studied by the univariate linear regression or quantile regression. Values of $p < 0.05$ were considered significant. Statistical analyses were performed using the statistical package for social science (SPSS, IBM, Armonk, NY, USA), version 26.0.

3. Results

3.1. Characterization of the Obese Population with Gut Dysbiosis

A total of twenty patients (14 females, mean age 46.4 ± 5.7 years-old; and 6 males, mean age 41.0 ± 12.1 years-old) with mostly class-I obesity were included in this pilot study (Table 1). At baseline, their body weight and the body mass index (BMI) were 87.8 ± 8.4 kg and 32.2 (5.3) kg/m^2, respectively. According with the established pathophysiological parameters of blood pressure and glycemia [26,27], they were in the limit of normotension and normoglycemia. Their lipid profile was also slightly altered [28], showing a minor elevation of triglycerides, total cholesterol, and LDL-cholesterol, whereas HDL-cholesterol was in the normal range.

Table 1. Distribution of age, gender, and baseline blood pressure, glycemic and lipid profile between groups.

	Total Population ($n = 20$)	PENS-Diet ($n = 10$)	PENS-Diet + Probiotics ($n = 10$)	T(df)/U Value	p Value
Age (years)	44.7 ± 8.2	45.2 ± 8.9	44.3 ± 7.8	0.24	0.813
Females/Males	14/6	7/3	7/3	-	>0.999
Body weight (kg)	87.8 ± 8.4	84.6 ± 5.1	91.1 ± 10.1	−1.82 (18)	0.085
BMI (kg/m^2)	32.2 (5.3)	32.2 (2.76)	33.0 (6.82)	48.0	0.912
Systolic blood pressure (mmHg)	137.5 (20.0)	140.0 (20.0)	130.0 (22.5)	41.5	0.529
Diastolic blood pressure (mmHg)	80.0 (8.75)	80.0 (6.25)	80.0 (10.0)	46.0	0.796
Fasting glucose (mg/dL)	95.5 (24.5)	96.5 (29.7)	95.5 (20.2)	48.0	0.912
A1C (%)	5.5 ± 0.7	5.4 ± 0.7	5.6 ± 0.7	−0.61 (18)	0.544
Triglycerides (mg/dL)	148.5 (60.7)	156.0 (96.2)	147.0 (42.5)	49.5	>0.999
Total cholesterol (mg/dL)	199.9 ± 44.0	204.9 ± 52.4	195.0 ± 35.9	0.49 (18)	0.628
LDL-cholesterol (mg/dL)	102.0 (57.0)	114.6 (79.0)	107.0 (44.2)	48.0	0.912
HDL-cholesterol (mg/dL)	45.0 (55.1)	47.7 (22.7)	44.5 (15.0)	38.0	0.393

BMI, A1C, LDL, and HDL, as the body mass index, glycated hemoglobin, and low- and high-density lipoprotein, respectively. T and U values are also shown. Df, as degrees of freedom.

In addition, this obese cohort with a potential low risk of metabolic and cardiovascular disease showed an altered composition and distribution of bacterial gut microbiota. By directed qPCR analysis of fecal samples, we evaluated the presence of muconutritive, immunomodulatory, and proteolytic bacteria. We observed an overall decrease in bacteria number, with a reduction in Firmicutes and mostly Bacteroidetes phylum (8.3 and 7.5 log NGC/g, respectively), compared to reference parameters (Table 2). Among Firmicutes, *Faecalibacterium sp* and *Enterococcus spp* were lessened. In the Bacteroidetes phylum, there was a notorious diminution of *Bacteroides spp*. Thus, the ratio of Firmicutes/Bacteroidetes was 0.5, which was over the reference range. In contrast, these patients showed normal levels of the Proteobacteria and Fusobacteria phyla (Table 2), but a robust decrease in the Actinobacteria and Verrucomicrobia phyla, particularly in the *Bifidobacterium spp* and *Akkermansia muciniphila*, respectively. As expected, these data suggest that obese patients exhibited gut dysbiosis with a significant alteration in the number and distribution of, particularly, muconutritive and immunomodulatory bacteria.

Table 2. Gut microbiota in obese patients.

	Total Population (log NGC/g)	PENS-Diet (n = 10)	PENS-Diet + Probiotics (n = 10)	T(df)/U Value	p Value	Reference Range (log NGC/g)
Firmicutes phylum	**8.3 ± 0.86**	8.2 ± 0.94	8.4 ± 0.81	−0.49 (18)	0.630	8.5–11.0
Lactobacillus spp	4.9 ± 1.13	4.8 ± 1.47	5.0 ± 0.7	−0.5 (18)	0.619	4.5–7.0
Faecalibacterium sp	**6.2 ± 1.09**	6.0 ± 1.25	6.5 ± 0.89	−1.04 (18)	0.308	7.0–9.0
Roseburia spp	6.7 (1.08)	6.6 (1.75)	6.9 (0.85)	33.5	0.218	6.5–8.5
Bacillus sp	1.9 ± 0.82	2.0 ± 1.0	1.9 ± 0.67	0.27 (18)	0.979	0–4.0
Staphylococcus spp	3.0 ± 0.62	3.1 ± 0.64	2.9 ± 0.62	0.67 (18)	0.509	2.5–5.0
Veillonella spp	4.5 ± 0.86	4.4 ± 1.06	4.6 ± 0.63	−0.61 (18)	0.547	4.5–7.0
Clostridium (Cocc)	8.2 (1.05)	7.9 (1.7)	8.4 (0.9)	28.5	0.105	7.0–9.0
Clostridium (Perf)	3.8 ± 1.19	3.7 ± 1.51	3.9 ± 0.83	−0.23 (18)	0.814	0–5.0
Enterococcus spp	**5.9 (1.20)**	5.6 (1.67)	6.2 (1.05)	28.5	0.105	6.0–8.5
Bacteroidetes phylum	**7.5 (1.63)**	8.1 (1.87)	7.5 (1.0)	40.0	0.481	8.0–11.0
Prevotella spp	6.7 (3.7)	5.1 (4.1)	7.3 (4.5)	47.5	0.853	5.0–8.5
Bacteroides spp	**7.1 ± 1.26**	7.4 ± 1.16	6.7 ± 1.33	1.18 (18)	0.252	7.5–9.0
Firmicutes/Bacteroidetes	**0.5 ± 0.4**	0.5 ± 0.4	0.46 ± 0.3	0.37 (18)	0.714	0.1–0.3
Proteobacteria phylum	5.7 (1.89)	6.0 (1.37)	5.0 (1.29)	39.0	0.436	3.0–7.0
Escherichia coli	4.5 ± 1,81	4.5 ± 1.79	4.6 ± 1.92	−0.18 (18)	0.859	4.5–7.0
Pseudomonas spp	1.0 (1.45)	1.0 (1.42)	1.0 (1.5)	45.5	0.739	0–4.0
Campylobacter spp	1.0 (<0.001)	1.0 (<0.001)	1.0 (0.73)	45.0	0.739	0–3.5
Helicobacter spp	2.4 (2.1)	1.9 (2.2)	2.4 (1.95)	48.0	0.912	0–3.5
Fusobacteria phylum	2.79 ± 1.24	2.42 ± 1.26	3.16 ± 1.15	−1.36 (18)	0.188	0–4.5
Fusobacterium nucleatum	2.79 ± 1.24	2.42 ± 1.26	3.16 ± 1.15	−1.36 (18)	0.188	0–4.5
Actinobacteria phylum	**4.41 ± 2.28**	4.34 ± 2.78	4.48 ± 1.79	−0.14 (18)	0.891	6.5–9.0
Bifidobacterium spp	**3.85 ± 1.96**	3.8 ± 2.4	3.9 ± 1.6	−0.11 (18)	0.913	5.5–7.5
Verrucomicrobia phylum	**2.6 (3.65)**	1.8 (2.3)	3.7 (3.47)	30.0	0.143	5.5–9.0
Akkermansia muciniphila	**2.4 (3.33)**	1.7 (2.1)	3.4 (3.2)	29.0	0.123	5.0–8.5

Relevant bacteria phyla; Firmicutes and Bacteriodetes, and its ratio, and Proteobacteria, Fusobacteria, Actinobacteria, and Verrumicrobia, were evaluated in fecal samples before anti-obesity treatments. The reference ranges for the bacteria phyla were obtained from fecal samples of a control population (see Methodology and Supplementary Materials Figure S1). T and U values are shown. Df, as degrees of freedom. In bold, bacteria levels outside the reference ranges. NGC/g: number of gene copies per gram of feces.

3.2. Reduction of the Body Weight and CV Risk Factors by PENS-Diet +/− Probiotics

Since patients displayed an elevated BMI with altered microbiota, we next examined the effect of an anti-obesity strategy based on satiety neurostimulation and intake of a hypocaloric diet (PENS-Diet), with or without administration of multistrain probiotics. Patients were randomly divided into two groups (n = 10, each), with no significant differences in age, gender, body weight, BMI, blood pressure, glycemia, and lipid profile (Table 1). Gut microbiota was also akin in both groups (Table 2). Thus, before interventions, anthropomorphic characteristics and microbiota distribution were similar between groups. After ten weeks, patients with a PENS-Diet showed significant reductions in body weight and BMI (Table 3). BMI was reduced by 13% and dropped into the overweight range (28.0 kg/m^2). PENS-Diet also decreased systolic and diastolic blood pressure, fasting glucose, triglycerides, and total cholesterol. Interestingly, patients with a PENS-Diet + probiotics exhibited a similar effect by ameliorating 20% of body weight and BMI (26.3 kg/m^2), as well as blood pressure, fasting glucose, A1C, and triglycerides. Moreover, no adverse effects were found in both groups of subjects.

By further comparison between both therapeutic approaches (Table 4), PENS-Diet + probiotics unveiled a significantly higher weight loss (16.2 vs. 11.1 kg, respectively; p = 0.022) and total weight loss (%TWL) (17.5 vs. 12.9%, respectively; p = 0.02) than the PENS-Diet intervention. The excess BMI lost (%EBMIL) was also significantly higher (84.2 vs. 57.0%, respectively; p = 0.021) after probiotics. Moreover, plasma A1C, triglycerides and HDL-cholesterol levels were more reduced (−0.46 vs. −0.05 mg/dL, p = 0.032; −47.0 vs. −8.5 mg/dL, p = 0.002; and 10.5 vs. 0.05 mg/dL, p = 0.005, respectively) (Table 4). These data suggest that an administration of multistrain probiotics to a PENS therapy under hypocaloric diets could further decrease the body weight, glycemia, and dyslipidemia in obese patients. In this regard, we tested the potential associations between probiotics and the body weight parameters, A1C, and lipid levels. By univariate linear regression, probiotics administration was significantly associated with the difference of WL, %TWL, %EBMIL, and A1C. Similarly, by quantile regression, probiotics was associated with the difference of TG and HDL (Figure 1A). Indeed, probiotics showed a positive association with WL, %TWL, %EBMIL, and HDL, while it was negative with A1C and TG (Figure 1B).

Table 3. Weight loss and improvement of blood pressure, glycemia, and dyslipidemia after PENS-Diet or PENS-Diet + probiotics interventions.

	Baseline	+ PENS-Diet	T(df)/W Value	p Value
Body weight (kg)	84.6 ± 5.1	73.5 ± 3.7	7.91 (9)	<0.001
BMI (kg/m^2)	32.2 (2.76)	28.0 (1.6)	0.00	0.005
Systolic blood pressure (mmHg)	140.0 (20.0)	120.0 (2.5)	0.00	0.018
Diastolic blood pressure (mmHg)	80.0 (6.25)	70.0 (20.0)	7.5	0.038
Fasting glucose (mg/dL)	96.5 (29.7)	88.5 (25.0)	0.00	0.005
A1C (%)	5.4 ± 0.7	5.3 ± 0.5	0.36 (9)	0.723
Triglycerides (mg/dL)	156.0 (96.2)	138.5 (80.9)	0.00	0.005
Total cholesterol (mg/dL)	204.9 ± 52.4	195.9 ± 46.5	1.75 (9)	0.004
LDL-cholesterol (mg/dL)	114.6 (79.0)	132.5 (78.25)	21.0	0.507
HDL-cholesterol (mg/dL)	47.7 (22.7)	51.5 (24.9)	5.0	0.798
	Baseline	+PENS-Diet + probiotics	T(df)/W value	p value
Body weight (kg)	91.1 ± 10.1	74.9 ± 6.7	11.09 (9)	<0.001
BMI (kg/m^2)	33.0 (6.82)	26.3 (4.3)	0.00	0.005
Systolic blood pressure (mmHg)	130.0 (22.5)	120.0 (12.5)	0.00	0.011
Diastolic blood pressure (mmHg)	80.0 (10.0)	80.0 (15.0)	0.00	0.041
Fasting glucose (mg/dL)	95.5 (20.2)	84.0 (11.5)	6.00	0.028
A1C (%)	5.6 ± 0.7	5.1 ± 0.4	3.63 (9)	0.012
Triglycerides (mg/dL)	147.0 (42.5)	85.5 (38.7)	0.0	0.005
Total cholesterol (mg/dL)	195.0 ± 35.9	176.5 ± 47.2	1.75 (9)	0.113
LDL-cholesterol (mg/dL)	107.0 (44.2)	100.0 (46.2)	13.0	0.139
HDL-cholesterol (mg/dL)	44.5 (15.0)	57.0 (20.0)	10	0.074

The body weight, BMI, systolic and diastolic blood pressures, fasting glucose, A1C, and lipid profiles were analyzed after ten weeks of anti-obesity approaches. In bold are the statistically significant data. Variables with normal distribution were compared using Student's t test for paired samples, whereas variables with non-normal distribution were compared using the Wilcoxon Signed Rank test. T and W values are shown. Df, as degrees of freedom. $p < 0.05$ was considered significant. BMI, A1C, LDL, and HDL, as the body mass index, glycated hemoglobin, and low- and high-density lipoprotein, respectively.

Table 4. Differences in weight loss, blood pressure, and plasma parameters between PENS-Diet and PENS-Diet + probiotics.

	+PENS-Diet	+PENS-Diet + Probiotics	T(df)/U-Value	p Value
WL (kg)	11.1 ± 4.4	16.2 ± 4.6	2.51 (18)	0.022
%TWL	12.9 ± 4.5	17.5 ± 3.5	−2.54 (18)	0.020
%EBMIL	57.0 ± 12.3	84.2 ± 29.5	−2.28 (18)	0.021
Dif. Systolic blood pressure (mmHg)	−12.5 (22.5)	−10.0 (12.5)	43.0	0.631
Dif. Diastolic blood pressure (mmHg)	−10.0 (10.0)	−2.5 (10.0)	24.0	0.052
Dif. Fasting glucose (mg/dL)	−7.0 (11.0)	−13.0 (16.5)	31.0	0.165
Dif. A1C (%)	−0.05 ± 0.4	−0.46± 0.4	2.32 (18)	0.032
Dif. Triglycerides (mg/dL)	−8.5 (26.0)	−47.0 (63.75)	11.0	0.002
Dif. Total cholesterol (mg/dL)	−9.0 ± 7.4	−18.5 ± 33.3	0.87 (18)	0.391
Dif. LDL-cholesterol (mg/dL)	0.5 (42.75)	−18.0 (25.5)	26.0	0.075
Dif. HDL-cholesterol (mg/dL)	0.05 (6.8)	10.5 (12)	14.00	0.005

The weight loss and percentages of TWL and EBMIL, systolic and diastolic blood pressure, and plasma glucose and lipids (triglycerides, total cholesterol, LDL-c and HDL-c) were compared between both groups of patients. In bold, the statistically significant data. Variables with a normal distribution were compared using Student's t-test for independent samples, while those with a non-normal distribution were compared using the Mann–Whitney U test. T and U values are also shown. Df, as degrees of freedom. $p < 0.05$ was considered significant. WL, %TWL and %EBMIL, as weight loss, percent of total weight loss, and the percentage excess BMI loss, respectively. A1C, LDL, and HDL, as glycated hemoglobin, and low- and high-density lipoprotein, respectively.

	+ PENS-Diet	+ PENS-Diet + Probiotics	Coefficient	p Value	95% CI	R Squared
WL (kg)	11.1 ± 4.4	16.2 ± 4.6	5.08	**0.022**	0.83 to 9.33	0.259
%TWL	12.9 ± 4.5	17.5 ± 3.5	4.565	**0.020**	0.80 to 8.33	0.265
%EBMIL	57.0 ± 12.3	84.2 ± 29.5	53.42	**0.021**	4.32 to 102.5	0.225
Dif. A1C (%)	−0.05 ± 0.4	−0.46 ± 0.4	−0.41	**0.032**	−0.79 to −0.039	0.230
Dif. Triglycerides (mg/dL)	−8.5 (26.0)	−47 (63.75)	−53.0	**0.014**	−93.93 to −12.06	-
Dif. HDL-cholesterol (mg/dL)	0.05 (6.8)	10.5 (12)	14.7	**0.036**	1.03 to 28.4	-

(A)

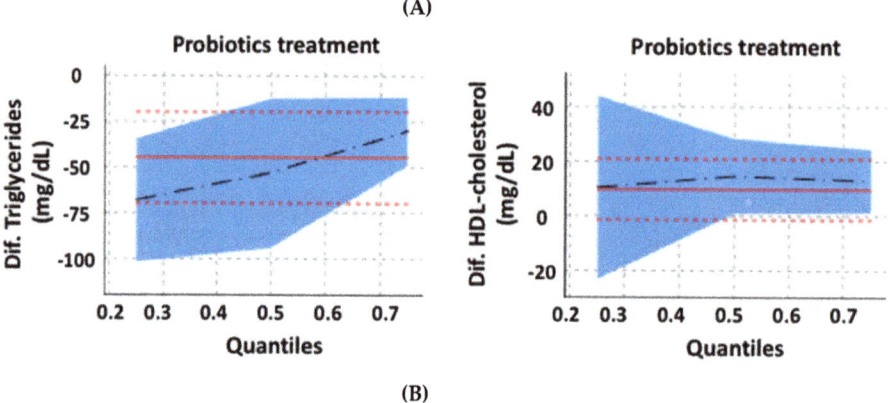

(B)

Figure 1. Associations for probiotics and the body weight, glycemia, and dyslipidemia in obese patients. By univariate linear regression, the probiotics administration was significantly associated with WL, %TWL, %EBMIL, and A1C, whereas by a quantile regression, probiotics were associated with TG and HDL (**A**). In bold, the statistically significant data. Probiotics exhibited a positive association with WL, %TWL, %EBMIL, and HDL, while it was negative with A1C and TG (**B**). The associations between variables with a normal distribution were studied by a univariate linear regression, while those with non-normal distribution were studied by a quantile regression. WL, %TWL and %EBMIL, as weight loss, percent of total weight loss, and the percentage excess BMI loss, respectively. A1C and HDL, as glycated hemoglobin, and high-density lipoprotein, respectively.

3.3. Microbiota Modifications after PENS-Diet +/− Probiotics

Alterations in human obesity, glycemia, and lipidemia could parallel changes in gut microbiota [29]. In fact, PENS-Diet showed a tendency to enrich some specific bacteria (i.e., *Prevotella spp*, *Bifidobacterium spp*) and to improve the Firmicutes/Bacteroidetes ratio (Table 5). However, PENS-Diet + probiotics was able to increase *Prevotella spp* (+1.3%, $p = 0.05$) and further reduce the Firmicutes/Bacteroidetes ratio (0.10).

This intervention also stimulated *Bifidobacterium spp* (+51.2%; $p = 0.005$) and *Akkermansia muciniphila* (+41.1%, $p = 0.033$) growth (Table 5). Thus, an addition of probiotics to anti-obesity intervention with a PENS-Diet may help to attenuate the altered Firmicutes/Bacteroidetes ratio in an obese gut, and to enrich its content of *Prevotella spp*, and mostly, Actinobacteria *(Bifidobacterium spp)* and Verrucomicrobia *(Akkermansia muciniphila)* bacteria.

Table 5. Bacterial differences after PENS-Diet or PENS-Diet + probiotics interventions.

	Baseline	+ PENS-Diet	*p* Value	Baseline	+PENS-Diet + Probiotics	*p* Value	T *(df)/U *	*p* *
Prevotella spp	5.10 (4.1)	5.25 (2.9)	>0.999	7.30 (4.5)	7.40 (2.5)	0.05	20.5	**0.023**
Bifidobacterium spp	3.80 ± 2.4	3.90 ± 2.1	0.911	3.90 ± 1.6	5.90 ± 0.9	**0.005**	−2.27 (18)	**0.036**
Akkermansia muciniphila	1.70 (2.1)	1.50 (2.6)	0.151	3.40 (3.2)	4.80 (1.7)	**0.033**	13.5	**0.004**
Firmicutes/Bacteroidetes	0.50 ± 0.4	0.40 ± 0.3	0.480	0.46 ± 0.3	0.10 ± 0.5	**0.019**	2.17 (18)	**0.043**

Prevotella spp, *Bifidobacterium spp*, and *Akkermansia muciniphila* levels (log NGC/g) in obese patients after PENS-Diet or PENS-Diet + probiotics. The ratio of Firmicutes/Bacteroidetes is also shown for both strategies. Variables with a normal distribution were compared using Student's t test for independent and paired samples, whereas variables with non-normal distribution were compared using the Mann–Whitney U test for independent samples and Wilcoxon Signed Rank test for related samples. $p < 0.05$ was considered significant. T * and U *, as T-value and U-value between PENS-Diet + probiotics and PENS-Diet interventions. Df, as degrees of freedom. *p* *, as *p* value between PENS-Diet + probiotics and PENS-Diet interventions. In bold, the statistically significant data.

4. Discussion

The great majority of obese subjects are in the class I obese category, which considerably increases morbidity and public health expenses. In the US Centers for Disease Control and Prevention [30], epidemiological data indicate that approximately 2/3 of obese men and 50% of obese women are in this group. Although the mortality rate within class I obesity is similar to normal weight, the risk of developing T2DM, hypertension, dyslipidemia, metabolic syndrome, obstructive sleep apnea, cancer, and non-alcoholic fatty liver disease is notoriously elevated [31]. Therefore, the evidence calls attention to finding more effective and safe therapies for these patients. In this regard, PENS of dermatome T6 has been proposed as an alternative to pharmacological products and surgical procedures to decrease appetite and weight loss, allowing a better compliance of hypocaloric diets. PENS was initially applied to morbidly obese patients awaiting bariatric surgery, in order to reduce the pre-surgery body weight [10]. Later, we and others extended this technique to patients with overweight and mild-to-moderate obesity. PENS or the hypocaloric diet induced by themselves a significant but slight reduction in body weight (3.6 and 5.6 kg, respectively). However, the combination of both PENS and a diet revealed a mean of weight loss over 10–14 kg, with maintained effects for at least one year after therapy [8,9,32]. Now, in class I obese individuals, we show that ten weeks of PENS-Diet displayed a similar reduction in body weight (11.1 kg) and an improvement of blood pressure and the glycemic and lipid profiles. These effects could be justified by the caloric restriction and by the neurostimulation of the gastric wall and promotion of early satiety [9]. However, an alteration in gut microbiota could have also played a key role. In this regard, the etiopathogenetic of obesity is multifactorial and data from literature suggest a contribution of intestinal dysbiosis in obesity development [33]. Our obese subjects unveiled a microbiota alteration, with a reduction of muconutritive and immunomodulatory bacteria such as *Akkermansia muciniphila*, *Faecalibacterium sp*, and *Bifidobacterium spp*. In consonance, the Firmicutes/Bacteroidetes ratio was considerably elevated. Importantly, these variations in microbiota may have influenced on obesity development [34,35]. However, PENS-Diet tended to enrich *Prevotella spp* and consequently, the balance of Firmicutes/Bacteroidetes was slightly lessened. The amelioration of this ratio has been frequently linked with an improvement of weight loss and intestinal inflammation and permeabilization [36], and although a precise taxonomic characterization of the bacteria would have been discerned between species, *Prevotella spp* can lead to beneficial effects on mucin regulation, glucose metabolism, and hepatic glycogen storage [37]. Undoubtedly, several lifestyle factors (e.g., smoking, sedentarism, stress, circadian rhythms, personal hygiene, ovarian cycle) may have also altered intestinal microbiota. In this sense, a 20% rate of menopause (without hormonal supplementation) was described in both groups of patients.

In this line, the addition of a multistrain probiotic to the PENS-Diet could have further enhanced these favorable effects. Adomelle® is formulated by *Lactobacillus plantarum LP115*, *Bifidobacterium brevis B3*, and *Lactobacillus acidophilus LA14*. Supplementation of *L. plantarum* in humans and mice induced a body fat decrease and muscle mass increase, enhancing energy harvest and anti-fatigue effects [38,39]. In obese mice, *L. plantarum* also reduced insulin resistance, plasma triglycerides and proinflammatory factors [40]. *L. acidophilus*, when combined with phenolic compounds or other probiotics, induced weight loss in overweight adults [41]. Moreover, it promoted a significant improvement of glucose homeostasis and cholesterol metabolism in obese mice, by gene downregulation of glucose transporters, cholesterol precursors, and immune factors [42]. Finally, administration of *B. breve-B3* ameliorated the body fat in obese individuals and rats due to its ability to conjugate linoleic acid from diets [43,44]. In our study, the addition of these probiotics to the PENS-Diet further improved the body weight, plasma A1C, triglycerides, and HDL-cholesterol. Moreover, a clear tendency was found for fasting glucose, TC and LDL-cholesterol, which could reach statistical significance in a larger group of patients. Previous randomized controlled trials showed that administration of probiotics alone slightly reduced the body weight and BMI (−0.55 kg and −0.3 kg/m^2, respectively) in parallel with fasting glucose (−0.35 mg/dL) and lipids (total cholesterol, −0.43 mg/dL and LDL-cholesterol, −0.41 mg/dL) [19]. Particularly, single probiotics such as *Lactobacillus gasseri*, *Bifidobacterium animalis*, and *Pediococcus pentosaceus* achieved higher benefits than multiple probiotics (i.e., combinations of *Bifidobacterium spp.*, *Lactobacillus spp.*, and/or *Lactococcus spp.*) Thus, a combination of diverse anti-obesity strategies could lead to better outcomes against obesity. In particular, probiotics may induce summative effects when administered together with PENS and a hypocaloric diet. In fact, this triple intervention exhibited a synergic action on reduction of body weight and cardiovascular risk factors. Likely, the promotion of early satiety induced by PENS could be helped by the ingestion of a salutary diet of low caloric intake, and by the balance of healthy microbiota. In this sense, the addition of probiotics further enhanced *Prevotella spp*, *Bifidobacterium spp*, and *Akkermansia muciniphila*, promoting a more muconutritive and immunomodulatory microbiota. *Bifidobacterium spp* have been demonstrated to be positive for the gastrointestinal barrier function and for immunoregulation [45]. By increasing the abundance of *Bifidobacterium spp* (i.e., with prebiotic oligofructose), gut permeability was reduced in obese mice, in correlation with a decrease in LPS and inflammatory markers [46]. In these animals, when combined with *L. acidophilus*, *Bifidobacterium spp* also enriched microbiota composition [47]. Moreover, *Bifidobacterium spp* produced lactate, which is transformed into butyrate by butyrate-producing bacteria in the intestine (i.e., *Prevotella ruminicola*) [48]. These SCFAs play a crucial role in cardiovascular homeostasis and lipid and glucose metabolism by supplying energy and producing glucagon-like peptide-1, peptide YY, and leptin [49]. Furthermore, butyrate induces mucin synthesis and protects intestine integrity by increasing tight junction assembly. In addition, *A. muciniphila* can also regulate gut permeability [50]. Its abundance was inversely correlated with adipose tissue inflammation and insulin resistance in mice and humans [51,52]. In obese hyperlipidemic mice, *A. muciniphila* also improved metabolic endotoxemia, vascular inflammation, and atherosclerotic lesions [53]. Altogether, the enrichment of the muconutritive and immunomodulatory bacteria observed in our patients could also participate in the improvement of their plasma metabolic and cardiovascular factors, and in the attenuation of their body weight.

Limitations of the Study

In this pilot study, we evaluated the addition of probiotics to an anti-obesity strategy with the PENS-Diet. Probiotics administration further reduced body weight, but its effect on the waist circumference was not evaluated. The abdominal obesity might be affected by microbiota changes, and its quantification would also add key information on the risk of cardiovascular disease. In addition, since multiple factors could influence the effects of probiotics, our data should be taken with care.

Unknown comorbidities or habits may alter bacterial distribution and probiotics action. Furthermore, different physical levels and skills could have affected the practice of daily exercise and subsequent weight loss in patients. A personalized control of these practices by an exercise specialist might also improve the adherence and outcomes of this work. Finally, for a group of subjects who follow only a diet regime, PENS intervention or probiotics intake could offer interesting and comparative data about potential changes in microbiota distribution. Therefore, all these variables will be considered in a future study. In this line, the estimation of the sample size per group of obese patients will be at least thirty (two-side significance level; $\alpha = 0.05$ and power $1 - \beta = 0.8$), following the published formula [54]. According to previous works, the difference of BMI among treatments would be at least 3.0 ± 4.87 kg/m^2 [55,56].

5. Conclusions

A Mediterranean-like hypocaloric diet helped to decrease the body weight, and associated hyperglycemia/hyperlipidemia and blood pressure in class-I obese patients intervened with PENS. However, the addition of *Lactobacillus plantarum LP115*, *Bifidobacterium brevis B3*, and *Lactobacillus acidophilus LA14*) promoted a positive influence on anti-obesogenic gut bacteria by increasing muconutritive (*Akkermansia muciniphila*) and immunomodulatory (*Bifidobacterium spp*) microbiota, and Bacteroidetes phylum (*Prevotella spp*). Consequently, the Firmicutes/Bacteroidetes ratio was further reduced, and these changes could be mediating, at least in part, the further improvement of the body weight and plasma A1C, triglycerides, and HDL-cholesterol. Therefore, a combined strategy of a hypocaloric diet, PENS and probiotics administration may promote summative effects against obesity and related comorbidities (i.e., cardiovascular diseases). Nevertheless, larger studies are needed to analyze the direct actions and interactions of these strategies on gut microbiota.

Supplementary Materials: The following are available online at http://www.mdpi.com/1660-4601/17/19/7239/s1, Figure S1. Gut bacteria in control subjects. Fecal samples from one hundred age- and sex-matched non-obese, normoglycemic, and normolipidemic voluntaries without known cardiovascular, malignant and digestive diseases were analyzed to estimate the control ranges for each bacteria. NGC/g: number of gene copies per gram of feces.

Author Contributions: M.C.-Y. and T.H. processed and analyzed the fecal samples. M.G.-A. acquired and interpreted the microbiota data. A.M.H. and C.L. provided the probiotics and diet recommendations to patients. J.L.-C. performed the statistics analysis. O.L. and J.R.-T. designed the study and wrote the manuscript. All authors have read and agreed to the published version of the manuscript.

Funding: This research did not receive any specific grant from funding agencies in the public, commercial, or not-for-profit sectors. L.-C.J. is a predoctoral fellow of Universidad Autónoma Madrid (FPI contract).

Acknowledgments: Authors want to thank Bromatech for the provision of probiotics Adomelle® and for dealing with the costs of microbiota analysis.

Conflicts of Interest: The authors declare no conflict of interest.

References

1. Chooi, Y.C.; Ding, C.; Magkos, F. The epidemiology of obesity. *Metab. Clin. Exp.* **2019**, *92*, 6–10. [CrossRef] [PubMed]
2. World Health Organization. *Obesity: Preventing and Managing the Global Epidemic*; Report of a WHO consultation; World Health Organization Technical Report Series; World Health Organization: Geneva, Switzerland, 2000; Volume 894, pp. 1–253.
3. Su, X.; Peng, D. Emerging functions of adipokines in linking the development of obesity and cardiovascular diseases. *Mol. Biol. Rep.* **2020**. [CrossRef] [PubMed]
4. Weinstock, A.; Silva, H.M.; Moore, K.J.; Schmidt, A.M.; Fisher, E.A. Leukocyte heterogeneity in adipose tissue, including in obesity. *Circ. Res.* **2020**, *126*, 1590–1612. [CrossRef] [PubMed]
5. Kyle, T.K.; Dhurandhar, E.J.; Allison, D.B. Regarding obesity as a disease: Evolving policies and their implications. *Endocrinol. Metab. Clin. N. Am.* **2016**, *45*, 511–520. [CrossRef]
6. Normand, M.P.; Gibson, J.L. Behavioral approaches to weight management for health and wellness. *Pediatr. Clin. N. Am.* **2020**, *67*, 537–546. [CrossRef]

7. Van Der Pal, F.; Van Balken, M.R.; Heesakkers, J.P.F.A.; Debruyne, F.M.; Bemelmans, B.L. Percutaneous tibial nerve stimulation in the treatment of refractory overactive bladder syndrome: Is maintenance treatment necessary? *BJU Int.* **2006**, *97*, 547–550. [CrossRef]
8. Ruiz-Tovar, J.; Llavero, C. Long-term effect of percutaneous electrical neurostimulation of dermatome T6 for Appetite reduction and weight loss in obese patients. *Surg. Laparosc. Endosc. Percutaneous Tech.* **2016**, *26*, 212–215. [CrossRef]
9. Ruiz-Tovar, J.; Llavero, C.; Smith, W. Percutaneous electrical neurostimulation of dermatome T6 for short-term weight loss in overweight and obese patients: Effect on ghrelin levels, glucose, lipid, and hormonal profile. *Surg. Laparosc. Endosc. Percutaneous Tech.* **2017**, *27*, 241–247. [CrossRef]
10. Ruiz-Tovar, J.; Oller, I.; Diez, M.; Zubiaga, L.; Arroyo, A.; Calpena, R. Percutaneous electrical neurostimulation of dermatome T6 for appetite reduction and weight loss in morbidly obese patients. *Obes. Surg.* **2013**, *24*, 205–211. [CrossRef]
11. Schroeder, B.O. Fight them or feed them: How the intestinal mucus layer manages the gut microbiota. *Gastroenterol. Rep. (Oxf.)* **2019**, *7*, 3–12. [CrossRef]
12. Lozupone, C.A.; Stombaugh, J.I.; Gordon, J.I.; Jansson, J.K.; Knight, R. Diversity, stability and resilience of the human gut microbiota. *Nature* **2012**, *489*, 220–230. [CrossRef]
13. Thursby, E.; Juge, N. Introduction to the human gut microbiota. *Biochem. J.* **2017**, *474*, 1823–1836. [CrossRef] [PubMed]
14. Sun, L.; Ma, L.; Ma, Y.; Zhang, F.; Zhao, C.; Nie, Y. Insights into the role of gut microbiota in obesity: Pathogenesis, mechanisms, and therapeutic perspectives. *Protein Cell* **2018**, *9*, 397–403. [CrossRef] [PubMed]
15. Tilg, H.; Moschen, A.R.; Kaser, A. Obesity and the Microbiota. *Gastroenterology* **2009**, *136*, 1476–1483. [CrossRef] [PubMed]
16. Duncan, S.H.; Lobley, G.; Holtrop, G.; Ince, J.; Johnstone, A.M.; Louis, P.; Flint, H. Human colonic microbiota associated with diet, obesity and weight loss. *Int. J. Obes. (Lond.)* **2008**, *32*, 1720–1724. [CrossRef] [PubMed]
17. Jumpertz, R.; Le, D.S.; Turnbaugh, P.J.; Trinidad, C.; Bogardus, C.; Gordon, J.; Krakoff, J. Energy-balance studies reveal associations between gut microbes, caloric load, and nutrient absorption in humans. *Am. J. Clin. Nutr.* **2011**, *94*, 58–65. [CrossRef] [PubMed]
18. Cerdó, T.; García-Santos, J.A.; Bermúdez, M.G.; Campoy, C. The Role of Probiotics and Prebiotics in the Prevention and Treatment of Obesity. Available online: https://www.ncbi.nlm.nih.gov/pmc/articles/PMC6470608/ (accessed on 14 February 2020).
19. Wang, Z.-B.; Xin, S.-S.; Ding, L.-N.; Ding, W.-Y.; Hou, Y.-L.; Liu, C.-Q.; Zhang, X. The potential role of probiotics in controlling overweight/obesity and associated metabolic parameters in adults: A systematic review and meta-analysis. *Evid. Based Complement. Altern. Med.* **2019**, *2019*, 3862971. [CrossRef]
20. Ajala, O.; English, P.; Pinkney, J. Systematic review and meta-analysis of different dietary approaches to the management of type 2 diabetes. *Am. J. Clin. Nutr.* **2013**, *97*, 505–516. [CrossRef]
21. Mabire, L.; Mani, R.; Liu, L.; Mulligan, H.; Baxter, G.D. The influence of age, sex and body mass index on the effectiveness of brisk walking for obesity management in adults: A systematic review and meta-analysis. *J. Phys. Act. Health* **2017**, *14*, 389–407. [CrossRef]
22. Choo, J.M.; Leong, L.E.X.; Rogers, G.B. Sample storage conditions significantly influence faecal microbiome profiles. *Sci. Rep.* **2015**, *5*, 16350. [CrossRef]
23. Ramírez, E.; Picatoste, B.; González-Bris, A.; Oteo, M.; Cruz, F.; Caro-Vadillo, A.; Egido, J.; Tuñón, J.; Morcillo, M. Ángel; Lorenzo, O. Sitagliptin improved glucose assimilation in detriment of fatty-acid utilization in experimental type-II diabetes: Role of GLP-1 isoforms in Glut4 receptor trafficking. *Cardiovasc. Diabetol.* **2018**, *17*, 12. [CrossRef] [PubMed]
24. Ley, R.E.; Hamady, M.; Lozupone, C.; Turnbaugh, P.J.; Ramey, R.R.; Bircher, J.S.; Schlegel, M.L.; Tucker, T.A.; Schrenzel, M.D.; Knight, R.; et al. Evolution of mammals and their gut microbes. *Science* **2008**, *320*, 1647–1651. [CrossRef] [PubMed]
25. Cole, J.R. The Ribosomal Database Project (RDP-II): Sequences and tools for high-throughput rRNA analysis. *Nucleic Acids Res.* **2004**, *33*, D294–D296. [CrossRef] [PubMed]
26. Williams, B.; Mancia, G.; Spiering, W.; Agabiti Rosei, E.; Azizi, M.; Burnier, M.; Clement, D.L.; Coca, A.; de Simone, G.; Dominiczak, A.; et al. 2018 ESC/ESH Guidelines for the management of arterial hypertension. *Eur. Heart J.* **2018**, *39*, 3021–3104. [CrossRef] [PubMed]

27. American Diabetes Association. Glycemic targets: Standards of medical care in diabetes. *Diabetes Care* **2018**, *41*, S55–S64. [CrossRef]
28. Catapano, A.L.; Graham, I.; De Backer, G.; Wiklund, O.; Chapman, M.J.; Drexel, H.; Hoes, A.W.; Jennings, C.S.; Landmesser, U.; Pedersen, T.R.; et al. 2016 ESC/EAS guidelines for the management of dyslipidaemias. *Eur. Heart J.* **2016**, *37*, 2999–3058. [CrossRef]
29. Brahe, L.K.; Astrup, A.; Larsen, L.H. Can we prevent obesity-related metabolic diseases by dietary modulation of the gut microbiota? *Adv. Nutr.* **2016**, *7*, 90–101. [CrossRef]
30. CDC. Adult Overweight and Obesity. Available online: https://www.cdc.gov/obesity/adult/index.html (accessed on 5 February 2020).
31. Flegal, K.M.; Kit, B.K.; Orpana, H.M.; Graubard, B.I. Association of all-cause mortality with overweight and obesity using standard body mass index categories: A systematic review and meta-analysis. *JAMA* **2013**, *309*, 71–82. [CrossRef]
32. Abdel-Kadar, M. Percutaneous Electrical Neurostimulation (PENS) of dermatome t6 with an ambulatory self-applied patch vs PENS of dermatome T6 with conventional procedure: Effect on appetite and weight loss in moderately obese patients. *Obes. Surg.* **2016**, *26*, 2899–2905. [CrossRef]
33. Huang, X.; Fan, X.; Ying, J.; Chen, S. Emerging trends and research foci in gastrointestinal microbiome. *J. Transl. Med.* **2019**, *17*, 1–11. [CrossRef]
34. Grigorescu, I.; Dumitrascu, D. Implication of gut microbiota in diabetes mellitus and obesity. *Acta Endocrinol. (Buchar.)* **2016**, *12*, 206–214. [CrossRef] [PubMed]
35. Roselli, M.; Devirgiliis, C.; Zinno, P.; Guantario, B.; Finamore, A.; Rami, R.; Perozzi, G. Impact of supplementation with a food-derived microbial community on obesity-associated inflammation and gut microbiota composition. *Genes Nutr.* **2017**, *12*, 25. [CrossRef] [PubMed]
36. Montandon, S.A.; Jornayvaz, F.R. Effects of antidiabetic drugs on gut microbiota composition. *Genes* **2017**, *8*, 250. [CrossRef] [PubMed]
37. Kovatcheva-Datchary, P.; Nilsson, A.; Akrami, R.; Lee, Y.S.; De Vadder, F.; Arora, T.; Hallén, A.; Martens, E.; Björck, I.; Bäckhed, F. Dietary fiber-induced improvement in glucose metabolism is associated with increased abundance of prevotella. *Cell Metab.* **2015**, *22*, 971–982. [CrossRef] [PubMed]
38. Huang, W.-C.; Lee, M.-C.; Lee, C.-C.; Ng, K.-S.; Hsu, Y.-J.; Tsai, T.-Y.; Young, S.-L.; Lin, J.-S.; Huang, C.-C. Effect of lactobacillus plantarum TWK10 on exercise physiological adaptation, performance, and body composition in healthy humans. *Nutrients* **2019**, *11*, 2836. [CrossRef] [PubMed]
39. Chen, Y.-M.; Wei, L.; Chiu, Y.-S.; Hsu, Y.-J.; Tsai, T.-Y.; Wang, M.-F.; Huang, C.-C. Lactobacillus plantarum TWK10 supplementation improves exercise performance and increases muscle mass in mice. *Nutrients* **2016**, *8*, 205. [CrossRef] [PubMed]
40. Lee, E.; Jung, S.-R.; Lee, S.-Y.; Lee, N.-K.; Paik, H.-D.; Lim, S. Lactobacillus plantarum strain Ln4 attenuates diet-induced obesity, insulin resistance, and changes in hepatic mRNA levels associated with glucose and lipid metabolism. *Nutrients* **2018**, *10*, 643. [CrossRef]
41. Crovesy, L.; Ostrowski, M.; Ferreira, D.M.T.P.; Rosado, E.L.; Soares-Mota, M. Effect of Lactobacillus on body weight and body fat in overweight subjects: A systematic review of randomized controlled clinical trials. *Int. J. Obes. (Lond.)* **2017**, *41*, 1607–1614. [CrossRef]
42. Sun, Q.; Zhang, Y.; Li, Z.; Yan, H.; Li, J.; Wan, X. Mechanism analysis of improved glucose homeostasis and cholesterol metabolism in high-fat-induced obese mice treated with La-SJLH001 via transcriptomics and culturomics. *Food Funct.* **2019**, *10*, 3556–3566. [CrossRef]
43. Minami, J.-I.; Iwabuchi, N.; Tanaka, M.; Yamauchi, K.; Xiao, J.-Z.; Abe, F.; Sakane, N. Effects of Bifidobacterium breve B-3 on body fat reductions in pre-obese adults: A randomized, double-blind, placebo-controlled trial. *Biosci. Microbiota Food Health* **2018**, *37*, 67–75. [CrossRef] [PubMed]
44. Kondo, S.; Xiao, J.-Z.; Satoh, T.; Odamaki, T.; Takahashi, S.; Sugahara, H.; Yaeshima, T.; Iwatsuki, K.; Kamei, A.; Abe, K. Antiobesity effects ofBifidobacterium breveStrain B-3 Supplementation in a mouse model with high-fat diet-induced obesity. *Biosci. Biotechnol. Biochem.* **2010**, *74*, 1656–1661. [CrossRef] [PubMed]
45. He, F.; Morita, H.; Hashimoto, H.; Hosoda, M.; Kurisaki, J.-I.; Ouwehand, A.C.; Isolauri, E.; Benno, Y.; Salminen, S. Intestinal Bifidobacterium species induce varying cytokine production. *J. Allergy Clin. Immunol.* **2002**, *109*, 1035–1036. [CrossRef] [PubMed]

46. Cani, P.D.; Possemiers, S.; Van De Wiele, T.; Guiot, Y.; Everard, A.; Rottier, O.; Geurts, L.; Naslain, D.; Neyrinck, A.M.; Lambert, D.M.; et al. Changes in gut microbiota control inflammation in obese mice through a mechanism involving GLP-2-driven improvement of gut permeability. *Gut* **2009**, *58*, 1091–1103. [CrossRef] [PubMed]
47. Bubnov, R.V.; Babenko, L.; Lazarenko, L.; Mokrozub, V.V.; Demchenko, O.A.; Nechypurenko, O.V.; Spivak, M.Y. Comparative study of probiotic effects of Lactobacillus and Bifidobacteria strains on cholesterol levels, liver morphology and the gut microbiota in obese mice. *EPMA J.* **2017**, *8*, 357–376. [CrossRef]
48. Nagpal, R.; Wang, S.; Woods, L.C.S.; Seshie, O.; Chung, S.T.; Shively, C.A.; Register, T.C.; Craft, S.; McClain, D.A.; Yadav, H. Comparative Microbiome signatures and short-chain fatty acids in mouse, rat, non-human primate, and human feces. *Front. Microbiol.* **2018**, *9*, 2897. [CrossRef]
49. Lin, H.V.; Frassetto, A.; Kowalik, E.J.; Nawrocki, A.R.; Lu, M.M.; Kosinski, J.R.; Hubert, J.A.; Szeto, D.; Yao, X.; Forrest, G.; et al. Butyrate and propionate protect against diet-induced obesity and regulate gut hormones via free fatty acid receptor 3-independent mechanisms. *PLoS ONE* **2012**, *7*, e35240. [CrossRef]
50. Geerlings, S.Y.; Kostopoulos, I.; De Vos, W.M.; Belzer, C. Akkermansia muciniphila in the human gastrointestinal tract: When, where, and how? *Microorganisms* **2018**, *6*, 75. [CrossRef]
51. Everard, A.; Belzer, C.; Geurts, L.; Ouwerkerk, J.P.; Druart, C.; Bindels, L.B.; Guiot, Y.; Derrien, M.; Muccioli, G.G.; Delzenne, N.M.; et al. Cross-talk between Akkermansia muciniphila and intestinal epithelium controls diet-induced obesity. *Proc. Natl. Acad. Sci. USA* **2013**, *110*, 9066–9071. [CrossRef]
52. Shin, N.-R.; Lee, J.-C.; Lee, H.-Y.; Kim, M.-S.; Whon, T.W.; Lee, M.-S.; Bae, J.-W. An increase in the Akkermansia spp. population induced by metformin treatment improves glucose homeostasis in diet-induced obese mice. *Gut* **2013**, *63*, 727–735. [CrossRef]
53. Li, J.; Lin, S.; Vanhoutte, P.M.; Woo, C.W.; Xu, A. Akkermansia muciniphila protects against atherosclerosis by preventing metabolic endotoxemia-induced inflammation in Apoe-/- Mice. *Circulation* **2016**, *133*, 2434–2446. [CrossRef]
54. Clifton, L.; Birks, J.S.; Clifton, D. Comparing different ways of calculating sample size for two independent means: A worked example. *Contemp. Clin. Trials Commun.* **2018**, *13*, 100309. [CrossRef] [PubMed]
55. Giner-Bernal, L.; Ruiz-Tovar, J.; Violeta, J.; Mercader, M.; Miralles, J.; Calpena, R.; Arroyo, A. Plasma ghrelin levels after percutaneous electrical nerve stimulation of dermatome T6 for the treatment of obesity. *Endocrinol. Diabetes Nutr.* **2020**, *67*, 179–185. [CrossRef] [PubMed]
56. Sobaler, A.M.L.; Aparicio, A.; Aranceta-Bartrina, J.; Gil, Á.; González-Gross, M.; Serra-Majem, L.; Varela-Moreiras, G.; Ortega, R.M. Overweight and general and abdominal obesity in a representative sample of Spanish adults: Findings from the ANIBES study. *BioMed Res. Int.* **2016**, *2016*, 1–11. [CrossRef] [PubMed]

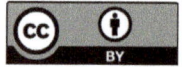

© 2020 by the authors. Licensee MDPI, Basel, Switzerland. This article is an open access article distributed under the terms and conditions of the Creative Commons Attribution (CC BY) license (http://creativecommons.org/licenses/by/4.0/).

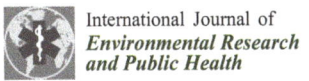

Review

Probiotic Supplements on Oncology Patients' Treatment-Related Side Effects: A Systematic Review of Randomized Controlled Trials

Miguel Rodriguez-Arrastia [1,2], Adrian Martinez-Ortigosa [3], Lola Rueda-Ruzafa [4,*], Ana Folch Ayora [1,2] and Carmen Ropero-Padilla [1,2]

[1] Faculty of Health Sciences, Pre-Department of Nursing, Jaume I University, Av. Sos Baynat, 12071 Castellon de la Plana, Spain; arrastia@uji.es (M.R.-A.); afolch@uji.es (A.F.A.); ropero@uji.es (C.R.-P.)
[2] Research Group CYS, Faculty of Health Sciences, Jaume I University, Av. Sos Baynat, 12071 Castello de la Plana, Spain
[3] Emergency Department, Miguel Servet University Hospital, Puerto de Isabel la Catolica, 50009 Zaragoza, Spain; adriaanortigosa@gmail.com
[4] Department of Functional Biology and Health Sciences, Faculty of Biology-CINBIO, Campus Lagoas-Marcosende, University of Vigo, 36310 Vigo, Spain
* Correspondence: lolarrzg@gmail.com

Abstract: Cancer affects more than 19.3 million people and has become the second leading cause of death worldwide. Chemo and radiotherapy, the most common procedures in these patients, often produce unpleasant treatment-related side effects that have a direct impact on the quality of life of these patients. However, innovative therapeutic strategies such as probiotics are being implemented to manage these complications. Thus, this study aimed to evaluate the efficacy of probiotics supplements as a therapeutic strategy in adult oncology treatment-related side effects. A systematic review of randomized controlled trials was conducted in PubMed, Scielo, ProQuest and OVID databases up to and including January 2021, following the PRISMA guidelines. The quality of the included studies was assessed by the Jadad Scale. Twenty clinical trials published between 1988 and 2020 were included in this review. Seventeen studies (85%) revealed predominantly positive results when using probiotics to reduce the incidence of treatment-related side effects in oncology patients, while three studies (15%) reported no impact in their findings. This study sheds some light on the significance of chemotherapy and radiotherapy in altering the composition of gut microbiota, where probiotic strains may play an important role in preventing or mitigating treatment-related side effects.

Keywords: drug therapy; gut microbiota; neoplasms; probiotics; radiotherapy; systematic review

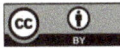

1. Introduction

According to the World Health Organization (WHO), cancer is the second leading cause of death, affecting more than 19.3 million people and claiming 10 million lives worldwide, and the number of new cases is expected to double by 2040 [1]. This disease is diagnosed differently in men and women, with one in every five people developing cancer at some point in their lives, resulting in the death of one in every eight men and one in every eleven women diagnosed with cancer. In this sense, breast, colorectal, lung, cervical, and thyroid cancer are the most common cancers in women, while lung and prostate cancer are the most common in men [2].

There are diverse therapeutic strategies to reduce cell proliferation and disease progression, with surgery, chemotherapy, radiotherapy, and, more recently, immunotherapy and hormone therapy being the most commonly used treatments [3,4]. These treatments have significant side effects, particularly chemotherapy and radiotherapy, which is why it is frequently necessary to use combination treatments to increase effectiveness, despite the fact that this strategy multiplies side effects [5]. As a result, cancer treatments have the greatest impact on cells with the highest rate of cell division, resulting in low cell counts in blood cells, which manifests as anemia, infections, and bleedings. Likewise, gastrointestinal cells are also altered, resulting in nausea, vomiting, diarrhea, taste disturbances, mucositis, and swallowing difficulties [6,7], which cause many patients to postpone or discontinue their treatments [8].

Chemo- and radiotherapy modify the composition of intestinal microbiota in a process known as dysbiosis, which is often associated with biochemistry and immunologic disorders in the gastrointestinal tract [9,10]. Multiple strategies are being developed to modify microbiota with the underlying idea of propelling this dysbiosis toward eubiosis or the hemostasis of the gut microbiota in order to prevent or inhibit cancer progression [11,12]. In this regard, it has been reported that paclitaxel, a mitosis inhibitor, is able to increase matrix metalloproteinase 9 (MMP9) and tumor necrosis factor-alpha (TNF-α) levels and alter bacterial diversity in female mice colon [13]. Probiotics, defined as live microorganisms that provide a health benefit to the host when administered in adequate amounts [14], have been shown to be effective in the management of diarrhea and constipation, as well as highly effective in the treatment of inflammatory bowel diseases by improving bowel function [15,16]. For example, a probiotic mixture improved altered intestinal tight junction levels in mice with dextran sodium sulfate (DSS)-induced colitis [17]. Consequently, probiotics containing one or more strains could indeed restore the composition of altered gut microbiota and improve certain parameters, leading to significant homeostasis in animal models of obesity, Parkinson's disease, and depression [15,18,19]. Similarly, immune function may improve after the administration of a probiotic combination. Treatment with Bifidobacterium longum, Lactobacillus lactis, and Enterococcus faecium significantly reduced the occurrence of radio- chemotherapy-induced oral mucositis, as well as increased CD4+, CD8+, and CD3+ T cells in oncological patients [20]. In that manner, 5-fluorouracil-induced intestinal mucositis has also shown an improvement after probiotic treatment by reducing TNF-α, IL-6, and IFN-γ levels in mice [21].

In this context, corticosteroids and antiemetics are key elements in oncology to be used prior to the administration of chemotherapy to avoid side effects [5]. However, relatively little is understood about including probiotics in this preventive regimen due to beneficial results in intestinal disorders and altered immunity, which could be of great interest in reducing certain oncology treatment-related side effects, such as diarrhea, mucositis, or constipation. Therefore, this review aims to evaluate the efficacy of probiotic supplements to ameliorate chemo- and radiotherapy-related side effects in adults.

2. Materials and Methods

2.1. Design

A systematic review of randomized controlled trials was undertaken in January 2021, following the Preferred Reporting Items for Systematic Reviews and Meta-Analyses (PRISMA) guidelines (Supplementary File 1) [22]. This review used a structured Patient–Intervention–Outcome (PIO) question as follows [23]: "In adult oncology patients (P), what is the efficacy of probiotics supplements (I) on treatment-related side effects (O)?" The protocol for this review was not registered.

2.2. Search Strategy

The electronic databases included PubMed, Scielo, ProQuest, and OVID, using natural and structured language in the following search strategy: (((((probiotics [Title/Abstract] OR probiotics [MeSH Terms]) OR lactobacillus [Title/Abstract]) OR bifidobacterium [Title/Abstract]) OR lactobacillus [MeSH Terms]) OR bifidobacterium [MeSH Terms]) AND ((((radiotherapy [Title/Abstract] OR chemotherapy [Title/Abstract]) OR chemotherapy [MeSH Terms]) OR radiotherapy [MeSH Terms]) OR radiation [Title/Abstract]). This search strategy was adapted for use across databases (Appendix A). "Randomized clinical trial", "humans", and "adult:19+ years" search filters were applied for this search strategy.

2.3. Selection Criteria

The following inclusion criteria were used: (i) randomized clinical trials, (ii) published in English or Spanish, (iii) related to the aim of the study; the use of probiotics supplements on adult oncology-related treatments and side effects; and (iv) published until January 2021. Likewise, the exclusion criteria included (i) studies on other pathologies than cancer or symptoms related to cancer treatments, (ii) symbiotics and other treatment combinations, (iii) re-publications, and (iv) studies with animals. No articles were excluded after quality appraisal.

2.4. Data Screening

Initially, the two authors (MR, AM) performed a first screening by titles and abstracts, following the selection criteria independently and in duplicate. Once a third author (CR) double-checked the screening and discussed any discrepancy, a full-text reading was performed for their quality appraisal by authors.

2.5. Quality Appraisal

The quality of selected articles was assessed by two researchers independently (MR, AM). Any disagreements on quality ratings were discussed with a third author (CR) and a consensus was reached. The Jadad Scale of Clinical Trials was used to assess the methodological quality of experimental human studies included. This is a scale with five simple items and it has known reliability and external validity. A score below 3 points indicate low quality based on (i) the quality of randomization, (ii) double blinding, and (iii) drop-outs extracted from each study [24].

2.6. Data Abstraction and Synthesis

Consecutively, the relevant data from the included studies were extracted and tabulated according to (i) authors, (ii) country, (iii) population, (iv) probiotic strains, (v) variables, (vi) measures, and (vii) main findings.

3. Results

3.1. Characteristics of Selected Studies

Firstly, a total of 402 articles were retrieved through databases searching (PubMed (n = 349), Scielo (n = 6), ProQuest (n = 29) and OVID (n = 18)), from which 68 papers were discarded by duplicity. After title, abstract, and full-text screening, a total of 314 articles were excluded following the selection criteria. Twenty studies were included in this review (Figure 1).

All trials and patients' characteristics are summarized in Table 1. On the whole, all individuals were treated using conventional cancer therapy methods, such as radiotherapy (n = 11, 55%), chemotherapy (n = 6, 30%), or both (n = 3, 15%). In some studies, sex was not specified (n = 2, 10%), and only women were included in studies dealing with specific carcinomas of the female reproductive tract (n = 4, 20%), such as endometrial, vaginal, uterine, and cervical cancers. The age range of the patients ranged from 18 to 75 years old (with a mean age of 57.41 years), enrolling a total of 2508 participants. All studies included were published between 1988 and 2020, and 15 studies (75%) were not registered in any clinical trial registry. Most of these studies were conducted in Asia (n = 9), Europe (n = 8), but also in America (n = 2) and Oceania (n = 1). As regards the use of probiotics, 10 of the selected studies (50%) used a single probiotic strain, while the remaining 10 (50%) used two or more probiotics combined. The presentation and forms of administration varied from study to study, with the most commonly used forms being capsules, gelatine, and yoghurt. The time of administration as well as the dose administered to the patients were also varied, which ranged from 1 to 24 weeks and 10^6 to 10^{11} CFU/day, respectively. Finally, 17 studies (85%) revealed predominantly positive results when using probiotics to reduce the incidence of treatment-related side effects in oncology patients, while three studies (15%) reported no impact in their findings.

Table 1. Overview of clinical selected articles.

Reference	Country (TN)	Population (n)	Probiotic Strains	Dose and Treatment Period	Variables	Measures	Main Findings
Gastrointestinal side effects							
Linn et al. (2019) [25]	Myanmar (TCTR20170314001)	54 cervical cancer patients	Single: *L. acidophilus* LA-5 plus *B. animalis* subsp. *lactis* BB-12	1.75×10^9 CFU/day 3 weeks	The incidence of RID, abdominal pain and use of anti-diarrheal	RID severity was assessed by the common terminology criteria for adverse events, and the severity of abdominal pain was assessed by the CTCAE	The incidence and severity grades of RID was significantly reduced, as well as abdominal pain and the use of anti-diarrheal drug
Golkhalkhali et al. (2018) [26]	Malaysia (IRCT2011061568141N1)	140 colorectal cancer patients	Multi: *L. acidophilus* BMC12130, *L. casei* BCMC12313, *L. lactis* BCMC12451, *B. bifidum* BCMC02290, *B. longum* BCMC02120 and *B. infantis* BCMC02129	3×10^{10} CFU/day 8 weeks	Effect of supplementation in QOL, chemotherapy side effects, and inflammatory markers in colorectal cancer	QOL was assessed by EORTC QLQ-C30 scale. CRP measure was used for the evaluation of inflammatory markers	Patients' QOL was improved, reducing certain inflammatory biomarkers and relieving diarrhea, nausea, and vomiting
Liu and Huang (2014) [27]	China	100 cancer patients	Multi: *B. infantis, L. acidophilus, E. faecalis* and *Bacillus cereus*	0.5×10^6 CFU/day 4 weeks	Efficacy, side effects, and difference between the two groups	Wexner Score was used to measure changes	Functional constipation during chemotherapy was effectively and safely treated
Demers et al. (2014) [28]	Canada	246 pelvic cancer patients	Multi: *L. acidophilus* LAC-361 and *B. longum* BB-536	1×10^{10} CFU/day 15 weeks	Severity of RID, intestinal pain, and the usage of anti-diarrheal medication	Diarrhea severity was evaluated by WHO grading scale and the abdominal pain according to NCI scale. Stool consistency was measured by Bristol scale	RID was reduced at the end of the treatment. Nutritional assessment appears to reduce global digestive symptomatology
Ki et al. (2013) [29]	USA	40 prostate cancer patients	Single: *L. acidophilus*	1×10^8 CFU/day 3 weeks	Rectal volume and volume change of the rectum	CT, MVCT, and PVCR for checking the percentage volume change of the rectum	*L. acidophilus* was effective for reducing excessive gas and exacerbated bloating or distension

Table 1. Cont.

Reference	Country (TN)	Population (n)	Probiotic Strains	Dose and Treatment Period	Variables	Measures	Main Findings
Holma et al. (2013) [30]	Finland	143 colorectal cancer patients	Single: L. rhamnosus GG ATCC 53103	1×10^9 CFU/day 24 weeks	Gastrointestinal symptoms during chemotherapy, methane production and fecal pH	Both fecal and breath samples were analyzed to assess methane production and its pH. Gastrointestinal symptoms and OLT were used to assess chemotherapy injuries	L. rhamnosus GG reduced diarrhea during chemo and did not affect significantly to methane production
Chitapanarux et al. (2010) [31]	China	63 cervical cancer patients	Multi: L. acidophilus plus B. bifidum	2×10^9 CFU/day 6 weeks	Incidence and severity of diarrhea, stool characteristics, and the use of anti-diarrheal medication	Stool consistency was analyzed in laboratory and hematological toxicities were measured by CTC	Incidence of RID and the usage of anti-diarrheal medication were reduced, while the stool consistency was improved
Giralt et al. (2008) [32]	Spain	85 endometrial adenocarcinoma patients	Multi: S. thermophilus, L. delbrueckii subsp. bulgaricus, and L. casei DN-114 001	1×10^8 CFU/day 6 weeks	Severity of RID, and inflammatory intestinal conditions	Diarrhea was measured by CTC. The fecal calprotectin was analyzed in laboratory, using an enzyme-linked immunoassay	The oral supplementation may result in a modest clinical benefit for stool consistency
Osterlund et al. (2007) [33]	Finland	150 colorectal cancer patients	Single: L. rhamnosus GG ATCC 53103	$1-2 \times 10^{10}$ CFU/day 24 weeks	Chemotherapy dose intensity and tolerability	A diary kept by the patients and by a physician was used to assess side effects	The frequency of severe 5-FU-based chemotherapy-related diarrhea was reduced
Delia et al. (2007) [34]	Italy	490 sigmoid, rectal, or cervical cancer patients	Multi: L. casei, L. plantarum, L. acidophilus, and L. delbrueckii subsp. thermophilus; B. longum, B. breve, and B. infantis; S. salivarius subsp. thermophilus	4.5×10^{11} CFU/day 4 weeks	Clinical symptoms after radiation therapy, concomitant medications, and AEs. Incidence and severity of RID	Daily bowel movements were monitored, and the severity of gastrointestinal toxicity was measured as WHO grading	This treatment constitutes a safe option to protect patients against RID even in the setting of intestinal inflammation

Table 1. Cont.

Reference	Country (TN)	Population (n)	Probiotic Strains	Dose and Treatment Period	Variables	Measures	Main Findings
Osterlund et al. (2004) [35]	Finland	150 colorectal cancer patients	Single: L. rhamnosus GG ATCC 53103	$1-2 \times 10^{10}$ CFU/day 24 weeks	Lactose intolerance, effect of probiotic, treatment-related toxicity, and nutritional status	OLT, symptom questionnaire, and Subjective Global Assessment of Nutritional Status questionnaire	L. rhamnosus GG had an impact on lactulose intolerance symptoms, but not in the frequency of hypolactasia
Urbancsek et al. (2001) [36]	Austria	205 cancer patients	Single: L. casei var. rhamnosus	1.5×10^9 CFU/day 1 week	Efficacy for treatment of diarrhea	Bowel movements, diarrhea grading, feces ratings by the investigator, and patient diarrhea ratings	Probiotic therapy produced a highly favorable benefit/risk ratio in RID
Salminen et al. (1988) [37]	Finland	24 cervix or uterus carcinoma patients	Single: L. acidophilus NCDO1748	2×10^9 CFU/day 6 weeks	Frequency and severity of intestinal side effects, the usage of anti-diarrheal medication	Data on diarrhea, abdominal pain, meteorism, flatulence, vomiting, defecation frequency and usage of anti-diarrheal medication was collected	L. acidophilus NCDO1748 appears to prevent RID, but increases the incidence of flatulence due to its substrate
Immune-related side effects							
Shao et al. (2014) [38]	China	46 ARE patients	Multi: B. lactobacillus and S. thermophilus	0.5×10^9 CFU/day 2 weeks	Nutritional status, abdominal pain, flatulence, and diarrhea	Level of serum albumin, prealbumin occurrence rate of abdominal pain, flatulence, diarrhea, and blood PCT in fast blood was measured	Patients' immune status was improved, and the tolerance of enteral nutrition could be better for the bowel function and the patients' rehabilitation
Inflammatory-related side effects							
De Sanctis et al. (2019) [39]	Italy (NCT01707641)	75 HNC patients	Single: L. brevis CD2	2×10^9 CFU/day 1 week	Incidence of severe oral mucositis and of requirement for enteral nutrition	Incidence and severity of treatment-related dysphagia; patient QOL; body weight loss during; the incidence and time-course of treatment-related pain	The effects of L. brevis CD2 were not able to confirm the beneficial in reducing OM in patients with HNC

Table 1. Cont.

Reference	Country (TTN)	Population (n)	Probiotic Strains	Dose and Treatment Period	Variables	Measures	Main Findings
Jiang et al. (2019) [20]	China	99 NC patients	Multi: B. longum, L. lactis and E. faecium	1×10^7 CFU/day 7 weeks	Patients' immunity status, composition and abundance of bacterial communities	Total bacterial genomic DNA extraction and high-throughput sequencing and efficacy at the end of treatment	Immune response was significantly increased and severity of OM was reduced
Sharma et al. (2012) [40]	India	200 HNC patients	Single: L. brevis CD2	2×10^9 CFU/day 4 weeks	Incidence and severity of OM and chemo-radiotherapy-related adverse effects	FACT-HN questionnaire was used for QOL. Saliva samples were collected for pro-inflammatory biomarkers	L. brevis CD2 proved to be safe and efficacious in reducing the incidence of severe OM
Performance status-related side effects							
Vesty et al. (2020) [41]	New Zealand (AC-TRN12617000710325)	17 HNC patients	Single: S. salivarius M18	3.5×10^9 CFU/day 4 weeks	Bacterial community networks and oral probiotic viability	Sample collection, oral health assessments, probiotic viability, DNA extraction and sequencing preparation, bioinformatic analyses, and network analyses were used	Oral probiotics to modulate host immune responses and microbial interactions is a promising mechanism to improve oral health
Doppalapudi et al. (2020) [42]	India (CTRI/2018/02/011812)	86 HNC patients	Multi: L. acidophilus, L. rhamnosus, B. longum and Saccharomyces boulardii	1.5×10^9 CFU/day 4 weeks	Difference in salivary count pre- and post-intervention, and prevalence at the end of treatment	Saliva samples were collected for isolation, count, and identification of Candida	The probiotic bacteria were effective in reducing oral Candida spp.
Masuno et al. (1991) [43]	USA	95 lung cancer patients	Single: L. casei LC9018	0.2×10^7 CFU/day 4 weeks	Median survival, common side effects, and changes in the severity of each symptom	CT scan and pleural fluid cytologic specimens were examined. Laboratory tests were performed	LC9018 appears to be a useful agent for the treatment of lung cancer and prevent pleural effusions

TTN: Trial number; CFU: Colony-forming unit; L.: Lactobacillus; B.: Bifidobacterium; E.: Enterococcus; S.: Streptococcus; RID: Radiation-induced diarrhea; CTCAE: Common Terminology Criteria for Adverse Events; QOL: Quality of life; EORTC: European Organization for Research and Treatment of Cancer; CRP: C-reactive protein; NCI: National Cancer Institute; CT: Computed tomographic; MVCT: Megavoltage computed tomography; PVCR: Percentage volume change of the rectum; OLT: Oral lactulose tolerance; CTC: Common Toxicity Criteria; AE: Adverse effects; ARE: Acute radiation enteritis; PCT: Procalcitonin; HNC: Head and neck cancer; NC: Nasopharyngeal carcinoma; OM: Oropharyngeal mucositis; FACT-HN: Functional Assessment of Cancer Therapy Head and Neck.

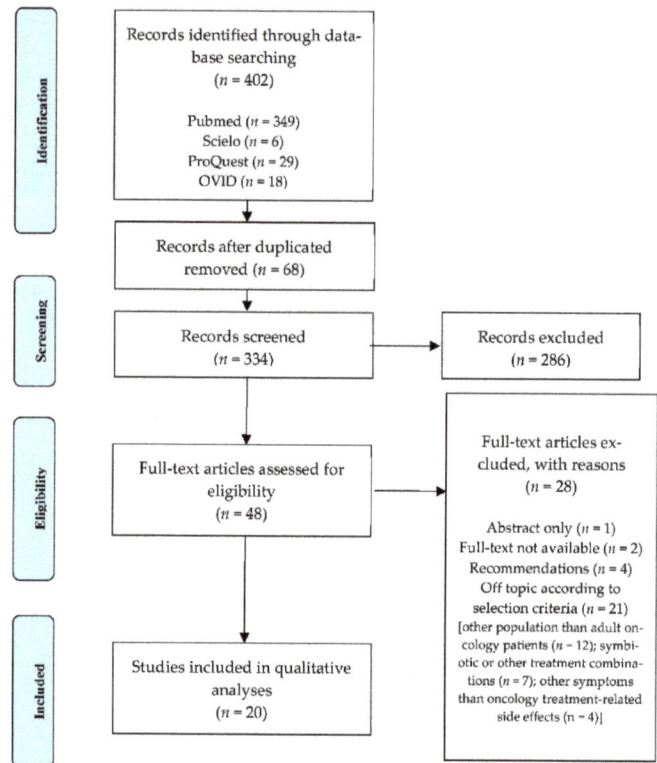

Figure 1. Flowchart depicting the article selection process.

The data synthesis revealed four categories related to the use of probiotic supplements for treatment-related side effects in clinical oncology. For that matter, these categories would study the effects of probiotic treatments for different treatment-related side effects in oncology such as gastrointestinal side effects, immune-related side effects, inflammatory side effects, and performance status-related side effects. These categories are described below.

3.2. Gastrointestinal Side Effects

Probiotics have been shown to be effective in the treatment of some common oncology treatment-related gastrointestinal adverse reactions, as demonstrated in 11 of 20 trials (55%) [25–31,33–36]. The main adverse effects identified and treated were mainly diarrhea, with other drawbacks being abdominal pain, nausea and vomiting, constipation, bloating, abdominal distension, and lactose intolerance caused by chemotherapy. The most commonly probiotic strains used along these studies were *Lactobacillus acidophilus*; *L. rhamnosus* GG ATCC 53103; and *L. casei* var. *rhamnosus*. Likewise, other probiotic strains used in combination were (*L. acidophilus* LA-5 along with *Bifidobacterium animalis* subsp. *lactis* BB-12), (*L. acidophilus* BMC12130, *L. casei* BCMC12313, *L. lactis* BCMC12451, *B. bifidum* BCMC02290, *B. longum* BCMC02120 and *B. infantis* BCMC02129), (*B. infantis*, *L. acidophilus*, *Enterococcus faecalis* and *Bacillus cereus*), (*L. acidophilus* LAC-361 and *B. longum* BB-536), (*L. acidophilus* plus *B. bifidum*), and (*L. casei*, *L. plantarum*, *L. acidophilus*, and *L. delbruekii* subsp. *thermophilus*; *B. longum*, *B. breve*, and *B. infantis*; *Streptococcus salivarius* subsp. *thermophilus*). The duration of treatment ranged from 1 to 24 weeks.

Conversely, 2 trials (10%) showed inconclusive results for their benefits to control stool consistency and flatulence, although their findings were promising to prevent radiotherapy-induced diarrhoea [32,37]. The probiotic strains used in these studies included: *L. acidophilus* NCDO1748, and (*S. thermophilus*, *L. delbrueckii* subsp. *bulgaricus*, and *L. casei* DN-114 001). The treatment for these studies ranged from 1 to 6 weeks and were observed only in women.

3.3. Immune-Related Side Effects

Despite having only one study [38], positive results of the probiotics on immune-related side effects have also been observed. A combination of probiotic strains (*Bifidobacterium*, *Lactobacillus* and *S. thermophilus*) was used for 1 to 2 weeks, in which patients improved their immune and nutritional status as well as rehabilitation, showing improved cellular immune parameters and tolerance to abdominal pain, bloating and diarrhoea. These authors used glutamine along with fish oil in their treatment as it has been shown to enhance epithelial cell growth and repair of intestinal mucous membrane, prevent bacterial translocation and reduce barrier injury, among others, which may actually be able to work synergistically with probiotics to protect the intestinal mucosa barrier and reduce permeability. In this manner, radiation-induced injuries may be alleviated by these probiotic strains, while other eco-nutrients feed the intestinal membrane.

3.4. Inflammatory-Related Side Effects

Impact on inflammatory-related side effects such as oral mucositis was also reported in three trials (15%). Among these studies, two trials [20,40] showed positive and effective results in reducing the severity of oral mucositis when using different probiotic strains: (*B. longum*, *L. lactis*, and *E. faecium*) and *L. brevis* CD2. The treatment period for these studies was from 1 to 7 weeks. However, De Sanctis et al. (2019) [39] did not notice any significant changes in the severity of oral mucositis with *L. brevis* CD2, although their treatment lasted only 1 week due to premature closure of patient accrual. While it is true that radio-chemotherapy-induced mucositis is a complex process and further prospective studies are needed to explore oral microbiota modulation in reducing its incidence, the findings of Jiang and collaborators (2019) [20] and Sharma and collaborators (2012) [40] strongly underpinned the probiotics used as a plausible strategy to manage mucositis-associated pain and reduce its incidence.

3.5. Performance Status-Related Side Effects

Concerning to the impact of probiotics in patients' general well-being and activities of daily life, three trials (15%) evaluated their effects over a 4-week treatment period [41–43]. Two of these studies used a single probiotic strain, *S. salivarius* M18 and *L. casei* LC9018 respectively, and the remaining study used a combination of *L. acidophilus*, *L. rhamnosus*, *B. longum*, and *Saccharomycesboulardii*. In line with the findings of Shao and collaborators (2014) [38], not only did Doppalapudi and collaborators (2020) [42] and Vesty and collaborators (2020) [41] observe clinical improvements driven by probiotic-induced changes in the oral microbiota but also a potential mechanism to improve these performance status-related side effects throughout other modulating host immune response and microbial interactions. Having said that, only one study [43] assessed the effect of probiotics in malignant pleural effusion, which is one of the most common complications in lung cancer. This complication can have a severe impact on patient performance and shortened survival, but interestingly, *L. casei* LC9018 has been shown to be a useful adjuvant in the treatment of this type of cancer and to prevent this complication.

3.6. Quality Assessment

On the Jadad Scale, the average quality of the analyzed studies was 3.75 (Figure 2). Its reporting quality varied from 2 (in four studies), 3 (in two studies), 4 (in nine studies), and 5 (in five studies), with none of them having an inappropriate reporting quality (lower than 1). At last, four of the studies reviewed received support from different manufacturers, indicating the possibility of a sponsorship bias [26,31,36,40].

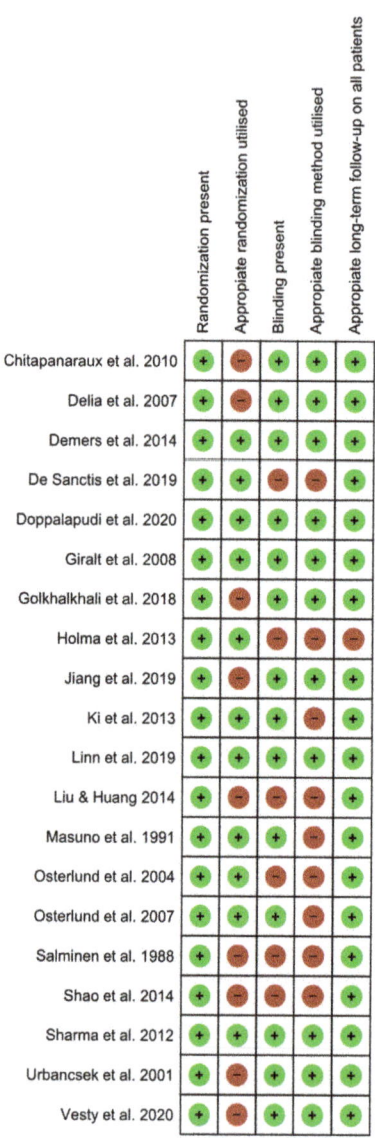

Figure 2. Risk of bias summary using the Jadad Scale for each included study.

4. Discussion

This review was aimed to evaluate the efficacy of probiotics supplements as a therapeutic strategy for treatment-related side effects in adult oncology patients. After analyzing 20 randomized controlled trials, our findings showed the beneficial effects that probiotic may have in a range of common treatment-related side effects, which have a direct impact of the oncology patients' quality of life. In this manner, 11 of 20 studies (55%) observed positive outcomes among gastrointestinal adverse effects management such as diarrhea, abdominal pain, nausea, and vomiting among others. Similarly, another six studies (30%) reported promising results in the control of immune and inflammatory responses, as well as other side effects related to their overall well-being and daily life activities. These findings further support the idea of previous reviews [44,45], suggesting that microbiota plays a key role in the pathogenesis of some treatment-related side effects, although further evidence is needed to determine their safety and accuracy [46,47].

The studies included in this review were heterogenous in the use of probiotic strains, where *Lactobacillus acidophilus* (LA-5, BMC12130, LAC-361, and NCDO1748) was the most widely used strain among other 15 different strains, both in single strain [29,37] and multiple strain trials [25–28,31,34,42]. This heterogeneity added to the number of cancers included may explain some of the between-studies variability of the results [47]. Another possible explanation may be the interindividual diversity of the microbiota composition, where personalized medicine might well contribute to predicting the most suitable probiotic strain for the individual [48]. In this vein, strong evidence suggests that the efficacy of probiotics is strain-specific as well as disease-specific, and therefore, these factors should be considered when recommending the best probiotic for the patient [49]. Furthermore, the duration of treatment may also have to be considered to demonstrate probiotic clinical position in the oncology of treatment-related side effects, 4 weeks being the most common duration of treatment among the studies included. These results are consistent with the findings of De Sanctis and collaborators (2019) [39], who stated that a probiotic treatment period of less than 4 weeks may not be sufficient to observe and confirm their beneficial effects. However, to date, there are not standardized procedures available on the minimum treatment duration for the selected probiotic strain in order to observe positive outcomes, as it requires time to promote gut microbiota re-shaping and, as a result, the beneficial effect [50].

In reference to the treatment-related side effects, authors such as Delia and collaborators (2007) [34], Golkhalkhali and collaborators (2018) [26], as well as Osterlund and collaborators (2007) [33] among others, concur that the use of probiotics and microbial cell preparations improves the intestinal immune barrier, particularly intestinal IgA responses. In line with the results of other studies, these probiotic strains are able to stabilize the intestinal microbial environment and improve the permeability of the intestinal barrier, leading to a reduction in inflammatory response and promoting changes in the intestinal flora [51,52]. This promotes an ideal environment for the growth of non-pathogenic bacteria, helping to protect epithelial cells, the process of apoptosis, and some cytoprotective processes [53]. Interestingly, similar results were found using probiotic strains such as *Lactobacillus*, *Bifidobacterium*, or *Streptococcus* along with other eco-nutrients such as glutamine and fish oil [38]. These results match those observed in recent preclinical studies [54,55], where the colonization of this bacteria genera enhanced the immune and anti-inflammatory response to radiation, forming an enteric–intestinal barrier that increased the thickness of the intestinal flora. Moreover, the optimization of the medium promotes the life of living microorganisms, which can restore the balance of a radiation-damaged microecosystem by repairing the intestinal membrane, inhibiting the growth of intestinal pathogens, and reducing endotoxin production [56]. These probiotic strains are antioxidant agents that act by eliminating free radicals produced by ionization and preventing lipid oxidation, thereby prioritizing the repair and regeneration of the cell membrane, DNA, and proteins, resulting in their high efficacy in reducing abdominal pain, flatulence, and diarrhea, as these authors highlight in their findings [38,56].

In accordance with these findings, Holma and collaborators (2013) [30] underline the importance of fecal pH and methane production in this type of patient, where intestinal microbiota plays a central role in the incidence of unpleasant side effects such as diarrhea and constipation, bloating, or abdominal inflammation. These results confirm the association between the higher production of elements such as methane and microbiota, where a higher production of methane is associated with a lower incidence of diarrhea and a methane deficiency is associated with a higher incidence of abdominal discomfort [57]. In this context, the results showed that the *L. rhamnosus* GG ATCC 53,103 strain did not alter the production of pH or methane, as opposed to studies such as Salminen and collaborators (1988) [37], in which *L. acidophilus* NCDO1748 was administered and increased flatulence was observed, pointing directly to the lactulose content as a non-absorbable substrate, a mechanism favoring the production of methane and probiotic absorption. In this sense, Osterlund and collaborators (2004) [35] provide information on lactose intolerance caused by low intestinal villus height in relation to its depth of treatment, resulting in malabsorption syndrome and therefore hindering the production of diarrhea, flatulence, and abdominal pain [58]. In line with the overall evidence, it is worth noting how adverse effects can be managed by modifying gut microbiota and methane production mechanisms [30,59]. Replacing lactulose with another non-absorbable substrate would not cause diarrhea and would, in turn, allow the amount of methane to be controlled to achieve balance in intestinal transit, vary the amount of substrate administered, and greatly improve or even reduce the number of treatment doses administered to patients [35,57].

On the other hand, oral mucositis and oral health stand as one of the most treated side effects as they significantly reduce the patients' quality of life [60]. In that matter, probiotics such as *B. longum* (BCMC02120, BB-536), *L. lactis* BCMC12451, *E. faecium*, and *L. brevis* CD2 have shown to reduce the incidence of severe oral mucositis by promoting the growth and protection of the bacterial flora and, as a result, decreasing the number of adverse effects, severity, and incidence of mucositis [20,40–42]. These findings are in agreement with those of Vesty and collaborators (2020) [41], who identified that using *S. salivarius* M18 improved patients' quality of life by reducing the number of oral infections (candidiasis) and adverse effects (mucositis, diarrhea) that these patients experienced after their treatments. However, recent research found that the effects of *L. brevis* CD2 were unable to confirm its beneficial impact for severe oral mucositis, though one possible explanation for these findings could be the premature closure of patient accrual [39]. Lastly, it is also interesting to note the effect of probiotics on other side effects of these patients such as pleural effusion, which can severely affect their performance status and even shorten their life expectancy. Only Masuno and collaborators (1991) [43] evaluated the use of the *L. casei* LC9018 strain against this complication, demonstrating promising results in controlling pleural effusions by reducing the number of malignant cells at the pleural level, which are supported by preclinical models [61,62].

Limitations

That being said, there are some limitations to bear in mind when interpreting the findings of this study. Fifteen of the analyzed studies were not registered, and therefore there may be a risk of reporting bias, whereas these studies are consistent trials on the Jadad Scale. On the other hand, heterogeneity in strains, length of treatment, and population could be confounding factors, and hence, generalizations should be made with caution. As a result of this heterogeneity in strains, interventions, and data collection methods, neither meta-analysis nor meta-regression were considered in this review. Given the small number of studies included, further work is still needed on the clinical position of probiotic supplements in adult oncology treatment-related side effects, in particular to determine the efficacy of individual probiotic strains, which could help to compare strains and lead more closely to preventive approaches.

As a whole, this review contributes to the existing literature, providing evidence of the current clinical position of probiotics supplements for some common treatment-related side effects in adult oncology patients. Despite the main findings of these studies concluded in terms of the safety and efficacy of probiotics supplements for the treatment or prevention of these side effects, further research with larger groups, specific strains, and duration of treatment is needed to conclude the beneficial effects for each of these side effects. More broadly, research is needed to determine the effects of individual and combined probiotic strains in order to draw confident conclusions about their benefits for both general oncology treatment-related side effects and specific cancers. Future research will be particularly interesting in determining how the use of probiotics and prebiotics may enhance the beneficial effect of the first to improve therapeutic responses in patients with cancer.

5. Conclusions

This study has shown that some probiotic strains (*L. acidophilus, L. casei, B. longum,* or *L. rhamnosus* among others) are a valid therapeutic strategy in some common treatment-related side effects in adult oncology patients, using both single or multiple strain combinations for at least 4 weeks of treatment. The beneficial variation between the different strains in the selected studies has been similar, which is why all of them represent a possible strategy for complications such as gastrointestinal side effects, immune or inflammatory side effects, and performance status-related side effects. Furthermore, despite its exploratory nature, this study provides some insight into the importance of chemotherapy and radiotherapy, inducing major changes in the composition of microbiota, where these probiotic strains may play an important role to prevent or treat such complications.

Implications for Clinical Practice

Common treatment-related side effects such as diarrhea, vomiting, mucositis, or abdominal pain are unpleasant for patients who have to undergo chemo- or radiotherapy treatments. Although more research is clearly needed, it has been shown that the gut microbiota plays a key role in immunity, and therefore, probiotics could be considered as a potential therapeutic strategy for treating and preventing these complications in immunocompromised cancer patients. Certain probiotic strains (e.g., *Lactobacillus* or *Bifidobacterium*) have shown to be safe and effective for some of these effects secondary to chemo- and radiotherapy, but also to significantly enhance immune response in these patients. Rather than concluding on this topic, this review provides a common ground to explore more in detail the use of certain probiotic strains for common side effects such as pleural effusions, which have a profound impact on the quality of life and life expectancy of these patients.

Supplementary Materials: The following are available online at https://www.mdpi.com/1660-4601/18/8/4265/s1, Supplementary File 1.

Author Contributions: Conceptualization: M.R.-A., A.M.-O., C.R.-P.; methodology: M.R.-A., C.R.-P.; investigation: A.M.-O., L.R.-R., A.F.A., C.R.-P.; validation: M.R.-A., A.M.-O., C.R.-P.; formal analysis: M.R.-A., A.M.-O., C.R.-P.; writing—original draft: M.R.-A., C.R.-P.; writing—review and editing: A.M.-O., L.R.-R., A.F.A.; visualization: A.M.-O., L.R.-R., A.F.A.; supervision: C.R.-P.; project administration: M.R.-A., C.R.-P. All authors have read and agreed to the published version of the manuscript.

Funding: This research received no external funding.

Institutional Review Board Statement: Not applicable.

Informed Consent Statement: Not applicable.

Data Availability Statement: The dataset used and/or analyzed in this study is available from the corresponding author on reasonable request.

Conflicts of Interest: The authors declare no conflict of interest.

Appendix A

Table 1. Search strategies for each database used.

	Pubmed	Scielo	Proquest	Ovid
Probiotics	(((((probiotics [Title/Abstract] OR probiotics [MeSH Terms]) OR lactobacillus [Title/Abstract]) OR bifidobacterium [Title/Abstract]) OR lactobacillus [MeSH Terms]) OR bifidobacterium [MeSH Terms])	((ti:probiotics OR ab:probiotics OR kw:probiotics) OR (ti:lactobacillus OR ab:lactobacillus OR kw:probiotics) OR (ti:bifidobacterium OR ab:bifidobacterium OR kw:bifidobacterium))	((((AB,TI(probiotics) OR MESH(probiotics)) OR AB,TI(lactobacillus)) OR AB,TI(bifidobacterium)) OR MESH(lactobacillus) OR MESH(bifidobacterium))	((probiotics OR lactobacillus) OR bifidobacterium)

Table 1. Cont.

	Pubmed	Scielo	Proquest	Ovid
Oncology treatments	AND ((((radiotherapy [Title/Abstract] OR chemotherapy [Title/Abstract]) OR chemotherapy [MeSH Terms]) OR radiotherapy [MeSH Terms]) OR radiation [Title/Abstract])	AND ((((ti:chemotherapy OR ab:chemotherapy OR kw:chemotherapy) OR (ti:radiotherapy OR ab:radiotherapy OR kw:radiotherapy)) OR (ti:radiation OR ab:radiation OR kw:radiation))	AND (((AB,TI(chemotherapy) OR AB,TI(radiotherapy)) OR MESH(chemotherapy)) OR MESH(radiotherapy))	((chemotherapy OR radiotherapy) OR radiation)

References

1. World Health Organization (WHO). *Global Health Estimates 2020: Deaths by Cause, Age, Sex, by Country and by Region, 2000–2019*; WHO: Geneva, Switzerland, 2020.
2. Sung, H.; Ferlay, J.; Siegel, R.L.; Laversanne, M.; Soerjomataram, I.; Jemal, A.; Bray, F. Global Cancer Statistics 2020: GLOBOCAN Estimates of Incidence and Mortality Worldwide for 36 Cancers in 185 Countries. *CA Cancer J. Clin.* **2021**. [CrossRef]
3. Gervais, R.; Le Caer, H.; Monnet, I.; Falchero, L.; Baize, N.; Olivero, G.; Thomas, P.; Berard, H.; Auliac, J.B.; Chouaid, C. Second-Line Oral Chemotherapy (Lomustine, Cyclophosphamide, Etoposide) versus Intravenous Therapy (Cyclophosphamide, Doxorubicin, and Vincristine) in Patients with Relapsed Small Cell Lung Cancer: A Randomized Phase II Study of GFPC 0501. *Clin. Lung Cancer* **2015**, *16*, 100–105. [CrossRef]
4. Wang, S.L.; Fang, H.; Song, Y.W.; Wang, W.H.; Hu, C.; Liu, Y.P.; Jin, J.; Liu, X.F.; Yu, Z.H.; Ren, H.; et al. Hypofractionated versus Conventional Fractionated Postmastectomy Radiotherapy for Patients with High-Risk Breast Cancer: A Randomised, Non-Inferiority, Open-Label, Phase 3 Trial. *Lancet Oncol.* **2019**, *20*, 352–360. [CrossRef]
5. Link, W. *Principles of Cancer Treatment and Anticancer Drug Development*, 1st ed.; Springer Nature: Geneva, Switzerland, 2020; ISBN 978-3-030-18724-8.
6. Kayl, A.E.; Meyers, C.A. Side-Effects of Chemotherapy and Quality of Life in Ovarian and Breast Cancer Patients. *Curr. Opin. Obstet. Gynecol.* **2006**, *18*, 24–28. [CrossRef]
7. Mazzotti, E.; Antonini Cappellini, G.C.; Buconovo, S.; Morese, R.; Scoppola, A.; Sebastiani, C.; Marchetti, P. Treatment-Related Side Effects and Quality of Life in Cancer Patients. *Support. Care Cancer* **2012**, *20*, 2553–2557. [CrossRef] [PubMed]
8. Hanna, T.P.; King, W.D.; Thibodeau, S.; Jalink, M.; Paulin, G.A.; Harvey-Jones, E.; O'Sullivan, D.E.; Booth, C.M.; Sullivan, R.; Aggarwal, A. Mortality Due to Cancer Treatment Delay: Systematic Review and Meta-Analysis. *BMJ* **2020**, *371*, m4087. [CrossRef] [PubMed]
9. Goubet, A.-G.; Daillère, R.; Routy, B.; Derosa, L.M.; Roberti, P.; Zitvogel, L. The Impact of the Intestinal Microbiota in Therapeutic Responses against Cancer. *C. R. Biol.* **2018**, *341*, 284–289. [CrossRef] [PubMed]
10. Álvarez, J.; Fernández Real, J.M.; Guarner, F.; Gueimonde, M.; Rodríguez, J.M.; Saenz de Pipaon, M.; Sanz, Y. Gut Microbes and Health. *Gastroenterol. Hepatol.* **2021**. [CrossRef]
11. Parida, S.; Sharma, D. The Microbiome and Cancer: Creating Friendly Neighborhoods and Removing the Foes Within. *Cancer Res.* **2021**, *81*, 790–800. [CrossRef] [PubMed]
12. Sehrawat, N.; Yadav, M.; Singh, M.; Kumar, V.; Sharma, V.R.; Sharma, A.K. Probiotics in Microbiome Ecological Balance Providing a Therapeutic Window against Cancer. *Semin. Cancer Biol.* **2021**, *70*, 24–36. [CrossRef]
13. Loman, B.R.; Jordan, K.R.; Haynes, B.; Bailey, M.T.; Pyter, L.M. Chemotherapy-Induced Neuroinflammation Is Associated with Disrupted Colonic and Bacterial Homeostasis in Female Mice. *Sci. Rep.* **2019**, *9*, 1–16. [CrossRef] [PubMed]
14. WHO. *Report of the Joint FAO/WHO Expert Consultation on Evaluation of Health and Nutritional Properties of Probiotics in Food Including Powder Milk with Live Lactic Acid Bacteria, Córdoba, Argentina, 1–4 October 2001*; Food and Agriculture Organization of the United Nations: Rome, Italy, 2001.
15. Cassani, E.; Privitera, G.; Pezzoli, G.; Pusani, C.; Madio, C.; Iorio, L.; Barichella, M. Use of Probiotics for the Treatment of Constipation in Parkinson's Disease Patients. *Min. Gastroenterol. Dietol.* **2011**, *57*, 117–121.
16. Fox, M.J.; Ahuja, K.D.K.; Robertson, I.K.; Ball, M.J.; Eri, R.D. Can Probiotic Yogurt Prevent Diarrhoea in Children on Antibiotics? A Double-Blind, Randomised, Placebo-Controlled Study. *BMJ Open* **2015**, *5*. [CrossRef] [PubMed]
17. Mennigen, R.; Nolte, K.; Rijcken, E.; Utech, M.; Loeffler, B.; Senninger, N.; Bruewer, M. Probiotic Mixture VSL#3 Protects the Epithelial Barrier by Maintaining Tight Junction Protein Expression and Preventing Apoptosis in a Murine Model of Colitis. *Am. J. Physiol. Gastrointest. Liver Physiol.* **2009**, *296*, 1140–1149. [CrossRef]
18. Lee, S.; Kirkland, R.; Grunewald, Z.I.; Sun, Q.; Wicker, L.; de La Serre, C.B. Beneficial Effects of Non-Encapsulated or Encapsulated Probiotic Supplementation on Microbiota Composition, Intestinal Barrier Functions, Inflammatory Profiles, and Glucose Tolerance in High Fat Fed Rats. *Nutrients* **2019**, *11*, 1975. [CrossRef]

19. Messaoudi, M.; Violle, N.; Bisson, J.F.; Desor, D.; Javelot, H.; Rougeot, C. Beneficial Psychological Effects of a Probiotic Formulation (Lactobacillus Helveticus R0052 and Bifidobacterium Longum R0175) in Healthy Human Volunteers. *Gut Microb.* **2011**, *2*, 256–261. [CrossRef]
20. Jiang, C.; Wang, H.; Xia, C.; Dong, Q.; Chen, E.; Qiu, Y.; Su, Y.; Xie, H.; Zeng, L.; Kuang, J.; et al. A Randomized, Double-Blind, Placebo-Controlled Trial of Probiotics to Reduce the Severity of Oral Mucositis Induced by Chemoradiotherapy for Patients with Nasopharyngeal Carcinoma. *Cancer* **2019**, *125*, 1081–1090. [CrossRef]
21. Yeung, C.-Y.; Chan, W.-T.; Jiang, C.-B.; Cheng, M.-L.; Liu, C.-Y.; Chang, S.-W.; Chiau, J.-S.C.; Lee, H.-C. Amelioration of Chemotherapy-Induced Intestinal Mucositis by Orally Administered Probiotics in a Mouse Model. *PLoS ONE* **2015**, *10*, e0138746. [CrossRef] [PubMed]
22. Moher, D.; Liberati, A.; Tetzlaff, J.; Altman, D.G.; Group, T.P. Preferred Reporting Items for Systematic Reviews and Meta-Analyses: The PRISMA Statement. *PLoS Med.* **2009**, *6*, e1000097. [CrossRef]
23. Stone, P.W. Popping the (PICO) Question in Research and Evidence-Based Practice. *Appl. Nurs. Res.* **2002**, *15*, 197–198. [CrossRef] [PubMed]
24. Jadad, A.R.; Moore, R.A.; Carroll, D.; Jenkinson, C.; Reynolds, D.J.; Gavaghan, D.J.; McQuay, H.J. Assessing the Quality of Reports of Randomized Clinical Trials: Is Blinding Necessary? *Control. Clin. Trials* **1996**, *17*, 1–12. [CrossRef]
25. Linn, Y.H.; Thu, K.K.; Win, N.H.H. Effect of Probiotics for the Prevention of Acute Radiation-Induced Diarrhoea Among Cervical Cancer Patients: A Randomized Double-Blind Placebo-Controlled Study. *Prob. Antimicrob. Proteins* **2019**, *11*, 638–647. [CrossRef]
26. Golkhalkhali, B.; Rajandram, R.; Paliany, A.S.; Ho, G.F.; Wan Ishak, W.Z.; Johari, C.S.; Chin, K.F. Strain-Specific Probiotic (Microbial Cell Preparation) and Omega-3 Fatty Acid in Modulating Quality of Life and Inflammatory Markers in Colorectal Cancer Patients: A Randomized Controlled Trial. *Asia Pac. J. Clin. Oncol.* **2018**, *14*, 179–191. [CrossRef] [PubMed]
27. Liu, J.; Huang, X.-E. Efficacy of Bifidobacterium Tetragenous Viable Bacteria Tablets for Cancer Patients with Functional Constipation. *Asian Pac. J. Cancer Prev.* **2014**, *15*, 10241–10244. [CrossRef] [PubMed]
28. Demers, M.; Dagnault, A.; Desjardins, J. A Randomized Double-Blind Controlled Trial: Impact of Probiotics on Diarrhea in Patients Treated with Pelvic Radiation. *Clin. Nutr.* **2014**, *33*, 761–767. [CrossRef] [PubMed]
29. Ki, Y.; Kim, W.; Nam, J.; Kim, D.; Lee, J.; Park, D.; Jeon, H.; Ha, H.; Kim, T.; Kim, D. Probiotics for Rectal Volume Variation during Radiation Therapy for Prostate Cancer. *Int. J. Radiat. Oncol. Biol. Phys.* **2013**, *87*, 646–650. [CrossRef] [PubMed]
30. Holma, R.; Korpela, R.; Sairanen, U.; Blom, M.; Rautio, M.; Poussa, T.; Saxelin, M.; Osterlund, P. Colonic Methane Production Modifies Gastrointestinal Toxicity Associated with Adjuvant 5-Fluorouracil Chemotherapy for Colorectal Cancer. *J. Clin. Gastroenterol.* **2013**, *47*, 45–51. [CrossRef] [PubMed]
31. Chitapanarux, I.; Chitapanarux, T.; Traisathit, P.; Kudumpee, S.; Tharavichitkul, E.; Lorvidhaya, V. Randomized Controlled Trial of Live Lactobacillus Acidophilus plus Bifidobacterium Bifidum in Prophylaxis of Diarrhea during Radiotherapy in Cervical Cancer Patients. *Radiat. Oncol.* **2010**, *5*, 31. [CrossRef]
32. Giralt, J.; Regadera, J.P.; Verges, R.; Romero, J.; de la Fuente, I.; Biete, A.; Villoria, J.; Cobo, J.M.; Guarner, F. Effects of Probiotic Lactobacillus Casei DN-114 001 in Prevention of Radiation-Induced Diarrhea: Results from Multicenter, Randomized, Placebo-Controlled Nutritional Trial. *Int. J. Radiat. Oncol. Biol. Phys.* **2008**, *71*, 1213–1219. [CrossRef]
33. Osterlund, P.; Ruotsalainen, T.; Korpela, R.; Saxelin, M.; Ollus, A.; Valta, P.; Kouri, M.; Elomaa, I.; Joensuu, H. Lactobacillus Supplementation for Diarrhoea Related to Chemotherapy of Colorectal Cancer: A Randomised Study. *Br. J. Cancer* **2007**, *97*, 1028–1034. [CrossRef]
34. Delia, P.; Sansotta, G.; Donato, V.; Frosina, P.; Messina, G.; De Renzis, C.; Famularo, G. Use of Probiotics for Prevention of Radiation-Induced Diarrhea. *World J. Gastroenterol.* **2007**, *13*, 912–915. [CrossRef]
35. Osterlund, P.; Ruotsalainen, T.; Peuhkuri, K.; Korpela, R.; Ollus, A.; Ikonen, M.; Joensuu, H.; Elomaa, I. Lactose Intolerance Associated with Adjuvant 5-Fluorouracil-Based Chemotherapy for Colorectal Cancer. *Clin. Gastroenterol. Hepatol.* **2004**, *2*, 696–703. [CrossRef]
36. Urbancsek, H.; Kazar, T.; Mezes, I.; Neumann, K. Results of a Double-Blind, Randomized Study to Evaluate the Efficacy and Safety of Antibiophilus in Patients with Radiation-Induced Diarrhoea. *Eur. J. Gastroenterol. Hepatol.* **2001**, *13*, 391–396. [CrossRef] [PubMed]
37. Salminen, E.; Elomaa, I.; Minkkinen, J.; Vapaatalo, H.; Salminen, S. Preservation of Intestinal Integrity during Radiotherapy Using Live Lactobacillus Acidophilus Cultures. *Clin. Radiol.* **1988**, *39*, 435–437. [CrossRef]
38. Shao, F.; Xin, F.-Z.; Yang, C.-G.; Yang, D.-G.; Mi, Y.-T.; Yu, J.-X.; Li, G.-Y. The Impact of Microbial Immune Enteral Nutrition on the Patients with Acute Radiation Enteritis in Bowel Function and Immune Status. *Cell Biochem. Biophys.* **2014**, *69*, 357–361. [CrossRef] [PubMed]
39. De Sanctis, V.; Belgioia, L.; Cante, D.; La Porta, M.R.; Caspiani, O.; Guarnaccia, R.; Argenone, A.; Muto, P.; Musio, D.; DE Felice, F.; et al. Lactobacillus Brevis CD2 for Prevention of Oral Mucositis in Patients With Head and Neck Tumors: A Multicentric Randomized Study. *Anticancer Res.* **2019**, *39*, 1935–1942. [CrossRef]
40. Sharma, A.; Rath, G.K.; Chaudhary, S.P.; Thakar, A.; Mohanti, B.K.; Bahadur, S. Lactobacillus Brevis CD2 Lozenges Reduce Radiation- and Chemotherapy-Induced Mucositis in Patients with Head and Neck Cancer: A Randomized Double-Blind Placebo-Controlled Study. *Eur. J. Cancer* **2012**, *48*, 875–881. [CrossRef] [PubMed]

41. Vesty, A.; Gear, K.; Boutell, S.; Taylor, M.W.; Douglas, R.G.; Biswas, K. Randomised, Double-Blind, Placebo-Controlled Trial of Oral Probiotic Streptococcus Salivarius M18 on Head and Neck Cancer Patients Post-Radiotherapy: A Pilot Study. *Sci. Rep.* **2020**, *10*, 13201. [CrossRef]
42. Doppalapudi, R.; Vundavalli, S.; Prabhat, M.P. Effect of Probiotic Bacteria on Oral Candida in Head- and Neck-Radiotherapy Patients: A Randomized Clinical Trial. *J. Cancer Res. Ther.* **2020**, *16*, 470–477. [CrossRef]
43. Masuno, T.; Kishimoto, S.; Ogura, T.; Honma, T.; Niitani, H.; Fukuoka, M.; Ogawa, N. A Comparative Trial of LC9018 plus Doxorubicin and Doxorubicin Alone for the Treatment of Malignant Pleural Effusion Secondary to Lung Cancer. *Cancer* **1991**, *68*, 1495–1500. [CrossRef]
44. Sun, J.-R.; Kong, C.-F.; Qu, X.-K.; Deng, C.; Lou, Y.-N.; Jia, L.-Q. Efficacy and Safety of Probiotics in Irritable Bowel Syndrome: A Systematic Review and Meta-Analysis. *Saudi J. Gastroenterol.* **2020**, *26*, 66–77. [CrossRef] [PubMed]
45. Touchefeu, Y.; Montassier, E.; Nieman, K.; Gastinne, T.; Potel, G.; Bruley des Varannes, S.; Le Vacon, F.; de La Cochetière, M.F. Systematic Review: The Role of the Gut Microbiota in Chemotherapy- or Radiation-Induced Gastrointestinal Mucositis-Current Evidence and Potential Clinical Applications. *Alim. Pharmacol. Ther.* **2014**, *40*, 409–421. [CrossRef] [PubMed]
46. Hassan, H.; Rompola, M.; Glaser, A.W.; Kinsey, S.E.; Phillips, R.S. Systematic Review and Meta-Analysis Investigating the Efficacy and Safety of Probiotics in People with Cancer. *Support Care Cancer* **2018**, *26*, 2503–2509. [CrossRef] [PubMed]
47. Redman, M.G.; Ward, E.J.; Phillips, R.S. The Efficacy and Safety of Probiotics in People with Cancer: A Systematic Review. *Ann. Oncol.* **2014**, *25*, 1919–1929. [CrossRef] [PubMed]
48. Cammarota, G.; Ianiro, G.; Ahern, A.; Carbone, C.; Temko, A.; Claesson, M.J.; Gasbarrini, A.; Tortora, G. Gut Microbiome, Big Data and Machine Learning to Promote Precision Medicine for Cancer. *Nat. Rev. Gastroenterol. Hepatol.* **2020**, *17*, 635–648. [CrossRef]
49. McFarland, L.V.; Evans, C.T.; Goldstein, E.J.C. Strain-Specificity and Disease-Specificity of Probiotic Efficacy: A Systematic Review and Meta-Analysis. *Front. Med.* **2018**, *5*. [CrossRef]
50. Tilocca, B.; Burbach, K.; Heyer, C.M.E.; Hoelzle, L.E.; Mosenthin, R.; Stefanski, V.; Camarinha-Silva, A.; Seifert, J. Dietary Changes in Nutritional Studies Shape the Structural and Functional Composition of the Pigs' Fecal Microbiome—From Days to Weeks. *Microbiome* **2017**, *5*, 144. [CrossRef]
51. Maldonado-Galdeano, C.; Cazorla, S.I.; Lemme Dumit, J.M.; Vélez, E.; Perdigón, G. Beneficial Effects of Probiotic Consumption on the Immune System. *ANM* **2019**, *74*, 115–124. [CrossRef]
52. Saputro, I.D.; Putra, O.N.; Pebrianton, H. Suharjono, null Effects of Probiotic Administration on IGA and IL-6 Level in Severe Burn Patients: A Randomized Trial. *Ann. Burns Fire Dis.* **2019**, *32*, 70–76.
53. Isolauri, E.; Kirjavainen, P.V.; Salminen, S. Probiotics: A Role in the Treatment of Intestinal Infection and Inflammation? *Gut* **2002**, *50* (Suppl. 3), III54–III59. [CrossRef] [PubMed]
54. Yao, P.; Tan, F.; Gao, H.; Wang, L.; Yang, T.; Cheng, Y. Effects of Probiotics on Toll-like Receptor Expression in Ulcerative Colitis Rats Induced by 2,4,6-trinitro-benzene Sulfonic Acid. *Mol. Med. Rep.* **2017**, *15*, 1973–1980. [CrossRef]
55. Zhu, F.; Jiang, Z.; Li, H.-W. Intestinal Probiotics in Relieving Clinical Symptoms of Severe Hand, Foot, and Mouth Disease and Potential Mechanism Analysis. *Eur. Rev. Med. Pharmacol. Sci.* **2017**, *21*, 4214–4218. [PubMed]
56. Haussner, F.; Chakraborty, S.; Halbgebauer, R.; Huber-Lang, M. Challenge to the Intestinal Mucosa During Sepsis. *Front. Immunol.* **2019**, *10*. [CrossRef] [PubMed]
57. Kaźmierczak-Siedlecka, K.; Daca, A.; Fic, M.; van de Wetering, T.; Folwarski, M.; Makarewicz, W. Therapeutic Methods of Gut Microbiota Modification in Colorectal Cancer Management–Fecal Microbiota Transplantation, Prebiotics, Probiotics, and Synbiotics. *Gut Microb.* **2020**, *11*, 1518–1530. [CrossRef] [PubMed]
58. Holma, R.; Laatikainen, R.; Orell, H.; Joensuu, H.; Peuhkuri, K.; Poussa, T.; Korpela, R.; Österlund, P. Consumption of Lactose, Other FODMAPs and Diarrhoea during Adjuvant 5-Fluorouracil Chemotherapy for Colorectal Cancer. *Nutrients* **2020**, *12*, 407. [CrossRef] [PubMed]
59. Rana, S.V. Importance of Methanogenic Flora in Intestinal Toxicity during 5-Fluorouracil Therapy for Colon Cancer. *J. Clin. Gastroenterol.* **2013**, *47*, 9–11. [CrossRef] [PubMed]
60. Curra, M.; Soares Junior, L.A.V.; Martins, M.D.; da Silva Santos, P.S. Chemotherapy Protocols and Incidence of Oral Mucositis. An Integrative Review. *Einstein* **2018**, *16*, eRW4007. [CrossRef] [PubMed]
61. Tohgo, A.; Tanaka, N.G.; Okada, H.; Osada, Y. Effect of Combined Intrapleural Administration of Lactobacillus Casei (LC9018) and Adriamycin on Experimental Malignant Pleurisy in Mice. *Jpn. J. Cancer Res.* **1989**, *80*, 1238–1245. [CrossRef]
62. Yasutake, N.; Matsuzaki, T.; Kimura, K.; Hashimoto, S.; Yokokura, T.; Yoshikai, Y. The Role of Tumor Necrosis Factor (TNF)-Alpha in the Antitumor Effect of Intrapleural Injection of Lactobacillus Casei Strain Shirota in Mice. *Med. Microbiol. Immunol.* **1999**, *188*, 9–14. [CrossRef]

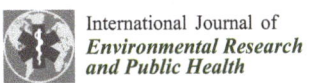

Article

Effect of Simulated Gastrointestinal Tract Conditions on Survivability of Probiotic Bacteria Present in Commercial Preparations

Lidia Stasiak-Różańska *, Anna Berthold-Pluta, Antoni Stanisław Pluta, Krzysztof Dasiewicz and Monika Garbowska

Department of Food Technology and Assessment, Institute of Food Sciences, Warsaw University of Life Sciences-SGGW, Nowoursynowska St. 166, 02-787 Warsaw, Poland; anna_berthold@sggw.edu.pl (A.B.-P.); antoni_pluta@sggw.edu.pl (A.S.P.); krzysztof_dasiewicz@sggw.edu.pl (K.D.); monika_garbowska@sggw.edu.pl (M.G.)
* Correspondence: lidia_stasiak_rozanska@sggw.edu.pl; Tel.: +48-225-937-539

Abstract: Probiotics are recommended, among others, in the diet of children who are under antibiotic therapy, or that suffer from food allergies or travel diarrhea, etc. In the case of toddlers taking probiotic preparations, it is highly recommended to first remove the special capsule, which normally protects probiotic strains against hard conditions in the gastrointestinal tract. Otherwise, the toddler may choke. This removal can impair probiotic survival and reduce its efficacy in a toddler's organism. The aim of this study was to evaluate the survivability of five strains of lactic acid bacteria from the commercial probiotics available on the Polish market under simulated conditions of the gastrointestinal tract. Five probiotics (each including one of these strains: *Bifidobacterium* BB-12, *Lactobacillus (Lb.) rhamnosus* GG, *Lb. casei*, *Lb. acidophilus*, *Lb. plantarum*) were protective capsule deprived, added in a food matrix (chicken–vegetable soup) and subjected under simulated conditions of the gastric and gastrointestinal passage. Strain survivability and possibility to growth were evaluated. Obtained results showed that, among all analyzed commercial probiotic strains, the *Lb. plantarum* was the most resistant to the applied conditions of the culture medium. They showed a noticeable growth under both in vitro gastric conditions at pH 4.0 and 5.0, as well as in vitro intestinal conditions at all tested concentrations of bile salts.

Keywords: probiotics; resistance; survivability; gastrointestinal passage; gut

1. Introduction

The definition of "probiotic" provided by the International Scientific Association of Probiotics and Prebiotics states that probiotics are "live microorganisms that, when administered in adequate amounts, confer a health benefit on the host" [1]. The best known and the most thoroughly investigated probiotic strains are representatives of *Lactobacillus (Lb.)* and *Bifidobacterium* genera [2–4]. The role of probiotics is to, i.a., alleviate symptoms of lactose intolerance, ameliorate outcomes of food allergies, and reduce cholesterol concentration in blood [5–7]. The administration of probiotic preparations is recommended, e.g., during and after antibiotic therapy to aid the reconstruction of natural enteric microflora [8–10].

It is estimated that from 11 to 30% of children treated with antibiotics (mainly β-lactam ones and vancomycin) suffer from intestinal discomfort and diarrheas [11–13]. Diarrhea is especially dangerous for small children/toddlers as it may cause malfunction of the water–electrolyte balance of their bodies within a short period of time [14]. Sometimes, however, children suffer from post-antibiotic diarrhea despite their diet supplementation with probiotic strains [15]. This is, probably, caused by reduced survivability of individual probiotic strains under varying conditions of the alimentary tract. Oral administration of at least 10^7 cells of a probiotic strain per milliliter or gram of food should ensure a positive

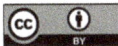

effect to the host even when some of them do not survive the unfavorable conditions of the gastrointestinal passage [16]. Most of the commercial probiotics are registered as "dietary supplements" and therefore do not have to comply with quality requirements obligatory for drugs [17]. After oral administration, the probiotic strains are exposed to low pH of the stomach and bile salts in the enteral section of the alimentary tract of the host. Many of them often fail to survive conditions of the passage [18,19]. Metabolic and biochemical activity of probiotics during gastrointestinal passage can be sustained through earlier encapsulation of their cells [20,21]. However, probiotic preparation producers recommend removal of the protective capsule before giving it to toddlers and making a suspension of probiotic powder with water to avoid choking or strangulation during swallow. Such information can be found on preparation leaflets. Another means of protecting probiotics against adverse effects of the gastrointestinal conditions is their administration together with a prebiotic [22]. The best known and the most commonly used prebiotics include inulin and oligofructose [23].

The aim of this study was to examine the survivability and possibility to growth of strains obtained from commercial probiotic preparations (without protective capsule) under conditions simulating gastrointestinal tract.

2. Materials and Methods

2.1. Commercial Probiotic Preparations

The study was conducted with 5 commercial preparations, available on the Polish market, which contained lyophilized cells of one-strain of probiotic bacteria, namely:

Preparation 1—*Lactobacillus rhamnosus* GG ATCC 53103 (3×10^9 CFU/one dose, 4.5×10^9 CFU/g);

Preparation 2—*Bifidobacterium* BB-12 (4×10^9 CFU/one dose, 1.7×10^{10} CFU/g);

Preparation 3—*Lactobacillus casei* (4×10^8 CFU/one dose, 2.1×10^9 CFU/g);

Preparation 4—*Lactobacillus acidophilus* (2×10^9 CFU/one dose, 3.1×10^{10} CFU/g);

Preparation 5—*Lactobacillus plantarum* (4×10^8 CFU/one dose, 1.8×10^9 CFU/g).

In the case of preparations 3, 4 and 5, producers did not provide any information about the number of strain or its origin. This information is a trade secret. Preparation 2 contained a prebiotic in the form of fructooligosaccharide (FOS), whereas preparations 3 and 4 contained inulin, and preparations 1 and 5 did not contain prebiotic. The preparations originated from various Polish producers and were registered as dietary supplements. Their production dates were similar. Preparation 1 was in the form of a lyophilizate in a paper sachet, whereas the other preparations were encapsulated in gelatin capsules. Preparation 1 was poured out of the sachet prior to testing. All gelatin capsules (which normally protect probiotics from outside the GIT environment) from preparations 2, 3, 4, and 5 were removed before using probiotic preparations in experiments; this is typically the intake procedure for probiotic preparations for toddlers (12–18 months) to avoid choking.

2.2. Growth Media and Solutions

MRS broth (Sigma-Aldrich, St. Louis, MO, USA), agar 15 gL^{-1} (for seeding step), pH 6.2. The broth was sterilized at a temperature of 121 °C for 15 min.

Gastric electrolyte solution (GES) [24,25], composed of [gL^{-1}]: NaCl 4.8, NaHCO$_3$ 1.56, KCl 2.2, CaCl$_2$ 0.22, pepsin 1. The solution was sterilized at a temperature of 121 °C for 20 min; after sterilization GES was supplemented with a filter sterile pepsin solution in water (P6887; Sigma-Aldrich, 0.22 µL, Sartorius Poland Sp. z o o.) to final concentration 1 gL^{-1}.

Double-concentrated J broth ($2 \times JB$) [24], was composed of [gL^{-1}]: peptone 10, yeast extract 30, K$_2$HPO$_4$ 6, glucose 4. The broth was sterilized at a temperature of 121 °C for 20 min. Glucose solution was filtered (filter pore diameter—0.22 µm, Sartorius Poland Sp. z o o.) and added to $2 \times JB$ after sterilization. Bile salts were subjected to mild sterilization (117 °C, 10 min) and added to sterilized $2 \times JB$. Concentration of bile salts (Sigma-Aldrich, B8631) was adjusted to 1%, 2%, and 3%.

Chicken–vegetable soup (CVS) composed of [gL^{-1}]: chicken breast fillet 200, onion 35, carrot 100, celery root 30, and parsley root 65. The CVS was prepared in a Termomix Vorwerc cooker, at a temperature of 100 °C, for 60 min, with a mixing rate knob in position 1. The CVS was filtered (filter pore diameter—0.45 µm).

Spring water was recommended for small children, sterilized at temperature 121 °C for 20 min.

Lactobacillus and *Bifidobacterium* BB-12 were enumerated by the pour plate technique on MRS and MRS modified by adding 0.2% (*w/v*) lithium chloride and 0.3% (*w/v*) sodium propionate (MRS-LP), respectively [26].

2.3. Study Design and Culture Conditions

The experiment was divided into three stages: control cultures, stomach stage, and gastrointestinal stage.

To observe how tested bacteria react in optimal conditions (control), *Lactobacillus* was incubated in MRS broth, while *Bifidobacterium* on MRS-LP, deemed optimal for their growth, was adjusted to pH 6.2 either with HCl 5M or with NaOH 1M at a temperature of 37 °C, for 48 h. In order to limit the access of oxygen to the *Bifidobacterium*, cultures were carried out without shaking and, additionally, the access of air was cut off with a layer of water agar. Incubations in MRS adjusted to pH 2.0, 3.0, 4.0 or 5.0 in the same growth conditions were also performed to have a positive control of probiotics growth. In the tested preparations, the initial number of viable cells of the probiotic strain was initially determined by inoculating petri dishes with MRS medium (preparations 1, 3, 4 and 5, respectively) and with MRS-LP Agar medium (preparation 2). The obtained results were expressed as CFU/g of each preparation (2.1.).

To simulate conditions occurring in the stomach, 100 mL of GES was mixed with 100 mL of CVS and 100 mL of sterile spring water containing 1 dose of a given probiotic preparation (1, 2, 3, 4 or 5). Each of the five mixtures was cultured at final pH 2.0, 3.0, 4.0, and 5.0; temperature 37 °C, for 3 h (Figure 1). The acidity of the solutions was adjusted using the HCl 5M.

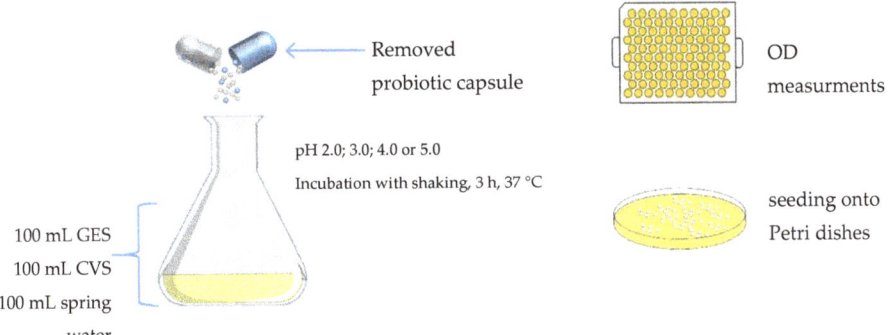

Figure 1. Scheme of the variants tested under gastric stage of experiment (GES—gastric electrolyte solution, CVS—chicken–vegetable soup).

The gastrointestinal stage consisted of mixing 100 mL of GES with 100 mL of CVS and 100 mL of spring water suspension containing a given probiotic, at final pH 3.0. The mixture was shaken in a reciprocating shaker 50 rpm, at 37 °C for 30 min (stomach stage) [27]. Afterwards, the suspension was mixed with 2 × JB (1:1, v/v). Survivability of all preparations was examined in the presence of bile salts with concentrations of 1, 2 or 3 (%), at 37 °C for 6 h; the final pH of mixture medium was 5.5 (regulated using NaOH 1M) (Figure 2).

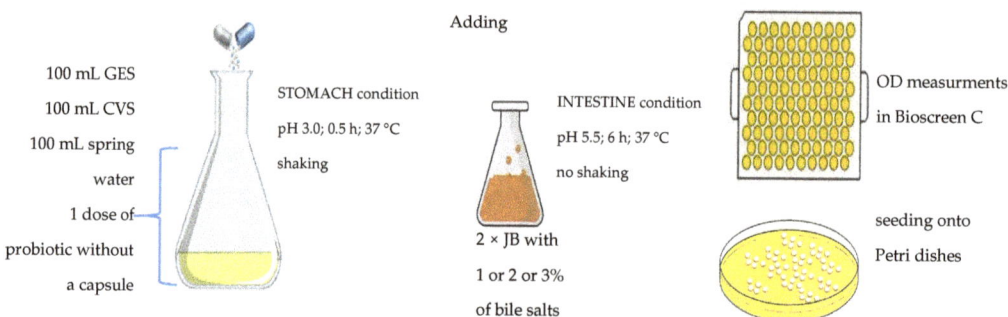

Figure 2. Scheme of the variants tested under gastrointestinal stage of experiment, (GES—gastric electrolyte solution, CVS—chicken–vegetable soup, 2 × JB—2 × concentrated J broth).

Optical density (OD) of individual cultures of probiotic preparations was measured every 30 min in a Bioscreen C MBR apparatus with the length of wave λ = 600 nm. Each culture variant was conducted in three independent replications. Simultaneously the count of bacteria on MRS Agar pH 6.3 (*Lactobacillus*) and MRS-LP Agar pH 6.3 (BB-12) plates was determined. Incubation was provided in anaerobic jars containing AnaeroGen® (Argenta, Poland) [26]. The samples for spread on petri dishes was taken from time points: 0; 12; 24; 36 and 48 h for MRS conditions, 0; 1; 2; 3 h for gastric stage, 0; 2; 4; 6 h for gastrointestinal stage. In each variant of the experiment, three independent series of replicates were performed for each analyzed sample inoculated into petri dishes, differentiated by the type of preparation (1; 2; 3; 4; 5), variant type (MRS control, stomach, gastrointestinal (GI), pH (2.0; 3.0; 4.0; 5.0 or 6.2) or bile salt concentration (1%; 2%; 3%) and measuring point (h) 0; 12; 24; 36; 48 for MRS stage, 0; 1; 2; 3 for stomach, 0; 2; 4; 6 for GI. In the case of the optical density (OD) measurement in Bioscreen Apparatus, measurements were made every 30 min for each individual sample, and each sample variant was performed in three independent measurement series.

2.4. Calculation of Coefficient of Specific Growth Rate

The coefficient of the specific growth rate (μ) in time (t) was calculated from the formula: $\mu(t) = (\ln OD_f - \ln OD_i) / (t_f - t_i)$, where: OD_f—final OD in the log phase, OD_i—initial OD in the log phase, t_f—time of log phase termination, t_i—time of log phase onset [28].

2.5. Statistical Analysis

Results obtained were subjected to statistical analysis using StatGraphicPlus 4.1. software Statgraphics Centurion software (Version 17.1.12, Gambit Centrum Oprogramowania i Szkoleń Ltd., Kraków, Poland). Analysis of variance (ANOVA) was conducted. The Tukey test was applied to compare the significance of differences between mean values at a significance level of α = 0.05. Mean values from three replicates (n = 3) were also calculated, and the standard deviation was added to the mean as ± SD.

3. Results

3.1. Survivability and Growth of Bacteria Present in Commercial Probiotic Preparations in MRS Broth

Bacteria were cultured in the MRS broth deemed optimal for the growth of LAB and bifidobacteria [29–31] to observe how they react in optimal conditions.

Curves of changes in optical density (OD, λ = 600 nm) during culture of commercial preparations of probiotic bacteria in MRS broth with various pH values are shown on Figure 3. The viable cell counts of the tested probiotic bacteria determined by the plate method are illustrated in Table 1.

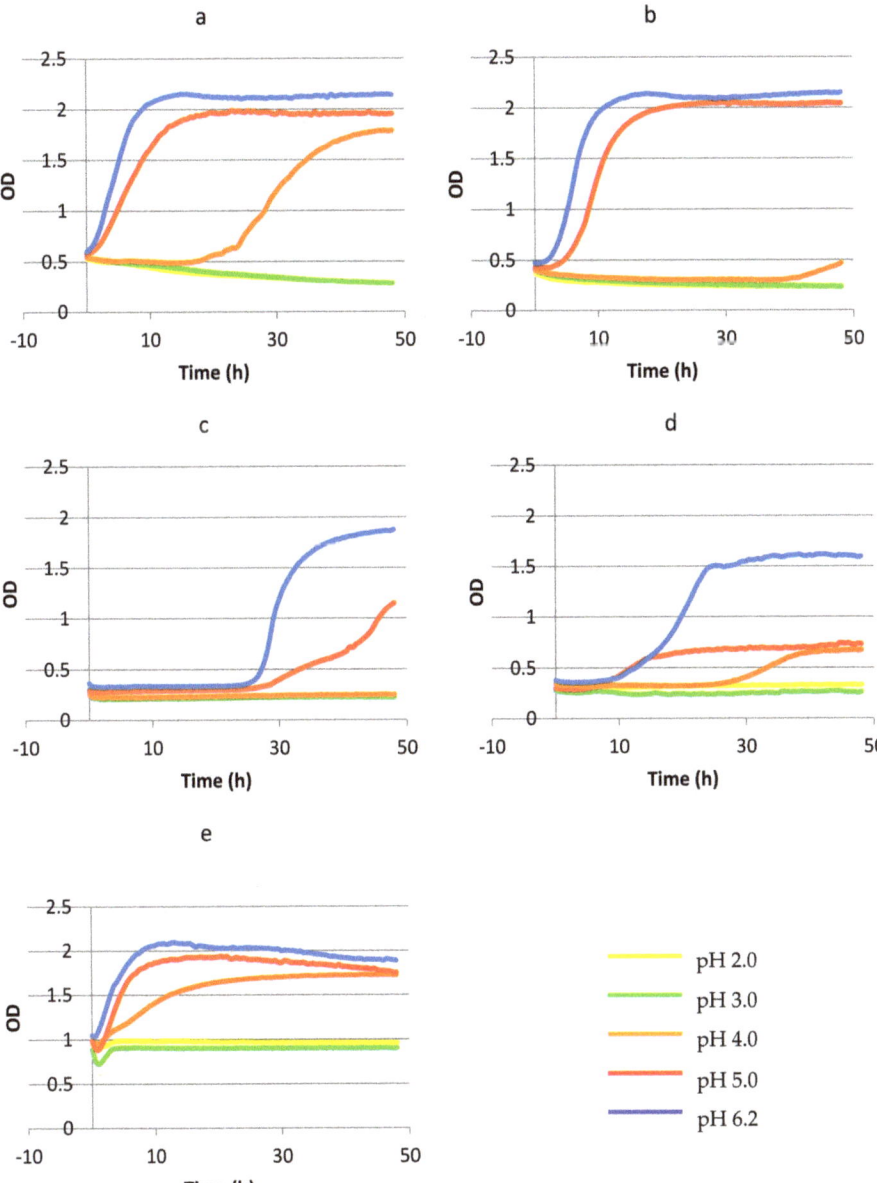

Figure 3. Changes in the optical density (OD$_{600}$) during culture of commercial probiotics preparations: (**a**) *Lb. rhamnosus* GG ATCC 53103; (**b**) *Bifidobacterium* BB-12; (**c**) *Lb. casei*; (**d**) *Lb. acidophilus*; (**e**) *Lb. plantarum* in MRS medium with different pH (2.0; 3.0; 4.0; 5.0; 6.2), ($p < 0.05$). The number of repeats for each treatment $n = 3$. Letters marked with the same color define a homogeneous group within one pH value among the tested variants of the experiment (a given color correlates with the pH value and a given letter correlates with a given homogeneous group within pH range).

Table 1. Growth of commercial probiotic strains (log CFU mL^{-1} ± SD) in MRS medium with different pH.

pH	Time of Incubation (h)				
	0	12	24	36	48
	Lb. rhamnosus GG				
2	7.76 ± 0.31	-	-	-	-
3	7.79 ± 0.11	-	-	-	-
4	7.79 ± 0.08	8.55 ± 0.11	8.83 ± 0.05	8.68 ± 0.13	9.02 ± 0.08
5	7.8 ± 0.15	9.59 ± 0.16	9.73 ± 0.12	9.88 ± 0.05	9.14 ± 0.11
6.2	7.81 ± 0.07	10.56 ± 0.03	10.03 ± 0.14	10.74 ± 0.21	10.01 ± 0.05
	Bifidobacterium BB-12				
2	6.74 ± 0.34	-	-	-	-
3	6.82 ± 0.11	-	-	-	-
4	7.13 ± 0.58	6.13 ± 0.17	5.93 ± 0.08	4.24 ± 0.31	5.46 ± 0.45
5	6.98 ± 0.27	8.61 ± 0.12	9.02 ± 0.20	9.57 ± 0.16	9.38 ± 0.14
6.2	7.23 ± 0.23	9.94 ± 0.11	9.98 ± 0.01	10.16 ± 0.14	10.22 ± 0.14
	Lb. casei				
2	6.12 ± 0.16	-	-	-	-
3	6.33 ± 0.19	5.16 ± 0.07	4.29 ± 0.00	-	-
4	6.14 ± 0.05	5.67 ± 0.00	5.82 ± 0.25	5.55 ± 0.01	5.12 ± 0.09
5	6.52 ± 0.08	6.41 ± 0.08	5.62 ± 0.09	6.85 ± 0.11	8.08 ± 0.09
6.2	6.42 ± 0.11	7.02 ± 0.16	7.16 ± 0.05	8.71 ± 0.05	9.13 ± 0.08
	Lb. acidophilus				
2	6.79 ± 0.13	-	-	-	-
3	6.89 ± 0.08	-	-	-	-
4	6.63 ± 0.11	6.51 ± 0.13	6.40 ± 0.14	6.82 ± 0.14	6.99 ± 0.21
5	6.92 ± 0.22	6.83 ± 0.02	7.94 ± 0.58	8.33 ± 0.05	8.17 ± 0.16
6.2	7.01 ± 0.22	8.64 ± 0.12	10.32 ± 0.15	10.13 ± 0.04	9.97 ± 0.14
	Lb. plantarum				
2	6.13 ± 0.39	-	-	-	-
3	6.29 ± 0.23	5.55 ± 0.08	4.17 ± 0.08	-	-
4	6.37 ± 0.25	7.36 ± 0.08	7.98 ± 0.01	9.17 ± 0.03	9.14 ± 0.24
5	6.22 ± 0.09	8.92 ± 0.08	9.28 ± 0.12	9.91 ± 0.09	9.68 ± 0.11
6.2	6.41 ± 0.03	9.32 ± 0.13	10.16 ± 0.08	10.28 ± 0.13	9.93 ± 0.03

"-"—no growth/less than 4 log CFU mL^{-1}.

The OD of *Lb.* GG culture in MRS broth with pH 2.0 and pH 3.0 was decreasing throughout the experiment (from the initial value of ca. 0.5 to the final value of ca. 0.36) (Figure 3). The results obtained using the plate method (Table 1) indicate that during the first 12 h of the experiment at pH 2.0 or 3.0, the number of *Lb.* GG decreased to less than 4 log CFU ml^{-1}. It was found that the other tested strains reacted in a similar way, except *Lb. casei* and *Lb. plantarum* in MRS with pH 3.0 (Table 1). The highest OD values were noted for this probiotic strain in MRS broth with pH 5.0 and pH 6.2 (Figure 3). The number of *Lb.* GG in the MRS with pH 5.0 after 48 h of the experiment increased by about 1.34 log order, while at the optimal pH (pH 6.2) by 2.2 log order.

The course of the growth curve plotted for the BB-12 strain at pH 4.0 indicated that the bacteria needed a lot of time to adapt to medium conditions before their cells began to divide (Figure 3). By the 36th hour of the experiment, a decrease in the number of strain BB-12 from the initial 7.13 log CFU mL^{-1} to 4.24 log CFU mL^{-1} was observed, while in the last twelve hours there was an increase in the number of bacteria by about one logarithmic order, which is also visible on the course of the OD curve (Figure 3). Only *Lb.* GG, *Lb. acidophilus* and *Lb. plantarum* strains showed an increase in cell number during incubation in MRS at pH 4.0 (Table 1).

Growth curves plotted for the BB-12 strain in MRS media with pH 5.0 and 6.2. had a similar course and indicated intensive cell proliferation (Figure 3). For all tested strains, the number of cells was increased during incubation in MRS at pH 5.0 and pH 6.2 (Table 1). The increase in the viable cell number at pH 5.0 was 1.25–3.46 log orders and at pH 6.0 about 3.0 log orders.

For most of the probiotic strains tested, the course of the growth curves was characteristic and included lag phase, log phase, and stationary phase. Worthy of notice is, however, that growth curves plotted for bacteria cultured under experimental conditions differed for each preparation (Figure 3).

Statistical analysis showed that there was not significant difference between the OD value of *L. rhamnosus* GG growing in MRS pH 2.0, 3.0, as well as in MRS pH 5.0 and 6.2 (Figure 3). It was also shown that in the case of the BB-12 strain growing in MRS, the same homologous group was for growth in pH 2.0, 3.0 and 4.0, and, simultaneously, the OD values for this strain cultivating in MRS pH 5.0 and 6.2 belonged to the same homologous group (Figure 3). An analogous situation was observed for the MRS culture of *Lb. casei* (Figure 3). However, in the case of cultivation with the use of an *Lb. acidophilus* strain, three homologous groups were observed—the first for growth in pH 2.0 and 3.0, second for pH 4.0 and the third for growth in pH 5.0 and 6.2 (Figure 3).

Selected lag phase and log phases, initial and maximal OD values, and coefficients of the specific growth rate of the analyzed probiotic preparations are summarized in Table 2.

Table 2. Selected lag and log phase lengths, initial and final OD$_{600}$ in log phase, and coefficient of specific growth rate for the bacteria present in commercial probiotic preparations tested in MRS medium.

Strain	Variant of Culture in MRS	Length of Lag Phase (h)	Length of Log Phase (h)	Initial OD$_{600}$ in Log Phase	Final OD$_{600}$ in Log Phase	Coefficient of Specific Growth Rate (μ) (h^{-1})
Lb. rhamnosus GG ATCC 53103	pH 4.0	19.0	29.0	0.53	1.78	0.042
	pH 5.0	0.5	19.0	0.59	1.97	0.063
	pH 6.2	0	16.0	0.56	2.15	0.084
Bifidobacterium BB-12	pH 5.0	3.0	16.5	0.44	2.05	0.093
	pH 6.2	2.5	12.0	0.54	2.13	0.114
Lb. casei	pH 5.0	24.5	35.0	0.30	1.55	0.047
	pH 6.2	24.5	20.0	0.35	1.85	0.083
Lb. acidophilus	pH 4.0	25.0	16.5	0.33	0.67	0.043
	pH 5.0	5.5	49.5	0.30	0.78	0.019
	pH 6.2	6.5	28.0	0.37	1.60	0.053
Lb. plantarum	pH 4.0	0	29.0	0.98	1.70	0.019
	pH 5.0	0	17.0	0.99	1.93	0.039
	pH 6.2	1.0	12.0	1.04	2.10	0.058

In the case of the *Lb. rhamnosus* GG ATCC 53103 strain, the highest value of the specific growth rate coefficient ($\mu = 0.084$) was determined in MRS broth with pH 6.2. The μ values computed for the culture of these bacteria in MRS broth with pH 4.0 and 5.0 reached 0.042 and 0.063, respectively. In the case of MRS broth with pH 4.0, bacterial cells needed 19 h to adapt to medium conditions, whereas in MRS broth with higher pH values (5.0 or 6.2), cells of this probiotic began proliferation immediately after culture initiation. The growth curve plotted for *Lb.* GG in the medium with pH 4.0 had the longest phase of logarithmic growth of 29 h, whereas at pH 5.0 and pH 6.2, the length of this phase reached 19 and 16 h, respectively. In MRS broth with pH 4.0 and pH 5.0, the final OD value increased three times, whereas in the medium with pH 6.2 the final OD value of culture increased nearly four times in comparison with initial OD (Table 2).

The value of the μ coefficient for the growth of BB-12 strain cells increased along with increasing active acidity of the culture medium ($\mu = 0.093$ at pH 5.0 and $\mu = 0.114$ at pH 6.2). The growth of the cells of this strain in the medium with pH 4.0 revealed a long, nearly 40 h phase of adaptation of the cells to conditions of the medium (Figure 3). In MRS broth with pH 5.0 and 6.2, the adaptation phase lasted ca. 3 h. The length of the logarithmic growth phase noted for BB-12 in pH 5.0 was 16.5 h and in pH 6.2 was 12 h (Table 2). The highest (4.7-fold) increase in OD value of BB-12 strain culture was observed in MRS broth with pH 5.0 (Table 2).

The *Lb. casei* strain showed no growth in MRS broth with pH 4.0 (Figure 3), whereas in MRS with pH 5.0 and 6.2 the length of lag phase was the same (24.5 h). The value of μ coefficient calculated for the culture incubated at pH 6.2 was higher by 0.036 compared to the culture incubated at pH 5.0 (Table 2).

The culture of the *Lb. acidophilus* strain was characterized by the highest value of the growth rate coefficient in MRS broth with pH 6.2 ($\mu = 0.053$). After cell introduction into the MRS broth with pH 4.0, the lag phase lasted ca. 25 h, whereas in the other media (with pH 5.0 and 6.2) it was definitely shorter and reached ca. 6 h. In MRS broth with pH 5.0, the final OD value increased 2.6-fold compared to the initial value (for comparison, in MRS broth with pH 6.2, the log phase lasted 28 h and OD increased over 4-fold) (Table 2).

No growth of the *Lb. plantarum* strain was observed in MRS broth with pH 2.0 and 3.0 (Table 1, Figure 3). The value of the μ coefficient determined for the *Lb. plantarum* strain cultured in MRS broth with pH 4.0, 5.0 and 6.2 reached 0.019, 0.039 and 0.058, respectively (Table 2). Cells of this strain started division immediately after culture onset, regardless of medium pH. The log phase lasted 29 h for the culture incubated at pH 4.0, as well as 17 and 12 h for cultures incubated at pH 5.0 and 6.2, respectively.

3.2. Survivability and Growth of Bacteria Present in Commercial Probiotic Preparations in a Food Matrix Simulating Gastric Passage

Food retention in the stomach usually lasts ca. 1–3 h [32] and liquid foods are retained. Once food has been ingested and its digestion has begun, pH value successively decreases [33,34].

Curves depicting changes in OD values during the incubation of the cultures of tested preparations in the medium simulating conditions likely to occur in the stomach of a small child after consumption of a chicken–vegetable soup (CVS), and after taking a probiotic preparation in a suspension of spring water, are shown on Figure 4. Changes in the cell number of the tested strains during incubation in the gastric medium are presented in Table 3.

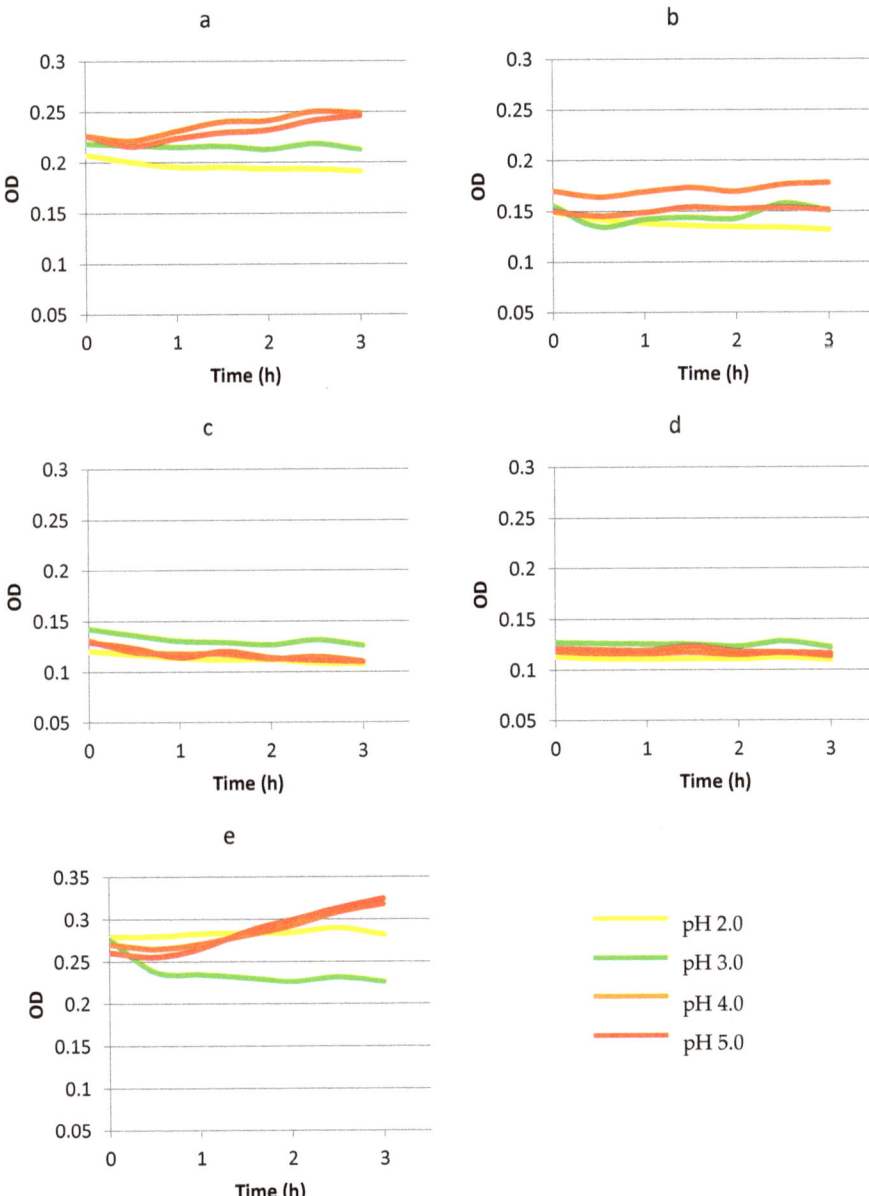

Figure 4. Changes in the optical density during culture of commercial probiotic strains in the food matrix under simulated condition of the gastric passage (**a**) *Lb. rhamnosus* GG ATCC 53103; (**b**) *Bifidobacterium* BB-12; (**c**) *Lb. casei*; (**d**) *Lb. acidophilus*; (**e**) *Lb. plantarum*, ($p < 0.05$). The number of repeats for each treatment $n = 3$. Letters marked with the same color define a homogeneous group within one pH value among the tested variants of the experiment (a given color correlates with the pH value and a given letter correlates with a given homogeneous group within pH range).

Table 3. Growth of commercial probiotic strains (log CFU mL^{-1} ± SD) in the food matrix under simulated condition of the gastric passage.

pH	Time of Incubation (h)			
	0	1	2	3
Lb. rhamnosus GG				
2.0	6.92 ± 0.17	5.19 ± 0.01	-	-
3.0	7.07 ± 0.04	5.72 ± 0.08	5.55 ± 0.17	5.63 ± 0.45
4.0	7.21 ± 0.00	6.64 ± 0.05	6.78 ± 0.13	6.33 ± 0.04
5.0	7.13 ± 0.34	6.96 ± 0.17	6.82 ± 0.09	6.80 ± 0.02
Bifidobacterium BB-12				
2.0	5.73 ± 0.28	4.62 ± 0.34	4.58 ± 0.05	4.70 ± 0.11
3.0	6.96 ± 0.00	7.13 ± 0.16	6.88 ± 0.00	6.86 ± 0.00
4.0	7.02 ± 0.13	6.32 ± 0.12	6.54 ± 0.15	6.38 ± 0.31
5.0	7.22 ± 0.13	7.16 ± 0.16	7.31 ± 0.03	7.18 ± 0.21
Lb. casei				
2.0	5.80 ± 0.08	-	-	-
3.0	6.29 ± 0.11	-	-	-
4.0	6.19 ± 0.54	5.37 ± 0.17	5.23 ± 0.14	4.22 ± 0.14
5.0	6.21 ± 0.35	5.98 ± 0.32	5.61 ± 0.17	4.92 ± 0.12
Lb. acidophilus				
2.0	6.24 ± 0.12	5.70 ± 0.05	5.30 ± 0.00	-
3.0	6.78 ± 0.12	5.99 ± 0.07	5.13 ± 0.05	-
4.0	6.88 ± 0.09	6.23 ± 0.13	6.19 ± 0.11	6.33 ± 0.03
5.0	7.02 ± 0.16	6.90 ± 0.12	6.96 ± 0.15	6.87 ± 0.02
Lb. plantarum				
2.0	6.68 ± 0.06	5.19 ± 0.08	5.22 ± 0.02	4.97 ± 0.17
3.0	7.18 ± 0.05	6.30 ± 0.16	6.41 ± 0.01	6.43 ± 0.25
4.0	7.20 ± 0.00	7.40 ± 0.12	7.32 ± 0.05	7.38 ± 0.16
5.0	7.31 ± 0.13	7.44 ± 0.01	7.27 ± 0.03	7.45 ± 0.00

"-"—no growth/less than 4 log.

Gastric fluids differed in pH values, which were higher at the beginning and lower at the end of digestion. Optical density of the culture of the *Lb.* GG strain decreased insignificantly at pH 2.0 and 3.0. Already active acidity of 4.0 and 5.0 enabled the growth of these bacteria; however, in both variants of culture the OD value increased by 0.02 on average (Figure 4). A reduction in the number of *Lb.* GG cells was observed during incubation regardless of the pH of the medium. In gastric medium with pH 2.0, after just 2 h of incubation, the *Lb.* GG number decreased to less than 4 log CFU mL^{-1}. BB-12, *Lb. casei* and *Lb. acidophilus* strains showed no growth during incubation, regardless of active acidity values, which was indicated by the course of curves depicting OD value changes in time of incubation (Figure 4). Among the commercial probiotic strains selected for this study, only *Lb. plantarum* showed significant growth in the GES and CSV medium at pH 4.0 and 5.0. In both cases, a 1.2-fold of increased OD (from the beginning till 3 h) was noticed. When analyzing changes in the number of cells of probiotic strains based on the results of the plate method (Table 3), it can be concluded that the *Lb. plantarum* strain was characterized by the highest resistance to low pH. In the gastric medium with pH 4.0 and pH 5.0, a slight increase in the cell number of this strain was noted (by 0.18 and 0.14 log order). In gastric medium with pH 2.0 at the last 3rd hour of the experiment, the number of *Lb. plantarum* was 4.97 log CFU mL^{-1}. Similar resistance was demonstrated only for strain BB-12.

3.3. Survivability of Commercial Probiotic Strains in a Food Matrix Simulating Gastrointestinal Passage

The passage of intestinal digesta through the section of the small intestine usually spans for 1–6 h [32]. No changes were observed in the optical density in any of the media simulating conditions occurring during digestion in the small intestine with BB-12, *Lb. rhamnosus*, *Lb. casei* and *Lb. acidophilus* strains (data not shown). The *Lb. plantarum* strain was the only one capable of proliferation under small intestine conditions, regardless of bile salts concentration (1%, 2% or 3%) (Figure 5). The log phases for *Lb. plantarum* took from 1.5 to 2 h for all tested concentrations of bile salts.

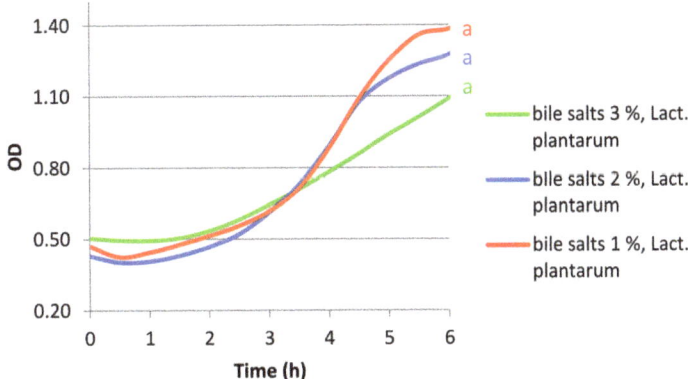

Figure 5. Changes in the optical density during culture of *Lb. plantarum* from commercial probiotic strains in the food matrix under simulated condition of the gastric and gastrointestinal passage; in this case it was only one homologous group signed *a* ($p < 0.05$). Each homogeneous group's corresponding pH was marked the same color as pH line axce.

The analysis of the initial and final OD values of the culture of the probiotic strain *Lb. plantarum* increased about 2-fold for concentration 1% and about 3-fold for the rest of the concentrations. The adaptation phase of the *Lb. plantarum* strain reached only 1.5 h regardless of bile concentrations.

Changes in the cell number of the tested strains during incubation in the food matrix under simulated condition of the gastrointestinal passage are presented in Table 4.

An increase in the number of cells was observed during incubation in the gastrointestinal medium irrespective of the amount of bile salt addition only in the case of *Lb. plantarum* strain. The number of *Lb. plantarum* in the gastrointestinal medium with 1% of bile after 6 h of the experiment increased by about 0.83 log order, while at 3% of bile by 0.29 order of magnitude in 1 mL. Some resistance to bile salts was found in the BB-12 strain. The final cell numbers of this strain after 6 h of incubation in gastrointestinal medium containing 1% and 2% of bile salts reached 6 log CFU mL^{-1}. Only in the medium with the highest tested content of bile salts (3%) was a slight reduction in the number of cells from the initial 6.17 to 5.86 log CFU mL^{-1} determined. The most sensitive to the presence of bile salts at the level of 3% were *Lb. casei* and *Lb.* GG strains (<4 log CFU mL^{-1} from the 2nd and 4th hour of incubation, respectively).

Table 4. Survival of commercial probiotic strains (log CFU mL^{-1} ± SD) in the food matrix under simulated condition of the gastrointestinal passage.

Bile Salts (%)	Time of Incubation (h)			
	0	2	4	6
Lb. rhamnosus GG				
1	6.13 ± 0.12	6.08 ± 0.26	5.86 ± 0.03	5.80 ± 0.37
2	6.21 ± 0.22	5.12 ± 0.00	4.87 ± 0.18	4.42 ± 0.17
3	6.06 ± 0.01	5.02 ± 0.12	-	-
Bifidobacterium BB-12				
1	6.32 ± 0.15	6.40 ± 0.03	6.18 ± 0.28	6.16 ± 0.22
2	6.38 ± 0.15	6.16 ± 0.2	5.97 ± 0.15	6.08 ± 0.12
3	6.17 ± 0.05	5.93 ± 0.09	5.90 ± 0.23	5.86 ± 0.06
Lb. casei				
1	5.30 ± 0.03	5.21 ± 0.14	4.44 ± 0.01	-
2	5.26 ± 0.12	5.07 ± 0.23	4.04 ± 0.00	-
3	5.01 ± 0.09	-	-	-
Lb. acidophilus				
1	6.65 ± 0.05	5.37 ± 0.00	5.16 ± 0.17	-
2	6.48 ± 0.03	5.02 ± 0.12	4.86 ± 0.03	4.71 ± 0.18
3	6.52 ± 0.22	5.12 ± 0.05	4.70 ± 0.05	-
Lb. plantarum				
1	5.63 ± 0.12	5.79 ± 0.28	5.84 ± 0.00	6.47 ± 0.02
2	5.72 ± 0.12	5.20 ± 0.02	5.63 ± 0.01	5.99 ± 0.33
3	5.48 ± 0.10	5.53 ± 0.01	5.70 ± 0.13	5.77 ± 0.00

"-"—no growth/less than 4 log.

4. Discussion

High variability of strains and unlimited possibilities of creating experimental conditions in scientific research significantly impair the comparison and discussion of results achieved in various studies [35]. There are several criteria, which need to be met to classify a strain as a "probiotic". The key ones among functional criteria include tolerance to gastric juice and bile, and capability of adhesion to colonic mucosa [36,37]. Probiotic bacterial strains have to survive unfavorable conditions encountered during their gastrointestinal passage to be able to colonize the colon and to exert a positive effect on consumer/host health [32]. However, as indicated in scientific research, not all strains classified as "probiotic" meet these criteria [38,39]. Both manufacturers of probiotic preparations and pediatricians exclude the administration of a probiotic preparation in the form of a gelatin capsule to young children. Giving toddlers a capsule is not advisable because they can easily choke by swallowing it. It is strictly recommended to remove the capsule and suspend probiotic with water and administrate it in this form. For this reason described, experiments showed results of survivability of strains lacking early protection against bile salts and low pH [40–43].

Lb. rhamnosus GG is a well-characterized probiotic strain [44]. It is a commensal, which colonizes the gastrointestinal tract in humans [45]. In 1985, *Lb.* GG was patented as a probiotic partly due to its resistance to low pH and to bile salts [46]. The exact mechanism of these bacteria effecting the organism of the host remains unknown; however, bacteria of the *Lb. rhamnosus* species are implied to exhibit antimicrobial, antiviral, and diarrhea-preventing properties [47,48]. Pitino et al. [34] demonstrated that *Lb. rhamnosus* strains isolated from cheese showed high survivability in MRS broth with pH 5.0 during simulated dynamic digestion in the stomach. In our study, the *Lb.* GG strain also showed growth in MRS broth with pH 5.0 (Figure 3, Table 1). In a clinical survey conducted by Hibberd et al. [48], in 73% of volunteers to whom *Lb. rhamnosus* was administered orally in a dose of 10^{10} CFU for 28 days, reduced numbers of these bacteria were detected in feces, i.e., from 1.4×10^3 to 1.3×10^8 CFU [48]. Other *Lb. rhamnosus* strains isolated from wine showed growth after 24 h incubation at pH 3.5, likewise *Lb. rhamnosus* isolated from meat [49]. Goldin et al. [44] proved that *Lb. rhamnosus* GG survived incubation in the medium with pH 3.0. Results of other studies indicate high resistance of this strain to a bile salt concentration of 1.5% [49]. In our study, the *Lb. rhamnosus* GG strain showed no growth at bile salt concentrations of 1, 2 or 3% (Table 4).

Bacteria of the genus *Bifidobacterium* possess the GRAS (Generally Recognised As Safe) status and constitute part of the natural microflora of the gastrointestinal tract of humans (likewise other probiotic bacteria, e.g., those from the genus *Lactobacillus*); therefore, they are often used as components of commercial dietary supplements [3] In our experiment, the BB-12 strain showed no growth either in MRS broth with pH 2.0 or with pH 3.0 (Figure 3b, Table 1). In MRS broth with pH 4.0, we observed the growth of BB-12 bacteria already after 36 h (Table 1). Analyses conducted in our study showed no growth of BB-12 strain under simulated gastrointestinal conditions. De Castro-Cislaghi et al. [30] observed a reduction in the cell count of the BB-12 strain in the presence of bile salts in the concentration of 1%, from the initial value of ca. 9.5 log CFU/g to ca. 9 log CFU/g after 3 h incubation. In addition, they demonstrated that resistance to various pH values and concentrations of bile salts is a variable, strain-specific feature.

Probiotic lactic bacteria of the species *Lb. casei* have been widely applied in the production of fermented foods [50]. The administration of lyophilized preparations of these bacteria is believed to reduce the blood level of cholesterol and to impair proliferation of cancer cells [51–53]. Apart from the *Lb. casei* strain, commercial preparation 3 tested in our study contained inulin, which was supposed to support its viability. Growth tests conducted in the model MRS culture medium demonstrated that the phase of cell adaptation to conditions of the culture medium was one of the longest in the case of this strain (ca. 25 h, Figure 3, Table 2). This was the only strain which showed no growth in MRS broth with pH 4.0 (Table 1). Cells of *Lb. casei* began to divide already at pH 5.0, although their adaptation phase was again one of the longest compared to the other strains (Figure 3, Table 2).

In our study, the *Lb. casei* strain showed no growth in conditions simulating the gastric and/or gastrointestinal passage (Tables 3 and 4). Dimitrellou et al. [32] demonstrated successive viability loss for the *Lb. casei* strain incubated in gastric media. After 3 h of incubation, they observed a decrease in the cell count of this strain by ca. 4.0 log CFU g^{-1} at the initial pH 2.0 and by 1.5 log CFU g^{-1} at pH 3.0. In addition, they showed the presence of bile salts in the concentration of 1 gL^{-1} to evoke *Lb. casei* cell count reduction by nearly 6 log CFU g^{-1} after 6 h of incubation. In turn, Mishra and Prasad [29] proved that all seven analyzed strains of *Lb. casei* survived incubation at pH 3.0, and two of them were viable once pH was decreased to the value of 2.0. All seven analyzed strains were viable after 12 h incubation in solutions with bile salt concentrations of 1 and 2%.

Bacteria of the *Lb. acidophilus* species naturally occur in the gastric tract of humans and animals [54]. In our study, the *Lb. acidophilus* NCFM strain (preparation 4) showed no growth under experimental gastro-intestinal conditions (Table 4).

Representatives of the *Lb. plantarum* species are also implied to exhibit probiotic traits. The *Lb. plantarum* NRRL-B4496 strain is one of the main probiotics used in fermented food products [55,56]. Multiple scientific works indicate this strain to be capable of inhibiting the growth of certain pathogens that induce diseases of the alimentary tract, e.g., *Helicobacter pylori* or *Listeria monocytogenes* [56–60].

Commercial probiotic preparations are often supplemented with prebiotics, the task of which is to increase the chances of probiotic strains for the survival of adverse conditions during gastrointestinal passage and to sustain their metabolic activity [3,61,62]. The most frequently used prebiotics include inulin [63,64], β-glucan, and fructooligosaccharides (FOS) [62,65,66].

Obtained results clearly show that, among all analyzed commercial probiotic strains, only the Lb. plantarum was the most resistant to the applied conditions of the culture medium. It showed a noticeable growth under both in vitro gastric conditions at pH 4.0 and 5.0, as well as in vitro intestinal conditions at all tested concentrations of bile salts. Interestingly, its preparations did not contain a prebiotic.

No OD changes of the tested commercial probiotics under the assumed experimental conditions does not have to indicate their incapability for surviving the in vivo gastrointestinal passage. However, obtained results from the plate count method show that the Lb. plantarum strain had the best capability for growth, which suggests it could proliferate in intestines also under in vivo conditions. Considering the fact that the tested probiotics were deprived of a gelatin capsule at the beginning of the experiment, it can be concluded that Lb. plantarum exhibited distinctive properties that allowed this strain to survive the simulated conditions of the passage. This is valuable knowledge, considering that exogenous probiotics share a limited capability for adhesion to cells of the intestinal epithelium and that their major part is excreted with feces.

The scheme of experiments, shown in this study, largely covers the simplified conditions during the gastrointestinal transit in the human body and does not include many factors. For some of the probiotic strains present in the tested preparations, there are literature data from several years ago showing their beneficial effect on the course and shortening of the duration of diarrhea of various origins [67]. The medical practice of using probiotic food supplements to children consists of administering them, for example, after or still during antibiotic therapy for the treatment of diarrheal disorders [67]. Recent data concerning the effect of probiotics on inflammation of gastroenteritis, which is often manifested by diarrhea, are different from those previously described. Freedman et al. [68] showed that administration of a probiotic product containing *Lactobacillus rhamnosus* R0011 and *L. helveticus* R0052, at a dose of 4.0×10^9 CFU/unit twice daily, did not reduce the incidence of diarrhea in children with gastroenteritis. Similarly, among preschool children with acute gastroenteritis, those who had taken *L. rhamnosus* GG did not show better outcomes than those children who had received placebo [69].

5. Conclusions

Results of our study show that among all analyzed probiotic bacteria from commercial preparations avaliable on Polish market, the Lb. plantarum was the most resistant to the applied conditions of the experiment. It showed a noticeable growth under both in vitro gastric conditions at pH 4.0 and 5.0, as well as in vitro intestinal conditions at all tested concentrations of bile salts. Interestingly, its preparations did not contain a prebiotic. In turn, preparation 2 (Bifidobacterium BB-12) contained FOS, which could affect its capability to grow under simulated conditions of the gastric passage (pH 4.0 and 5.0) and of the gastrointestinal passage at bile salts concentration of 10 gL^{-1}. The remaining preparations (preparation 3 – Lb. casei and preparation 4 – Lb. acidophilus) contained inulin which, however, didn't influence their cell proliferation capability during incubation under experimental conditions.

No growth of the tested commercial probiotics under the assumed experimental conditions does not have to indicate their incapability for surviving the in vivo gastrointestinal passage. However, study results show clearly that the Lb. plantarum strain had the best capability for growth, which suggests it could proliferate in intestines also under in vivo conditions. It is a valuable piece of information, considering that exogenous probiotics share a limited capability for adhesion to cells of the intestinal epithelium and that their major part is excreted with feces.

Author Contributions: Conceptualization, L.S.-R. and A.B.-P.; funding acquisition, L.S.-R., A.B.-P., A.S.P. and M.G.; investigation, L.S.-R.; Methodology, L.S.-R. and A.B.-P.; statistical analysis, M.G.; result interpretations, L.S.-R., A.B.-P., A.S.P., K.D. and M.G.; Writing—Original draft, L.S.-R.; Writing—Review and editing, L.S.-R., A.B.-P., A.S.P., K.D. and M.G. All authors have read and agreed to the published version of the manuscript.

Funding: This work had no financial support from any sponsors. This research did not receive any specific grant from funding agencies in the public, commercial or not-for-profit sectors. Funds received to cover publication costs come from scientific institutions in which the authors work.

Institutional Review Board Statement: Not applicable.

Informed Consent Statement: Not applicable.

Data Availability Statement: The data presented in this study are available on request from the corresponding author.

Conflicts of Interest: The authors declare no conflict of interest.

References

1. Hill, C.; Guarner, F.; Reid, G.; Gibson, G.R.; Merenstein, D.J.; Pot, B.; Morelli, L.; Canani, R.B.; Flint, H.J.; Salminen, S.; et al. Expert Consensus Document. The International Scientific Association for Probiotics and Prebiotics consensus statement on the scope and appropriate use of the term probiotic. *Nat. Rev. Gastroenterol. Hepatol.* **2014**, *11*, 506–514. [CrossRef]
2. Kligler, B.; Cohrssen, A. Probiotics. *Am. Fam. Physician* **2008**, *78*, 1073–1078.
3. Gomes, D.O.V.S.; Morais, M.B. Gut microbiota and the use of probiotics in constipation in children and adolescents: Systematic review. *Rev. Paul. Pediatr.* **2020**, *38*. [CrossRef]
4. Vandenplas, Y. Probiotics and prebiotics in infectious gastroenteritis. *Best. Pract. Res. Clin. Gastroenterol.* **2016**, *30*, 49–53. [CrossRef]
5. Khare, A.; Gaur, S. Cholesterol-Lowering Effects of Lactobacillus Species. *Curr. Microbiol.* **2020**, 1–7. [CrossRef]
6. Wieërs, G.; Belkhir, L.; Enaud, R.; Leclercq, S.; Philippart de Foy, J.M.; Dequenne, I.; Timay, P.; Cani, P.D. How Probiotics Affect the Microbiota. *Front. Cell. Infect. Microbiol.* **2020**, *9*, 454. [CrossRef]
7. Pratap, K.; Taki, A.C.; Johnston, E.B.; Lopata, A.L.; Kamath, S.D. A Comprehensive Review on Natural Bioactive Compounds and Probiotics as Potential Therapeutics in Food Allergy Treatment. *Front. Immunol.* **2020**, *11*, 996. [CrossRef] [PubMed]
8. Robertson, C.; Savva, G.M.; Clapuci, R.; Jones, J.; Maimouni, H.; Brown, E.; Minocha, A.; Hall, L.J.; Clarke, P. Incidence of necrotising enterocolitis before and after introducing routine prophylactic Lactobacillus and Bifidobacterium probiotics. *Arch. Dis. Child. Fetal Neonatal Ed.* **2020**, *105*, 380–386. [CrossRef] [PubMed]
9. Reid, G. Safe and efficacious probiotics: What are they? *Trends Microbiol.* **2006**, *14*, 348–352. [CrossRef] [PubMed]
10. Soccol, C.R.; Vandenberghe, L.P.S.; Spier, M.R.; Medeiros, A.B.P.; Yamaguishi, C.T.; Lindner, J.D.D.; Pandey, A.; Thomaz-Soccol, V. The Potential of Probiotics. *Food Technol. Biotechnol.* **2010**, *48*, 413–434.
11. Rui, X.; Ma, S.X.A. Retrospective study of probiotics for the treatment of children with antibiotic-associated diarrhea. *Medicine* **2020**, *99*, e20631. [CrossRef] [PubMed]
12. Kotowska, M.; Albrecht, P.; Szajewska, H. Saccharomyces boulardii in the prevention of antibiotic-associated diarrhoea in children: A randomized double-blind placebo-controlled trial. *Aliment. Pharmacol. Therapeut.* **2005**, *21*, 583–590. [CrossRef] [PubMed]
13. Fox, M.J.; Ahuja, K.D.K.; Robertson, I.K.; Ball, M.J.; Eri, R.D. Can probiotic yogurt prevent diarrhea in children on antibiotics? A doubleblind, randomised, placebo-controlled study. *BMJ Open* **2015**, *5*, e006474. [CrossRef] [PubMed]
14. Rouhani, S.; Griffin, N.W.; Yori, P.P.; Gehrig, J.L.; Olortegui, M.P.; Salas, M.S.; Trigoso, D.R.; Moulton, L.H.; Houpt, E.R.; Baratt, M.J.; et al. Diarrhea as a potential cause and consequence of reduced gut microbial diversity among undernourished children in Peru. *Clin. Infect. Dis.* **2020**, *71*, 989–999. [CrossRef] [PubMed]
15. Singhi, S.C.; Kumar, S. Probiotics in critically ill children. *F1000Research* **2016**, *5*. [CrossRef]
16. Venema, K.; Verhoeven, J.; Beckman, C.; Keller, D. Survival of a probiotic-containing product using capsule-within-capsule technology in an in vitro model of the stomach and small intestine (TIM-1). *Benef. Microbes* **2020**, 1–8. [CrossRef]
17. Temmerman, R.; Pot, B.; Huys, G.; Swings, J. Identification and antibiotic susceptibility of bacterial isolates from probiotic products. *Int. J. Food Microbiol.* **2003**, *81*, 1–10. [CrossRef]
18. Afzaal, M.; Saeed, F.; Saeed, M.; Ahmed, A.; Ateeq, H.; Nadeem, M.T.; Tufail, T. Survival and stability of free and encapsulated probiotic bacteria under simulated gastrointestinal conditions and in pasteurized grape juice. *J. Food Proc. Preserv.* **2020**, *44*, e14346. [CrossRef]
19. Klindt-Toldam, S.; Larsen, S.K.; Saaby, L.; Olsen, L.R.; Svenstrup, G.; Müllertz, A.; Knøchel, S.; Heimdal, H.; Nielsen, D.S.; Zielińska, D. Survival of Lactobacillus acidophilus NCFM® and Bifidobacterium lactis HN019 encapsulated in chocolate during in vitro simulated passage of the upper gastrointestinal tract. *LWT Food Sci. Technol.* **2016**, *74*, 404–410. [CrossRef]

20. Sultana, K.; Godward, G.; Reynolds, N.; Arumugaswamy, R.; Peiris, P.; Kailasapathy, K. Encapsulation of probiotic bacteria with alginate-starch and evaluation of survival in simulated gastrointestinal conditions and in yoghurt. *Int. J. Food Microbiol.* **2000**, *62*, 47–55. [CrossRef]
21. Huq, T.; Khan, A.; Khan, R.A.; Riedl, B.; Lacroix, M. Encapsulation of probiotic bacteria in biopolymeric system. *Critic. Rev. Food Sci. Nutr.* **2013**, *53*, 909–916. [CrossRef] [PubMed]
22. Gibson, G.R.; Scott, K.P.; Rastall, R.A.; Tuohy, K.M.; Hotchkiss, A.; Dubert-Ferrandon, A.; Gareau, M.; Murphy, E.F.; Saulnier, D.; Loh, G.; et al. Dietary prebiotics: Current status and new definition. *Food Sci. Technol. Bull. Func. Foods* **2010**, *7*, 1–19. [CrossRef]
23. Cardarelli, H.R.; Saad, S.M.I.; Gibson, G.R.; Vulevic, J. Functional petit-suisse cheese: Measure of the prebiotic effect. *Anaerobe* **2007**, *13*, 200–207. [CrossRef] [PubMed]
24. Clavel, T.; Carlin, F.; Lairon, D.; Nguyen-Then, C.; Schmitt, P. Survival of Bacillus cereus spores and vegetative cells in acid media simulating human stomach. *J Appl. Microbiol.* **2004**, *97*, 214–219. [CrossRef]
25. Berthold-Pluta, A.; Pluta, A.; Garbowska, M. The effect of selected factors on the survival of Bacillus cereus in the human gastrointestinal tract. *Microb. Pathog.* **2015**, *82*, 7–14. [CrossRef]
26. Vinderola, C.G.; Reinheimer, J.A. Enumeration of Lactobacillus casei in the presence of L. acidophilus, bifidobacteria and lactic starter bacteria in fermented dairy products. *Int. Dairy J.* **2000**, 271–275. [CrossRef]
27. Vamanu, E.; Pelinescu, D.; Marin, I.; Vamanu, A. Study of probiotic strains viability from PROBAC product in a single chamber gastrointestinal tract simulator. *Food Sci. Biotechnol.* **2012**, *21*, 979–985. [CrossRef]
28. Stasiak-Różańska, L.; Błażejak, S.; Gientka, I. Effect of glycerol and dihydroxyacetone concentration in the culture medium on the growth of acetic acid bacteria Gluconobacter oxydans ATCC 621. *Eur. Res. Technol.* **2014**, *239*, 453–461. [CrossRef]
29. Mishra, V.; Prasad, D.N. Application of in vitro methods for selection of Lactobacillus casei strains as potential probiotics. *Int. J. Food Microbiol.* **2005**, *103*, 109–115. [CrossRef]
30. De Castro-Cislaghi, F.P.; Silva, C.D.R.E.; Fritzen-Freire, C.B.; Lorentz, J.G.; St.Anna, E.S. Bifidobacterium Bb-12 microencapsulated by spray drying with whey: Survival under simulated gastrointestinal conditions, tolerance to NaCl, and viability during storage. *J. Food Eng.* **2012**, *113*, 186–193. [CrossRef]
31. Cabuk, B.; Harsa, S.T. Protection of Lactobacillus acidophilus NRRL-B 4495 under in vitro gastrointestinal conditions with whey protein/pullulan microcapsules. *J. Biosc. Bioeng.* **2015**, *120*, 650–656. [CrossRef] [PubMed]
32. Dimitrellou, D.; Kandylis, P.; Petrovic, T.; Dimitrijevic-Brankovic, S.I.; Levic, S.; Nedovic, V.; Kourkoutas, Y. Survival of spray dried microencapsulated Lactobacillus casei ATCC 393 in simulated gastrointestinal conditions and fermented milk. *LWT Food Sci. Technol.* **2016**, *71*, 169–174. [CrossRef]
33. Dressman, J.B.; Berardi, R.R.; Dermentzoglou, L.C.; Russell, T.L.; Schmaltz, S.P.; Barnett, J.L.; Jarvenpaa, K.M. Upper gastrointestinal (GI) pH in young, healthy men and women. *Pharm. Res.* **1990**, *7*, 756–761. [CrossRef] [PubMed]
34. Pitino, I.; Cinzia, L.R.; Giuseppina, M.; LoCurto, A.; Faulks, R.M.; LeMarc, Y.; Bisignano, C.; Caggia, C.; Wickham, M.S.J. Survival of Lactobacillus rhamnosus strains in the upper gastrointestinal tract. *Food Microbiol.* **2010**, *27*, 1121–1127. [CrossRef]
35. Villarreal, M.L.M.; Padilha, M.; Vieira, A.D.S.; Franco, B.D.G.M.; Martinez, R.C.R.; Saad, S.M.I. Advantageous direct quantification of viable closely related probiotics in petitsuisse cheeses under in vitro gastrointestinal conditions by propidium monoazide-qPCR. *PLoS ONE* **2013**, *8*, e82102. [CrossRef]
36. Shah, N.P. Health benefits of yogurt and fermented milks. In *Manufacturing Yogurt and Fermented Milks*, 1st ed.; Chandan, R.C., Ed.; Blackwell Publishing Professional: Minneapolis, MN, USA, 2006; pp. 327–340. ISBN 9780813823041.
37. Morelli, L. In vitro assessment of probiotic bacteria: From survival to functionality. *Int. Dairy J.* **2007**, *17*, 1278–1283. [CrossRef]
38. Rajam, R.; Karthik, P.; Parthasarathy, S.; Joseph, G.S.; Anandharamakrishnan, C. Effect of whey protein-alginate wall systems on survival of microencapsulated Lactobacillus plantarum in simulated gastrointestinal conditions. *J. Funct. Foods* **2012**, *4*, 891–898. [CrossRef]
39. Li, S.; Jiang, C.; Chen, X.; Wang, H.; Lin, J. Lactobacillus casei immobilized onto montmorillonite: Survivability in simulated gastrointestinal conditions, refrigeration and yogurt. *Food Res. Int.* **2014**, *64*, 822–830. [CrossRef]
40. Henker, J.; Laass, M.; Blokhin, B.M.; Bolbot, Y.K.; Maydannik, V.G.; Elze, M.; Wolff, C.; Schulze, J. The probiotic Escherichia coli strain Nissle 1917 (EcN) stops acute diarrhoea in infants and toddlers. *Eur. J. Pediatr.* **2007**, *166*, 311–318. [CrossRef]
41. Kent, R.M.; Doherty, S.B. Probiotic bacteria in infant formula and follow-up formula: Microencapsulation using milk and pea proteins to improve microbiological quality. *Food Res. Int.* **2004**, *64*, 567–576. [CrossRef]
42. Costa-Riberio, H.; Ribeiro, T.C.M.; Mattos, A.P.; Valois, S.S.; Neri, D.A.; Almeida, P.; Cerqueira, C.M.; Ramos, E.; Young, R.J.; Vanderhoof, J.A. Limitations of Probiotic Therapy in Acute, Severe Dehydrating Diarrhea. *J. Pediatr. Gastroentero. Nutr.* **2003**, *36*, 112–115. [CrossRef] [PubMed]
43. McFarland, L.V.; Elmer, G.W.; McFarland, M. Meta-analysis of probiotics for the prevention and treatment of acute pediatric diarrhea. *Int. J. Prob. Preb.* **2006**, *1*, 63–76.
44. Goldin, B.R.; Gorbach, S.L.; Saxelin, M.; Barakat, S.; Gualtieri, L.; Salminen, S. Survival of Lactobacillus species (strain GG) in human gastrointestinal tract. *Digest. Dis. Sci.* **1992**, *37*, 121–128. [CrossRef] [PubMed]
45. Korpela, R.; Moilanen, E.; Saxelin, M.; Vapaatalo, H. Lactobacillus rhamnosus GG (ATCC 53103) and platelet aggregation in vitro. *Int. J. Food Microbiol.* **1997**, *37*, 83–86. [CrossRef]
46. Gorbach, S.L.; Goldin, B.R. Lactobacillus Strains and Methods of Selection. US Patent 4839281 A, 1985.

47. Floch, M.H.; Walker, W.A.; Madsen, K.; Sanders, M.E.; Macfarlane, G.T.; Flint, H.J.; Dieleman, L.A.; Ringel, Y.; Guandalini, S.; Kelly, C.P.; et al. Recommendations for probiotic use-2011 update. *J. Clin. Gastroenterol.* **2011**, *45*, S168–S171. [CrossRef]
48. Hibberd, P.L.; Kleimola, L.; Fiorino, A.M.; Botelho, C.; Haverkamp, M.; Andreyewa, I.; Poutsiaka, D.; Fraser, C.; Solano-Aquilar, G.; Snydman, D.R. No evidence of harms of probiotic Lactobacillus rhamnosus GG ATCC 53103 in healthy elderly—A phase I open label study to assess safety, tolerability and cytokine responses. *PLoS ONE* **2012**, *9*, e113456. [CrossRef]
49. Reale, A.; Di Renzo, T.; Rossi, F.; Zotta, T.; Iacumin, L.; Preziuso, M.; Parente, E.; Sorrentino, E.; Coppola, R. Tolerance of Lactobacillus casei, Lactobacillus paracasei and Lactobacillus rhamnosus strains to stress factors encountered in food processing and in the gastro-intestinal tract. *LWT Food Sci. Technol.* **2015**, *60*, 721–728. [CrossRef]
50. Kourkoutas, Y.; Bosnea, L.; Taboukos, S.; Baras, C.; Lambrou, D.; Kanellaki, M. Probiotic cheese production using Lactobacillus casei cells immobilized on fruit pieces. *J. Dairy Sci.* **2006**, *89*, 1439–1451. [CrossRef]
51. Choi, S.S.; Kim, Y.; Han, K.S.; You, S.; Oh, S.; Kim, S.H. Effects of Lactobacillus strains on cancer cell proliferation and oxidative stress in vitro. *Lett. Appl. Microbiol.* **2006**, *42*, 452–458. [CrossRef]
52. Lye, H.S.; Rusul, G.; Liong, M.T. Removal of cholesterol by lactobacilli via incorporation and conversion to coprostanol. *J. Dairy Sci.* **2010**, *93*, 1383–1392. [CrossRef]
53. Xu, M.; Gagné-Bourque, F.; Dumont, M.-J.; Jabaji, S. Encapsulation of Lactobacillus casei ATCC 393 cells and evaluation of their survival after freeze-drying, storage and under gastrointestinal conditions. *J. Food Eng.* **2016**, *168*, 52–59. [CrossRef]
54. Gopal, P.K. Lactic Acid Bacteria: Lactobacillus spp.: Lactobacillus acidophilus. In *Encyclopedia of Dairy Sciences*, 2nd ed.; Fuquay, J.W., Fox, P.F., McSweeney, P.L.H., Eds.; Academic Press: Amsterdam, The Netherlands, 2011; Volume 3, pp. 91–95. ISBN 978-0-12-374402-9.
55. Fijan, S. Microorganisms with claimed probiotic properties: An overview of recent literature. *Int. J. Environ. Res. Public Health* **2014**, *11*, 4745–4767. [CrossRef]
56. Upadhyay, A. Investigating the Potential of Plant-Derived Antimicrobials and Probiotic Bacteria for Controlling Listeria Monocytogenes. Doctoral Thesis, University of Connecticut, Storrs, CT, USA, 2014. Available online: http://digitalcommons.uconn.edu/dissertations/326 (accessed on 2 November 2020).
57. Apostolidis, E.; Kwon, Y.I.; Shinde, R.; Ghaedian, R.; Shetty, K. Inhibition of Helicobacter pylori by fermented milk and soymilk using select lactic acid bacteria and link to enrichment of lactic acid and phenolic content. *Food Biotechnol.* **2011**, *25*, 58–76. [CrossRef]
58. Chen, X.; Liu, X.M.; Tian, F.; Zhang, Q.; Zhang, H.P.; Zhang, H.; Chen, W. Antagonistic Activities of Lactobacilli against Helicobacter pylori Growth and Infection in Human Gastric Epithelial Cells. *J. Food Sci.* **2012**, *77*, 9–14. [CrossRef]
59. Sunanliganon, C.; Thong-Ngam, D.; Tumwasorn, S.; Klaikeaw, N. Lactobacillus plantarum B7 inhibits Helicobacter pylori growth and attenuates gastric inflammation. *World J. Gastroenterol.* **2012**, *18*, 2472–8240. [CrossRef]
60. Ait, S.H.; Bendali, F.; Cudennec, B.; Drider, D. Anti-pathogenic and probiotic attributes of Lactobacillus salivarius and Lactobacillus plantarum strains isolated from feces of Algerian infants and adults. *Res. Microbiol.* **2017**, *168*, 244–254. [CrossRef]
61. Su, P.; Henriksson, A.; Mitchell, H. Prebiotics enhance survival and prolong the retention period of specific probiotic inocula in an in vivo murine model. *J. Appl. Microbiol.* **2007**, *106*, 2392–2400. [CrossRef]
62. Martinez, R.C.R.; Aynaou, A.E.; Albrecht, S.; Schols, H.A.; De Martinis, E.C.P.; Zoetendal, E.G.; Venema, K.; Saad, S.M.I.; Smidt, H. In vitro evaluation of gastrointestinal survival of Lactobacillus amylovorus DSM 16698 alone and combined with galactooligosaccharides, milk and/or Bifidobacterium animalis subsp. lactis Bb-12. *Int. J. Food Microbiol.* **2011**, *149*, 152–158. [CrossRef]
63. Donkor, O.N.; Nilmini, S.L.I.; Stolic, P.; Vasiljevic, T.; Shah, N.P. Survival and activity of selected probiotic organisms in set-type yoghurt during cold storage. *Int. Dairy J.* **2007**, *17*, 657–665. [CrossRef]
64. Hernandez-Hernandez, O.; Muthaiyan, A.; Moreno, F.J.; Montilla, A.; Sanz, M.L.; Ricke, S.C. Effect of prebiotic carbohydrates on the growth and tolerance of Lactobacillus. *Food Microbiol.* **2012**, *30*, 355–361. [CrossRef]
65. Perrin, S.; Grill, J.P.; Schneider, F. Effects of fructooligosaccharides and their monomeric components on bile salt resistance in three species of bifidobacteria. *J. Appl. Microbiol.* **2000**, *88*, 968–974. [CrossRef]
66. Charalampopoulos, D.; Pandiella, S.S.; Webb, C. Evaluation of the effect of malt, wheat and barley extracts on the viability of potentially probiotic lactic acid bacteria under acidic conditions. *Int. J. Food Microbiol.* **2003**, *82*, 133–141. [CrossRef]
67. Vandenplas, Y.; De Greef, E.; Hauser, B.; Devreker, T.; Veereman-Wauters, G. Probiotics and prebiotics in pediatric diarrheal disorders. *Expert Opin. Pharmacother.* **2013**, *14*, 397–409. [CrossRef]
68. Freedman, S.B.; Williamson-Urquhart, S.; Farion, K.J.; Gouin, S.; Willan, A.R.; Poonai, N.; Hurley, K.; Sherman, P.M.; Finkelstein, Y.; Lee, B.E. Multicenter trial of a combination probiotic for children with gastroenteritis. *N. Engl. J. Med.* **2018**, *379*, 2015–2026. [CrossRef]
69. Schnadower, D.; Tarr, P.I.; Casper, T.C. *Lactobacillus rhamnosus* GG versus placebo for acute gastroenteritis in children. *N. Engl. J. Med.* **2018**, *379*, 2002–2014. [CrossRef]

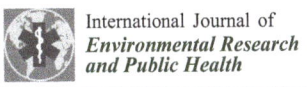

Article

Impact of Dietary Isoflavone Supplementation on the Fecal Microbiota and Its Metabolites in Postmenopausal Women

Lucía Guadamuro [1], M. Andrea Azcárate-Peril [2], Rafael Tojo [3], Baltasar Mayo [1,4] and Susana Delgado [1,4,*]

1. Instituto de Productos Lácteos de Asturias (IPLA-CSIC), Departament of Microbiology and Biochemistry of Dairy Products, Paseo Río Linares s/n, 33300 Villaviciosa, Spain; luciaguadamurogarcia@gmail.com (L.G.); baltasar.mayo@ipla.csic.es (B.M.)
2. Division of Gastroenterology and Hepatology, and Microbiome Core, School of Medicine, Department of Medicine, University of North Carolina (UNC), Chapel Hill, NC 2759, USA; azcarate@med.unc.edu
3. Gastroenterology Department, Cabueñes University Hospital, 33203 Gijón, Spain; tojorafael@uniovi.es
4. Instituto de Investigación Sanitaria del Principado de Asturias (ISPA), Avenida de Roma s/n, 33011 Oviedo, Spain
* Correspondence: sdelgado@ipla.csic.es

Abstract: Isoflavones are metabolized by components of the gut microbiota and can also modulate their composition and/or activity. This study aimed to analyze the modifications of the fecal microbial populations and their metabolites in menopausal women under dietary treatment with soy isoflavones for one month. Based on the level of urinary equol, the women had been stratified previously as equol-producers ($n = 3$) or as equol non-producers ($n = 5$). The composition of the fecal microbiota was assessed by high-throughput sequencing of 16S rRNA gene amplicons and the changes in fatty acid excretion in feces were analyzed by gas chromatography. A greater proportion of sequence reads of the genus *Slackia* was detected after isoflavone supplementation. Sequences of members of the family *Lachnospiraceae* and the genus *Pseudoflavonifractor* were significantly increased in samples from equol-producing women. Multivariable analysis showed that, after isoflavone treatment, the fecal microbial communities of equol producers were more like each other. Isoflavone supplementation increased the production of caproic acid, suggesting differential microbial activity, leading to a high fecal excretion of this compound. However, differences between equol producers and non-producers were not scored. These results may contribute to characterizing the modulating effect of isoflavones on the gut microbiota, which could lead to unravelling of their beneficial health effects.

Keywords: fecal microbiota; isoflavones; equol; pyrosequencing; menopause; fatty acids

1. Introduction

The existence of an inter-individual variability in response to diet and lifestyle interventions is widely accepted [1]. A complex interaction between diet, human genome, and the gut microbiome occurs and can determine the effects of dietary bioactives [2]. The gut microbiota is a critical component that can alter the absorption and metabolism of foods, and thus the final effects on human health. However, although a growing body of studies exists, the mechanisms underlying these processes are complex and not entirely understood. In this context, isoflavones-plant-derived polyphenols found at a relatively high concentration in soy and soy-derived products have been related to diverse health benefits such as the prevention of chronic diseases, including hormone dependent cancer, cardiovascular diseases, osteoporosis, and postmenopausal syndrome [3]. Although there is scientific evidence of the beneficial effects in counteracting symptoms like hot flushes and vasomotor reactions in menopausal women [4], the European Food Safety Authority (EFSA) has refuted health claims about the role of isoflavones in body functions [5]. The clinical effectiveness of ingested isoflavones might be due to their ability to be converted

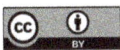

into active metabolites like equol [6,7]. This metabolite is the isoflavone-derived compound with the strongest estrogenic activity and antioxidant capacity, and is generated by specific members of the gut microbiota. Only some individuals harbor the microbiota required for the conversion into equol, resulting in different metabotypes: equol producers and non-producers [8]. Remarkably, compared with that in Asian populations (50–60%), the equol producer metabotype has a prevalence of 25–30% in Western populations [7].

Although the full range of intestinal bacteria involved in equol formation remains unknown [8,9], most of the equol-producing bacteria characterized so far are members of the family *Coriobacteriaceae* [10]. Additionally, the microorganisms responsible for equol production might differ across individuals [11–13].

Like other polyphenols, isoflavones are metabolized by components of the microbiota, and at the same time, they could also modulate the composition and/or activity of the intestinal microbial populations [14]. Analysis of intestinal microbiota modifications after isoflavone consumption could give clues as to the microorganisms involved in its metabolism. Some studies analyzed the effects of the isoflavone intake on the gut microbiota [15–19]. However, additional studies applying high-throughput approaches are still needed to determine low abundance microorganisms, like those probably involved in equol production.

This study aimed to determine changes in the intestinal microbiota induced by a 1-month period of isoflavone consumption and to explore changes related to the equol status metabotype. With this aim, high-throughput amplicon sequencing of the bacterial 16S rRNA gene was performed on fecal samples taken before and after isoflavone consumption by eight menopausal women (three equol producers and five equol non-producers). In addition, metabolite analysis of feces was performed using gas chromatography for determination of possible shifts in fatty acid excretion.

2. Materials and Methods

2.1. Human Volunteers

Ethical approval for this study was obtained from the Bioethics Subcommittee of the Spanish Research Council (Consejo Superior de Investigaciones Científicas or CSIC) and the Regional Ethics Committee for Clinical Research of the Health Service of Asturias (Servicio de Salud del Principado de Asturias) (approval number: 15/2011), in compliance with the Declaration of Helsinki. Fecal samples were provided, with written consent, by eight postmenopausal women recruited during a preceding study [18] at the Gynecology and Obstetrics Unit (in collaboration with the Gastroenterology Department) of Cabueñes Hospital (Gijón, Spain). The participants did not suffer from any infectious diseases or intestinal disorder. Additionally, they had not received antibiotics or any other medication for at least 6 months prior to the collection of samples. The women had been identified with an equol-producing metabotype (or not), based on the levels of urinary equol excretion [20]. For the present work, we selected three of the women (WC, WG, and WP) with an equol-producing phenotype (urine equol > 1000 nM as defined by Rowland et al. [21]) and five women (WE, WH, WF, WL, and WN) with a non-producing phenotype (excreted equol in urine ranging from 0 to 377 nM). Participants reported consuming a normo-type, Mediterranean diet and did not start following a vegetarian, vegan, or special diet during the intervention period. Supplementation consisted of a daily oral intake (80 mg/day) in the morning of a commercial dietary supplement (Fisiogen; Zambon, Bresso, Italy) rich in soy isoflavones (55–72% genistin/genistein, 28–45% other isoflavones) for one month.

2.2. Sample Collection

The study was conducted during the fall–winter seasons of 2011–2012. The volunteers provided samples of feces before treatment (basal, T0) and after one month (T1) of isoflavone supplementation. Fresh stools were collected in sterile plastic containers and kept under anaerobic conditions in jars containing Anaerocult A (Merck, Darmstadt,

Germany) for transporting to the laboratory within 2 h. Fecal samples were kept frozen at −80 °C until use.

2.3. Total Bacterial DNA Extraction

Fecal samples (0.2 g) were suspended in 1.8 mL of phosphate buffered saline (PBS) (pH 7.4). These suspensions were homogenized and centrifuged at 800 rpm for 5 min at 4 °C to eliminate insoluble material, and the supernatants were transferred to new tubes. These were then centrifuged again at 14,000 rpm for 5 min at 4 °C. Pelleted cells were suspended in 1 mL of PBS and lysed in an enzyme solution containing 20 mM TRIS-HCl pH 8.0, 2 mM EDTA, 1.20% Triton X-100, 20 mg/mL lysozyme (Merck), and 20 U mutanolysin (Sigma-Aldrich, Saint Louis, MO, USA). Total bacterial DNA was extracted following the protocol described by Zoetendal [22], and purified using the QIAamp DNA Stool Minikit (Qiagen, Hilden, Germany). Finally, the DNA was eluted in 100 µL of sterile molecular grade water (Sigma-Aldrich), and its concentration and quality were determined using an Epoch microvolume spectrophotometer (BioTek Instruments, Winooski, VT, USA).

2.4. Library Construction and Pyrosequencing

A segment of the 16S rRNA genes from the purified bacterial DNA were PCR-amplified using the universal primers Y1 (5′-TGGCTCAGGACGAACGCTGGCGGC-3′) (position 20–43 on the 16S rRNA gene of Escherichia coli) and Y2 (5′-CCTACTGCTGCCTCC CGTAGGAGT-3′) (positions 361–338). These primers amplify a 348 bp stretch of the prokaryotic rDNA embracing the V1 and V2 hypervariable regions. Further, 454-adaptors were included in both the forward (5′-CGTATCGCCTCCCTCGCGCCATCAG-3′) and reverse (5′-CTATGCGCCTTGCCAGCCCGCTCAG-3′) primers, followed by a 10 bp sample-specific barcode. Amplifications were performed using the NEBNext High-Fidelity 2x PCR Master Mix Kit (New England Biolabs., Ipswich, MA, USA) as follows: 95 °C for 5 min, 25 cycles of 94 °C for 30 s, 60 °C for 45 s, 72 °C for 30 s, and a final extension step at 72 °C for 5 min. The amplicons produced were purified using the GenElute PCR Clean-Up Kit (Sigma-Aldrich), and their concentration was measured in a Qubit fluorometer with dsDNA assay kits (Thermo Fisher Scientific Inc., Waltham, MA, USA).

An amplicon library was prepared for pyrosequencing by mixing equal amounts of amplicons from the different samples. Pooled amplicons were then sequenced using a 1/8 picotitre plate in a 454 Titanium Genome Sequencer (Roche, Indianapolis, IN, USA) in the UNC Microbiome Core (University of North Carolina, USA).

2.5. Sequence and Data Analysis

Raw sequences were denoised and filtered out of the original dataset. Filtering and trimming were performed using the Galaxy Web Server [23], employing the sliding window method. Only reads longer than 150 bp were used in further analysis. Chimeras were eliminated using the USEARCH v.6.0.307 clustering algorithm routine in de novo mode [24]. After demultiplexing, high quality rDNA sequences were classified taxonomically using the Ribosomal Database Project (RDP) Bayesian Classifier [25] with an 80% confidence threshold to obtain the taxonomic assignment and relative abundance of the different bacterial groups. "Genus" was the lowest taxonomic level contemplated. Sequences with at least 97% similarity were clustered into operational taxonomic units using the CD-Hit clustering method [26] and employed in the generation of rarefaction curves using a RarefactWin freeware (produced by S. Holland; http://strata.uga.edu/software/index.html). Different diversity indexes (Sobs, Chao, ACE, Jackknife, Shannon, Simpson) were calculated for each sample and compared between groups of women [27]. As diversity index values increase with sample size, normalization of sequencing effort in all samples was necessary to avoid biases in the results [28]. Thus, diversity indexes were normalized using the median number of sequences obtained in all samples as a scaling factor [29]. Weighted UniFrac analysis [30] was performed to assess the similarity of the microbial communities between samples and principal coordinates analysis (PCoA) was applied to the distance matrix for visualization.

2.6. Fatty Acids (FAs) Determination

One hundred microliters of a 1:10 dilution of feces (w/v) in PBS was supplemented with 100 µL of 2-ethyl butyric acid (Sigma-Aldrich, St. Louis, MO, USA) as an internal standard (1 mg/mL in methanol) and acidified with 100 µL of 20% formic acid (v/v). The acidic solution was then extracted with 1 mL of methanol and centrifuged for 10 min at 15,700× g. Supernatants were kept at −20 °C until analysis in a 6890 N gas chromatography (GC) apparatus (Agilent Technologies, Santa Clara, CA, USA) connected to a flame ionization detector (FID). All samples were analyzed in duplicate and FAs were quantified as previously described [31].

2.7. Statistical Analysis

Statistical analysis of data was performed using IBM SPSS 23 statistic software. The Mann–Whitney test for independent samples was performed to examine differences between equol producers and non-producers in terms of microbial groups, diversity indexes, and fecal FAs. The Wilcoxon signed-rank test for related samples was used to examine differences between before and after isoflavone supplementation. Alternatively, Student's t-test was used when normal distribution was confirmed using Saphiro-Wilk test. Two-tailed probability values of $p < 0.05$ were considered significant.

3. Results

3.1. Change in Fecal Microbiota Over Isoflavone Supplementation

After denoising, performing chimera checks, and trimming the reads by length (150–400 bp), a mean of 4756 (±875) high quality sequences was obtained. Taxonomic analysis grouped the sequences mainly into five phyla: *Firmicutes, Actinobacteria, Bacteroidetes, Proteobacteria,* and *Verrucomicrobia.* Fifty-two genera were identified, as well as five groups of clostridia (*Clostridium* cluster IV, cluster XI, cluster XIVa, cluster XVIII, and *Clostridium sensu stricto*) and two taxa with family-associated *incertae sedis* (*inc. sed.*) members (*Erysipelotrichaceae inc. sed.* and *Lachnospiraceae inc. sed.*). Taxonomic groups presenting at an abundance of <0.1% were designated as "others". A mean of 1813 sequences per sample remained unclassified.

Considerable differences were observed between the bacterial communities at T0 (before isoflavone supplementation) and T1 (one month after supplementation). Differences were noted at the family and genus levels (Figure 1). At the genus level, a significant ($p < 0.05$) increase in the relative abundance of the genus *Slackia* was observed at T1 (0.67%) versus T0 (0.27%). Although sequences of this genus were not detected in all women, when they were detected (WC, WG, WE, WL, and WN), their relative proportion increased after supplementation with soy isoflavones.

The supplementation with isoflavones significantly reduced alpha diversity in terms of Sobs and Shannon Indexes (Figure 2). The Sobs index reflects the number of observed species or "richness", while Shannon index weights the numbers of species by their relative evenness.

3.2. Differences in Microbial Groups Associated with the Equol Producer Status

UniFrac β-diversity analysis was done to assess the extent of similarity between microbial communities. UniFrac-based PCoA plots revealed a clear clustering between equol producing and non-producing women after isoflavone supplementation, while no clustering was observed at baseline (Figure 3).

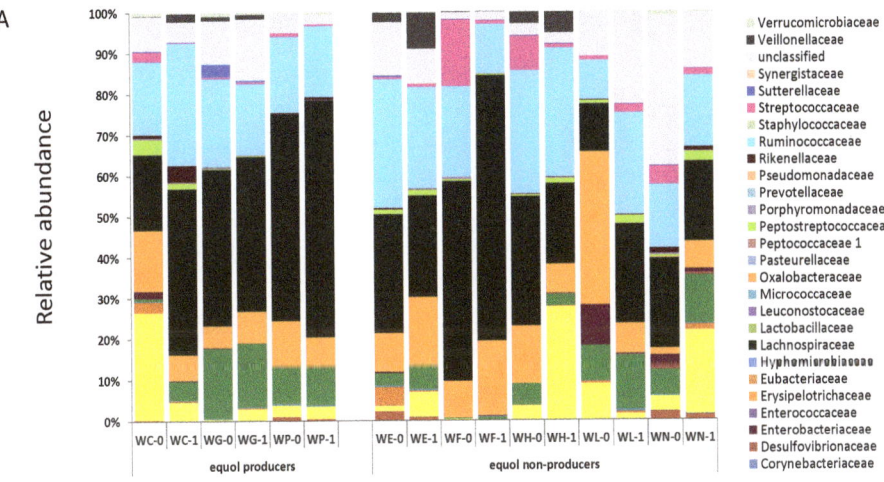

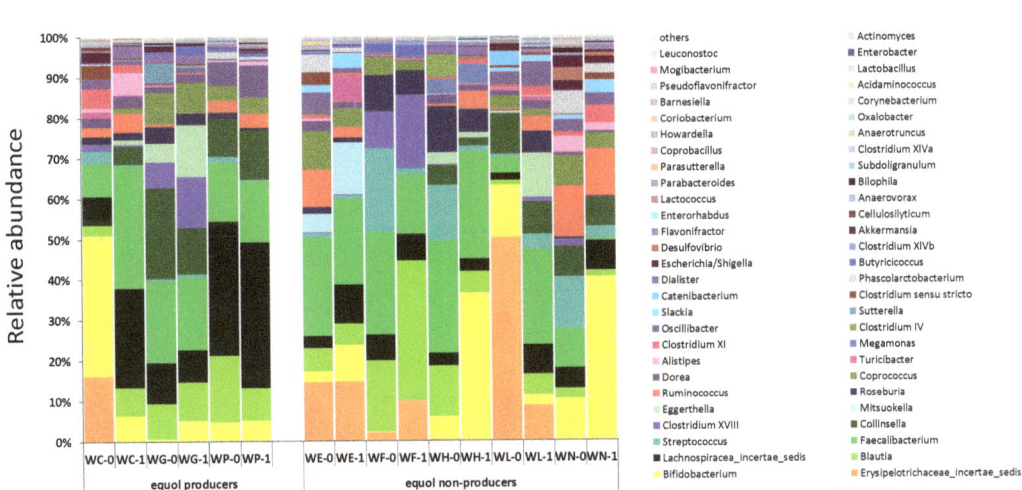

Figure 1. Changes in microbial composition with isoflavone supplementation. Microbial composition at the family (**A**) and genus (**B**) levels in fecal samples of eight menopausal women before (T0) and after one month (T1) of isoflavone supplementation presented as relative abundances (%).

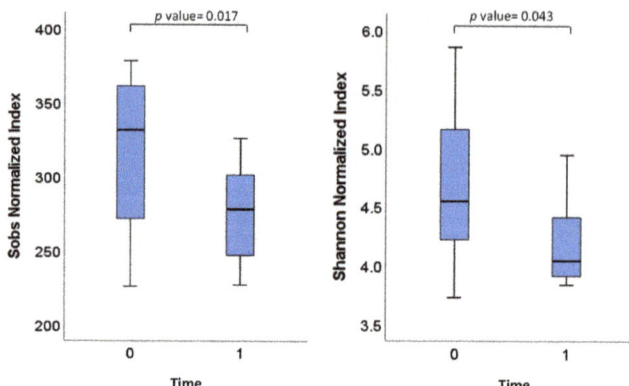

Figure 2. Comparison of Sobs and Shannon indexes before (T0) and after one month (T1) of isoflavone treatment in eight menopausal women. The lines inside the rectangles indicate the medians and the whiskers indicate the maximum and minimum values. Analysis was done using the nonparametric Wilcoxon signed-rank test to determine differences between T0 and T1.

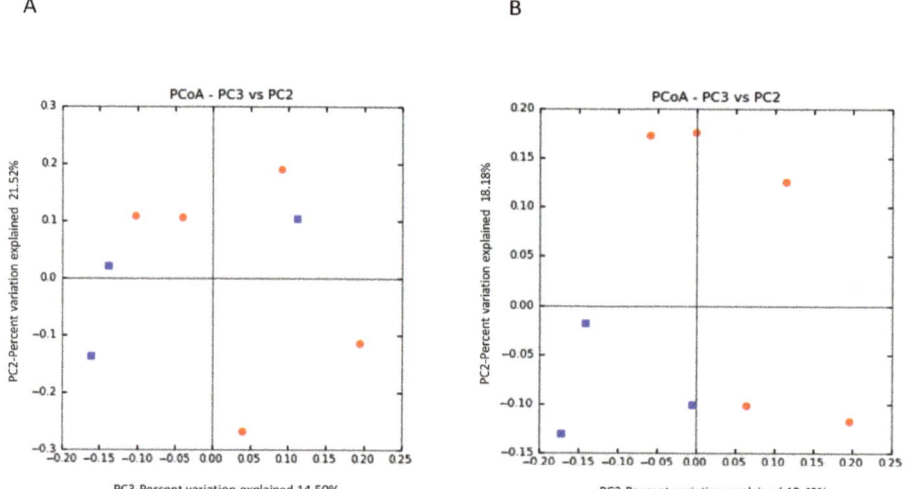

Figure 3. Weighted UniFrac principal coordinates analysis (PCoA) plots of fecal microbiota composition from the women in the study ($n = 8$) before soy isoflavone intervention (**A**), and after one month of daily supplementation (**B**). Subject color coding: red, equol non-producers ($n = 5$); blue, equol producers ($n = 3$).

Furthermore, comparison of fecal microbial composition between equol producers and non-producers revealed some differences. At T0, relative abundance (% sequences) of *Lachnospiraceae inc. sed.* taxa was significantly higher ($p = 0.025$) in the equol-producer group versus the non-producers (Table 1). While at T1, after one month of isoflavone consumption, the relative abundance of sequences belonging to the genera *Pseudoflavonifractor* and *Dorea* was greater in the equol-producing women.

Table 1. Fecal genera showing significant greater relative abundances (% sequences) in equol-producing women before (T0) and after (T1) the soy isoflavone intervention.

		% Relative Abundance [a]	
T0	p-Value [b]	Producers (n = 3)	Non-Producers (n = 5)
Lachnospiraceae incertae sedis	0.025	10.34 ± 7.99	2.26 ± 1.54
T1			
Dorea	0.025	2.66 ± 1.86	0.71 ± 0.46
Pseudoflavonifractor	0.022	0.10 ± 0.03	0.03 ± 0.04

[a] Mean relative abundance ± standard deviation. [b] Mann–Whitney test.

3.3. Differences in Fatty Acids (FAs) Associated with the Equol Producer Status

Fecal FAs remained stable after 1 month of isoflavone supplementation, except for caproic acid, which increased significantly after the intervention (Table 2). Regarding differences associated with the equol producing status, all FAs analysed showed higher concentrations in the equol non-producing women, but only isovaleric acid reached statistical significance (Table 3).

Table 2. Fecal fatty acids' (FAs) concentration before and after the isoflavone treatment of the eight menopausal women of the study.

Time	Acetic	Propionic	Isobutyric	Butyric	Isovaleric	Valeric	Caproic *
Basal (n = 8)	20.64 ± 12.99	7.51 ± 4.75	1.73 ± 0.49	9.62 ± 6.67	2.42 ± 0.93	2.27 ± 0.74	1.24 ± 0.34
1 month (n = 8)	23.67 ± 15.87	8.44 ± 3.6	1.61 ± 0.39	12.9 ± 7.85	2.01 ± 1.12	2.55 ± 1.27	1.64 ± 1.14

Key of statistical significance: * $p < 0.05$ versus basal sample (t = 0), Wilcoxon test.

Table 3. Differences in fecal FAs between equol producers and non-producers after isoflavone supplementation.

Equol Status	Acetic	Propionic	Isobutyric	Butyric	Isovaleric *	Valeric	Caproic
Producers (n = 3)	19.58 ± 12.12	7.96 ± 1.97	1.46 ± 0.11	10.94 ± 5.31	1.33 ± 1.01	2.32 ± 0.42	1.14 ± 0.23
Non-producers (n = 5)	26.13 ± 17.68	8.73 ± 4.34	1.71 ± 0.47	14.08 ± 9.01	2.42 ± 1.00	2.69 ± 1.58	1.94 ± 1.36

Key of statistical significance: * $p < 0.05$, Mann–Whitney test.

4. Discussion

Diet modulates the composition of the intestinal microbiota [32] and, in turn, gut microbiota metabolism can determine the final metabolites produced, and thus the corresponding effects on human health. Most studies, however, have focused on the effect of fat and fiber [33,34], while dietary microcomponents, like polyphenols, have received less attention [35]. Certainly, little is known about the influence of isoflavones on the microbial populations of the gut [15–19].

The use of high throughput sequencing techniques allows for the determination of gut members whose culture requirements are still unknown or are uncultivable—having estimated that they are 80% of the bacterial species found by molecular tools [36]. As previously suggested, different bacteria may contribute towards equol production [9,37], but these might be present in the gut in low abundance, making their detection difficult by other techniques. In this study, with the aim of identifying changes in gut microbiota composition associated with the ingestion of isoflavones, and related to the equol-producing metabotype, we selected and made use of fecal samples from eight menopausal women receiving daily isoflavone supplementation over one month. Among these women, we selected three equol-producers and five non-producers for comparative purposes.

In the present work, the abundance of the genera *Slackia* significantly increased after the isoflavone supplementation. This genus, belonging to the family *Coriobacteriaceae*, includes described equol-producing species and strains [38–40] and has been associated in vivo with isoflavone metabolism [17]. Additionally, bacteria belonging to the family *Lachnospiraceae* (*Dorea* and *inc. sed.*) increased in the postmenopausal women with an equol-producing metabotype. *Lachnospiraceae inc. sed.* has previously been reported to increase significantly with isoflavone treatment in a case report of an equol-producing woman [19], while *Dorea* has been associated with isoflavone metabolism in humans in several studies [17,41]. Enrichment of some of these bacteria belonging to the *Lachnospiraceae* family, as well as *Pseudoflavonifractor*, has also been seen in in vitro fecal cultures with isoflavones [42]. The family *Lachnospiraceae* has a very large presence in the human gut and has been linked to the production of butyric acid [43], a compound with beneficial effects on the gastrointestinal epithelium [44].

Supplementation with isoflavones for one month was shown to cause a decrease in the number of species (Sobs index) as well as in the species evenness (Shannon index). These effects have previously been observed with the use of other culture-independent techniques [18]. It has been suggested that isoflavones could provide a chemical environment that selects a subset of the initial bacterial communities [17,45]. Alternatively, isoflavones might have antimicrobial effects on certain intestinal bacterial populations, as has recently been reported on pure cultures of intestinal species [46]. When considering the two different metabotypes studied, no effect in the alpha diversity indexes was observed (data not shown). However, UniFrac analysis indicated a greater similarity of the microbial communities from equol-producing women after one month of isoflavone supplementation, suggesting that isoflavones enriches the gut with microbial species involved in the degradation of isoflavones and equol production.

The production of FAs (relevant gut bacterial metabolites) was carried out to determine their relationship with the consumption of isoflavones and the production of equol. Butyric, acetic, and propionic acids are the main short-chain fatty acids (SCFAs). They are produced in the proximal colon by bacterial fermentation of non-digestible carbohydrates [47] and exert anti-inflammatory and anticarcinogenic activities [48]. In contrast, medium-chain fatty acids (MCFAs), including caproic acid (CA), by favoring TH1 and TH17 differentiation [49], could antagonize the anti-inflammatory activities of SCFAs. Branched-chain fatty acids, such as isobutyric and isovaleric acids, are often associated with protein breakdown and have been less studied.

The current data reveal an increase in CA production after isoflavone supplementation, which indicates differential microbial activity leading to the production of this compound. CA derives from chain elongation reactions in which SCFAs are converted to MCFAs mainly using ethanol or lactate as an electron donor [50]. The elongation process is mediated by microorganisms through the reverse β-oxidation pathway. Whether *Slackia*, the bacterial species found to be increased after the consumption of isoflavones in this study, produces CA is not currently known. Alternatively, isoflavone consumption could stimulate the production of CA by other intestinal microorganisms. These possibilities, however, would require further study. Although studies are still controversial, CA has been related to inflammation-regulating effects. In some studies, diminishing of the production of inflammatory cytokines by CA has been reported [51], while inflammatory effects have been reported in others [49,52].

The concentration of isovaleric acid was higher in samples from the equol non-producing group ($n = 5$). This result partially agrees with the effect of isoflavones observed previously in fecal anaerobic batch cultures [42], where isovaleric acid was reported to increase in cultures inoculated with feces from equol producers ($n = 3$). This suggests that, regardless of the equol producing status, consumption of isoflavones might stimulate the production of this FA.

In this work, although limited to the small sample size, the description of specific gut microbial and FA changes with the ingestion of isoflavones is provided, contributing to the understanding of the modulation of the gut microorganisms and their activity by these polyphenols. However, more studies with greater numbers of people, and even different populations, are needed to confirm the effects of isoflavone intake on the gut ecosystem.

5. Conclusions

This study allowed the changes in fecal microbial communities caused by isoflavone supplementation for one month to be monitored in a group of menopausal women. Isoflavone consumption was associated with a significant increase in the relative abundance of the genus *Slackia*, to which strains that metabolise isoflavones and produce equol are the most studied in this respect. Moreover, the taxa *Pseudoflavonifractor*, *Dorea*, and *Lachnospiraceae incertae sedis* were found in greater proportions in equol-producing women. Fecal microbial communities of equol producers were more similar to each other after isoflavone treatment, a fact that was not observed among those of equol non-producers. However, distinctive differences in the excretion of fatty acids associated with the equol status (which might be related to inflammation) were not observed.

Author Contributions: S.D. and B.M. contributed with the conception and design of the study. L.G. performed bacterial DNA extraction, sequence data analysis, and statistics. S.D. performed library construction. R.T. carried out the recruitment and diagnoses of the women. M.A.A.-P. contributed with the high-throughput sequencing and analysis of the samples. S.D. and B.M. planned the experimental design of the study and contributed to the interpretation of the data. L.G. drafted the manuscript. B.M. and S.D. performed a critical revision of the manuscript. All authors have read and agreed to the published version of the manuscript.

Funding: The research was funded by the Spanish Ministry of Economy and Competitiveness (MINECO) (AGL-2014-57820-R) and Asturias Principality (GRUPIN14-137). The Microbiome Core Facility is supported in part by the NIH/National Institute of Diabetes and Digestive and Kidney Diseases grant P30 DK34987. L.G. was supported by a research contract of the FPI Program from MINECO (BES-2012-062502). S.D. was supported by a research contract from MINECO (RYC-2016-19726).

Institutional Review Board Statement: The study was conducted according to the guidelines of the Declaration of Helsinki, and approved by the Bioethics Subcommittee of the Spanish Research Council (Consejo Superior de Investigaciones Científicas or CSIC) and the Regional Ethics Committee for Clinical Research of the Health Service of Asturias (Servicio de Salud del Principado de Asturias) (approval number: 15/2011).

Informed Consent Statement: Informed consent was obtained from all subjects involved in the study.

Data Availability Statement: The raw data generated in this study can be found in the Sequence Read Archive (SRA) of the NCBI database. under accession numbers: SRR9855012-25, SRR6656999, and SRR6657000.

Acknowledgments: We would like to thank Ana Hernández and Jorge Rodríguez from IPLA-CSIC for their technical assistance in the chromatographic analysis of fecal acids.

Conflicts of Interest: The authors declare no conflict of interest. The funders had no role in the design of the study; in the collection, analyses, or interpretation of data; in the writing of the manuscript; or in the decision to publish the results.

References

1. Bashiardes, S.; Godneva, A.; Elinav, E.; Segal, E. Towards utilization of the human genome and microbiome for personalized nutrition. *Curr. Opin. Biotechnol.* **2018**, *51*, 57–63. [CrossRef] [PubMed]
2. Sonnenburg, J.L.; Bäckhed, F. Diet–microbiota interactions as moderators of human metabolism. *Nature* **2016**, *535*, 56–64. [CrossRef] [PubMed]
3. Zaheer, K.; Humayoun Akhtar, M. An updated review of dietary isoflavones: Nutrition, processing, bioavailability and impacts on human health. *Crit. Rev. Food Sci. Nutr.* **2017**, *57*, 1280–1293. [CrossRef] [PubMed]
4. Bolaños, R.; Del Castillo, A.; Francia, J. Soy isoflavones versus placebo in the treatment of climacteric vasomotor symptoms: Systematic review and meta-analysis. *Menopause* **2010**, *17*, 660–666. [CrossRef]

5. EFSA (European Food Science Authority). Scientific Opinion on the Substantiation of Health Claims Related to Soy Isoflavones and Maintenance of bone Mineral Density (ID 1655) and Reduction of Vasomotor Symptoms Associated with Menopause (ID 1654, 1704, 2140, 3093, 3154, 3590) (Further Assessment) Pursuant to Article 13(1) of Regulation (EC) No 1924/2006. *EFSA J.* **2012**. [CrossRef]
6. Atkinson, C.; Frankenfeld, C.L.; Lampe, J.W. Gut bacterial metabolism of the soy isoflavone daidzein: Exploring the relevance to human health. *Exp. Biol. Med.* **2005**, *230*, 155–170. [CrossRef]
7. Setchell, K.D.; Clerici, C. Equol: History, chemistry, and formation. *J. Nutr.* **2010**, *140*, 1355S–1362S. [CrossRef]
8. Tomás-Barberán, F.A.; González-Sarrías, A.; García-Villalba, R.; Núñez-Sánchez, M.A.; Selma, M.V.; García-Conesa, M.T.; Espín, J.C. Urolithins, the rescue of "old" metabolites to understand a "new" concept: Metabotypes as a nexus among phenolic metabolism, microbiota dysbiosis, and host health status. *Mol. Nutr. Food Res.* **2017**, *61*, 1500901. [CrossRef]
9. Kemperman, R.A.; Bolca, S.; Roger, L.C.; Vaughan, E.E. Novel approaches for analysing gut microbes and dietary polyphenols: Challenges and opportunities. *Microbiology* **2010**, *156*, 3224–3231. [CrossRef]
10. Clavel, T.; Lepage, P.; Charrier, C. The Family Coriobacteriaceae. In *The Prokaryotes*; Rosenberg, E., DeLong, E.F., Lory, S., Stackebrandt, E., Thompson, F., Eds.; Springer: Berlin/Heidelberg, Germany, 2014; pp. 201–238.
11. Kelly, G.E.; Joannou, G.E.; Reeder, A.Y.; Nelson, C.; Waring, M.A. The variable metabolic response to dietary isoflavones in humans. *Proc. Soc. Exp. Biol. Med.* **1995**, *208*, 40–43. [CrossRef]
12. Lampe, J.W.; Karr, S.C.; Hutchins, A.M.; Slavin, J.L. Urinary equol excretion with a soy challenge: Influence of habitual diet. *Proc. Soc. Exp. Biol. Med.* **1998**, *217*, 335–339. [CrossRef]
13. Arai, Y.; Uehara, M.; Sato, Y.; Kimira, M.; Eboshida, A.; Adlercreutz, H.; Watanabe, S. Comparison of isoflavones among dietary intake, plasma concentration and urinary excretion for accurate estimation of phytoestrogen intake. *J. Epidemiol.* **2000**, *10*, 127–135. [CrossRef] [PubMed]
14. Dueñas, M.; Muñoz-González, I.; Cueva, C.; Jiménez-Girón, A.; Sánchez-Patán, F.; Santos-Buelga, C.; Moreno-Arribas, M.; Bartolomé, B. A survey of modulation of gut microbiota by dietary polyphenols. *BioMed Res. Int.* **2015**, *2015*, 850902. [CrossRef] [PubMed]
15. Clavel, T.; Fallani, M.; Lepage, P.; Levenez, F.; Mathey, J.; Rochet, V.; Sérézat, M.; Sutren, M.; Henderson, G.; Bennetau-Pelissero, C.; et al. Isoflavones and functional foods alter the dominant intestinal microbiota in postmenopausal women. *J. Nutr.* **2005**, *135*, 2786–2792. [CrossRef]
16. Bolca, S.; Possemiers, S.; Herregat, A.; Huybrechts, I.; Heyerick, A.; De Vriese, S.; Verbruggen, M.; Depypere, H.; De Keukeleire, D.; Bracke, M.; et al. Microbial and dietary factors are associated with the equol producer phenotype in healthy postmenopausal women. *J. Nutr.* **2007**, *137*, 2242–2246. [CrossRef] [PubMed]
17. Nakatsu, C.H.; Armstrong, A.; Clavijo, A.P.; Martin, B.R.; Barnes, S.; Weaver, C.M. Fecal bacterial community changes associated with isoflavone metabolites in postmenopausal women after soy bar consumption. *PLoS ONE* **2014**, *9*, e108924. [CrossRef]
18. Guadamuro, L.; Delgado, S.; Redruello, B.; Flórez, A.B.; Suárez, A.; Martínez-Camblor, P.; Mayo, B. Equol status and changes in fecal microbiota in menopausal women receiving long-term treatment for menopause symptoms with a soy-isoflavone concentrate. *Front. Microbiol.* **2015**, *6*, 777. [CrossRef]
19. Guadamuro, L.; Azcárate-Peril, M.A.; Tojo, R.; Mayo, B.; Delgado, S. Use of high throughput amplicon sequencing and ethidium monoazide dye to track microbiota changes in an equol-producing menopausal woman receiving a long-term isoflavones treatment. *AIMS Microbiol.* **2019**, *5*, 102–116. [CrossRef]
20. Redruello, B.; Guadamuro, L.; Cuesta, I.; Álvarez-Buylla, J.R.; Mayo, B.; Delgado, S. A novel UHPLC method for the rapid and simultaneous determination of daidzein, genistein and equol in human urine. *J. Chromatogr. B* **2015**, *1005*, 1–8. [CrossRef]
21. Rowland, I.R.; Wiseman, H.; Sanders, T.A.; Adlercreutz, H.; Bowey, E.A. Interindividual variation in metabolism of soy isoflavones and lignans: Influence of habitual diet on equol production by the gut microflora. *Nutr. Cancer* **2000**, *36*, 27–32. [CrossRef] [PubMed]
22. Zoetendal, E.G.; Heilig, H.G.; Klaassens, E.S.; Booijink, C.C.; Kleerebezem, M.; Smidt, H.; De Vos, W.M. Isolation of DNA from bacterial samples of the human gastrointestinal tract. *Nat. Protoc.* **2006**, *1*, 870–873. [CrossRef] [PubMed]
23. Goecks, J.; Nekrutenko, A.; Taylor, J. Galaxy: A comprehensive approach for supporting accessible, reproducible, and transparent computational research in the life sciences. *Genome Biol.* **2010**, *11*, R86. [CrossRef]
24. Edgar, R.C.; Haas, B.J.; Clemente, J.C.; Quince, C.; Knight, R. UCHIME improves sensitivity and speed of chimera detection. *Bioinformatics* **2011**, *27*, 2194–2200. [CrossRef] [PubMed]
25. Wang, Q.; Garrity, G.M.; Tiedje, J.M.; Cole, J.R. Naive Bayesian classifier for rapid assignment of rRNA sequences into the new bacterial taxonomy. *Appl. Environ. Microbiol.* **2007**, *73*, 5261–5267. [CrossRef]
26. Li, W.; Godzik, A. Cd-hit: A fast program for clustering and comparing large sets of protein or nucleotide sequences. *Bioinformatics* **2006**, *22*, 1658–1659. [CrossRef]
27. Moreno, C.E.; Halffter, G. On the measure of sampling effort used in species accumulation curves. *J. Appl. Ecol.* **2001**, *38*, 487–490. [CrossRef]
28. Lemos, L.N.; Fulthorpe, R.R.; Triplett, E.W.; Roesch, L.F. Rethinking microbial diversity analysis in the high throughput sequencing era. *J. Microbiol. Methods* **2011**, *86*, 42–51. [CrossRef]

29. Dillies, M.A.; Rau, A.; Aubert, J.; Hennequet-Antier, C.; Jeanmougin, M.; Servant, N.; Keime, C.; Marot, G.; Castel, D.; Estelle, J.; et al. A comprehensive evaluation of normalization methods for Illumina high-throughput RNA sequencing data analysis. *Brief Bioinf.* **2013**, *14*, 671–683. [CrossRef]
30. Lozupone, C.A.; Knight, R. Unifrac: A new phylogenetic method for comparing microbial communities. *Appl. Envrion. Microbiol.* **2005**, *71*, 8228–8235. [CrossRef] [PubMed]
31. Salazar, N.; Gueimonde, M.; Hernández-Barranco, A.M.; Ruas-Madiedo, P.; de los Reyes-Gavilán, C.G. Exopolysaccharides produced by intestinal Bifidobacterium strains act as fermentable substrates for human intestinal bacteria. *Appl. Envrion. Microbiol.* **2008**, *74*, 4737–4745. [CrossRef]
32. Graf, D.; Di Cagno, R.; Fåk, F.; Flint, H.J.; Nyman, M.; Saarela, M.; Watzl, B. Contribution of diet to the composition of the human gut microbiota. *Microb. Ecol. Health Dis.* **2015**, *26*, 26164. [CrossRef]
33. David, L.A.; Maurice, C.F.; Carmody, R.N.; Gootenberg, D.B.; Button, J.E.; Wolfe, B.E.; Ling, A.V.; Devlin, A.S.; Varma, Y.; Fischbach, M.A.; et al. Diet rapidly and reproducibly alters the human gut microbiome. *Nature* **2014**, *505*, 559–563. [CrossRef]
34. Singh, R.K.; Chang, H.W.; Yan, D.; Lee, K.M.; Ucmak, D.; Wong, K.; Abrouk, M.; Farahnik, B.; Nakamura, M.; Zhu, T.H.; et al. Influence of diet on the gut microbiome and implications for human health. *J. Transl. Med.* **2017**, *15*, 73. [CrossRef]
35. Van Duynhoven, J.; Vaughan, E.E.; Jacobs, D.M.; Kemperman, R.A.; Van Velzen, E.J.; Gross, G.; Roger, L.C.; Possemiers, S.; Smilde, A.K.; Doré, J.; et al. Metabolic fate of polyphenols in the human superorganism. *Proc. Natl. Acad. Sci. USA* **2011**, *108*, 4531–4538. [CrossRef]
36. Turnbaugh, P.J.; Ley, R.E.; Hamady, M.; Fraser-Liggett, C.M.; Knight, R.; Gordon, J.I. The human microbiome project. *Nature* **2007**, *449*, 804–810. [CrossRef] [PubMed]
37. Vázquez, L.; Guadamuro, L.; Giganto, F.; Mayo, B.; Flórez, A.B. Development and use of a real-time quantitative PCR method for detecting and quantifying equol-producing bacteria in human faecal samples and slurry cultures. *Front. Microbiol.* **2017**, *8*, 1155. [CrossRef] [PubMed]
38. Jin, J.S.; Kitahara, M.; Sakamoto, M.; Hattori, M.; Benno, Y. Slackia equolifaciens sp. nov., a human intestinal bacterium capable of producing equol. *Int. J. Syst. Evol. Microbiol.* **2010**, *60*, 1721–1724. [CrossRef] [PubMed]
39. Matthies, A.; Loh, G.; Blaut, M.; Braune, A. Daidzein and genistein areconverted to equol and 5-hydroxy-equol by human intestinal Slackia isoflavoniconvertens in gnotobiotic rats. *J. Nutr.* **2012**, *142*, 40–46. [CrossRef]
40. Tsuji, H.; Moriyama, K.; Nomoto, K.; Akaza, H. Identification of an enzyme system for daidzein-to-equol conversion in *Slackia* sp. strain NATTS. *Appl. Environ. Microbiol.* **2012**, *78*, 1228–1236. [CrossRef] [PubMed]
41. Decroos, K.; Vanhemmens, S.; Cattoir, S.; Boon, N.; Verstraete, W. Isolation and characterisation of an equol-producing mixed microbial culture from a human faecal sample and its activity under gastrointestinal conditions. *Arch. Microbiol.* **2005**, *183*, 45–55. [CrossRef]
42. Guadamuro, L.; Dohrmann, A.B.; Tebbe, C.C.; Mayo, B.; Delgado, S. Bacterial communities and metabolic activity of faecal cultures from equol producer and non-producer menopausal women under treatment with soy isoflavones. *BMC Microbiol.* **2017**, *17*, 93. [CrossRef] [PubMed]
43. Meehan, C.J.; Beiko, R.G. A phylogenomic view of ecological specialization in the Lachnospiraceae, a family of digestive tract-associated bacteria. *Genome Biol. Evol.* **2014**, *6*, 703–713. [CrossRef] [PubMed]
44. Ríos-Covián, D.; Ruas-Madiedo, P.; Margolles, A.; Gueimonde, M.; de los Reyes-Gavilán, C.G.; Salazar, N. Intestinal short chain fatty acids and their link with diet and human health. *Front. Microbiol.* **2016**, *7*, 185. [CrossRef] [PubMed]
45. Clavel, T.; Mapesa, J.O. Phenolics in human nutrition: Importance of the intestinal microbiome for isoflavone and lignan bioavailability. In *Natural Products: Phytochemistry, Botany and Metabolism of Alkaloids, Phenolics and Terpenes*; Elsevier: Amsterdam, The Netherlands, 2013; pp. 2433–2463.
46. Vázquez, L.; Flórez, A.; Guadamuro, L.; Mayo, B. Effect of soy isoflavones on growth of representative bacterial species from the human gut. *Nutrients* **2017**, *9*, 727. [CrossRef]
47. Morrison, D.J.; Preston, T. Formation of short chain fatty acids by the gut microbiota and their impact on human metabolism. *Gut Microbes* **2016**, *7*, 189–200. [CrossRef] [PubMed]
48. Flint, H.J.; Duncan, S.H.; Scott, K.P.; Louis, P. Links between diet, gut microbiota composition and gut metabolism. *Proc. Nutr. Soc.* **2015**, *74*, 13–22. [CrossRef]
49. Schönfeld, P.; Wojtczak, L. Short- and medium-chain fatty acids in energy metabolism: The cellular perspective. *J. Lipid Res.* **2016**, *57*, 943–954. [CrossRef]
50. Crognale, S.; Braguglia, C.M.; Gallipoli, A.; Gianico, A.; Rossetti, S.; Montecchio, D. Direct Conversion of Food Waste Extract into Caproate: Metagenomics Assessment of Chain Elongation Process. *Microorganisms* **2021**, *9*, 327. [CrossRef]
51. El-Far, M.; Durand, M.; Turcotte, I.; Larouche-Anctil, E.; Sylla, M.; Zaidan, S.; Chartrand-Lefebvre, C.; Bunet, R.; Ramani, H.; Sadouni, M.; et al. Upregulated IL-32 expression and reduced gut short chain fatty acid caproic acid in people living with HIV with subclinical atherosclerosis. *Front. Immunol.* **2021**, *12*, 664371. [CrossRef]
52. De Preter, V.; Machiels, K.; Joossens, M.; Arijs, I.; Matthys, C.; Vermeire, S.; Rutgeerts, P.; Verbeke, K. Faecal metabolite profiling identifies medium-chain fatty acids as discriminating compounds in IBD. *Gut* **2015**, *64*, 447–458. [CrossRef]

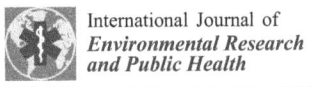

International Journal of
Environmental Research and Public Health

Article

Detection of Dysbiosis and Increased Intestinal Permeability in Brazilian Patients with Relapsing–Remitting Multiple Sclerosis

Felipe Papa Pellizoni [1,†], Aline Zazeri Leite [2,†], Nathália de Campos Rodrigues [3], Marcelo Jordão Ubaiz [1], Marina Ignácio Gonzaga [1], Nauyta Naomi Campos Takaoka [1], Vânia Sammartino Mariano [4], Wellington Pine Omori [5], Daniel Guariz Pinheiro [5], Euclides Matheucci Junior [6], Eleni Gomes [2] and Gislane Lelis Vilela de Oliveira [2,7,*]

1 Microbiome Study Group, School of Health Sciences Dr. Paulo Prata, Barretos 14785-002, Brazil; fppellizoni@gmail.com (F.P.P.); neuroclinicabarretos@uol.com.br (M.J.U.); marina.ignacio92@hotmail.com (M.I.G.); nauytatakaoka@gmail.com (N.N.C.T.)
2 Microbiology Program, Institute of Biosciences, Humanities and Exact Sciences, São Paulo State University, Sao Jose do Rio Preto 15054-000, Brazil; allline1@hotmail.com (A.Z.L.); eleni.gomes@unesp.br (E.G.)
3 DNA Consult Genetics and Biotechnology, Sao Carlos 13560-340, Brazil; nathdecampos@gmail.com
4 Barretos Cancer Hospital, Barretos 14784-400, Brazil; vaniasmariano@gmail.com
5 Department of Technology, School of Agricultural and Veterinarian Sciences, São Paulo State University (UNESP), Jaboticabal 14884-900, Brazil; wpomori@gmail.com (W.P.O.); dgpinheiro@gmail.com (D.G.P.)
6 Biotechnology Department, Sao Carlos Federal University, Sao Carlos 13565-905, Brazil; matheuccl@dnaconsult.com.br
7 Food Engineering and Technology Department, São Paulo State University (UNESP), Sao Jose do Rio Preto 15054-000, Brazil
* Correspondence: glelisvilela@gmail.com; Tel.: +55-17-3212-1058
† These authors contributed equally to this work.

Abstract: Dysbiosis, associated with barrier disruption and altered gut–brain communications, has been associated with multiple sclerosis (MS). In this study, we evaluated the gut microbiota in relapsing–remitting patients (RRMS) receiving disease-modifying therapies (DMTs) and correlated these data with diet, cytokines levels, and zonulin concentrations. Stool samples were used for 16S sequencing and real-time PCR. Serum was used for cytokine determination by flow cytometry, and zonulin quantification by ELISA. Pearson's chi-square, Mann–Whitney, and Spearman's correlation were used for statistical analyses. We detected differences in dietary habits, as well as in the gut microbiota in RRMS patients, with predominance of *Akkermansia muciniphila* and *Bacteroides vulgatus* and decreased *Bifidobacterium*. Interleukin-6 concentrations were decreased in treated patients, and we detected an increased intestinal permeability in RRMS patients when compared with controls. We conclude that diet plays an important role in the composition of the gut microbiota, and intestinal dysbiosis, detected in RRMS patients could be involved in increased intestinal permeability and affect the clinical response to DTMs. The future goal is to predict therapeutic responses based on individual microbiome analyses (personalized medicine) and propose dietary interventions and the use of probiotics or other microbiota modulators as adjuvant therapy to enhance the therapeutic efficacy of DMTs.

Keywords: autoimmunity; multiple sclerosis; gut microbiota; dysbiosis; inflammation; cytokines; intestinal permeability; disease modifying drugs

1. Introduction

Multiple sclerosis (MS) is a chronic inflammatory, neurodegenerative disease, mediated by autoimmune reactions against myelin proteins and gangliosides in white and grey matter of the brain and spinal cord, promoting physical disability, cognitive impairment, and decreased quality of life in young adults, aged between 20 and 40 years [1,2]. The incidence of MS is increasing worldwide and estimated to range from 5 to 300 per 100,000 individuals, affecting females three times more and having a significant socioeconomic impact, with financial burden to patients and to developed and developing economies [2,3].

The MS onset is clinically characterized as relapsing–remitting (RRMS), diagnosed in 85 to 90% of patients [1,4]. The relapses are due to blood–brain barrier breakdown and infiltration of T and B cells and myeloid cells into the central nervous system (CNS) parenchyma, which induces acute inflammation, detected as gadolinium-positive lesions in magnetic resonance imaging (MRI) [3]. Permanent neurological lesions and clinical disability evolve to a secondary progressive form, and few patients present a primary progressive course from disease onset [1]. Complex genetic–environmental interactions are hypothesized to be involved in MS development, including human leukocyte antigen (HLA) genes, Epstein–Barr virus infections, tobacco exposure, obesity, vitamin D deficiency, and alterations of the gut microbiota [1,5,6].

In homeostatic or eubiosis conditions, the gut microbiota is dominated by microorganisms that contribute to food digestion and fermentation, nutrient absorption, vitamin synthesis, epithelial cell maturation, gut barrier integrity, development and education of the immune system, protection against pathogens and inflammation, and regulation of host metabolism and CNS physiology [7–10]. Recently, it has become evident that the gut microbiota can affect neurologic processes through bidirectional communications, involving the enteric nervous system, the endocrine/immune systems, the gut microbiota, and their metabolites [10–13]. Neurotransmitters and short-chain fatty acids (SCFAs), derived from microbiota fermentation, can shape immune responses and impact behavior, memory, and neurodegenerative diseases [10,12,14,15]. Thus, alterations in function and diversity of the gut microbiota, known as dysbiosis, are associated with a dysregulation in these gut–brain connections, increased gut and blood–brain barrier permeability and neuroinflammation and can contribute to the development of inflammatory autoimmune diseases, including MS [16–19].

In MS animal models, when experimental autoimmune encephalomyelitis (EAE) was induced in germ-free mice, a decrease in inflammatory interferon-gamma (IFN-γ) and interleukin-(IL)-17A levels in the CNS was detected, as well as an increase in regulatory T cells (Treg) in the gut mucosa [20]. On the other hand, the colonization of EAE mice with segmented filamentous bacteria induced Th17 differentiation in the lamina propria and migration to the CNS, increasing neuroinflammation and disease severity [20,21]. The disease score ameliorated when germ-free EAE mice were colonized by *Bacteroides fragilis* containing polysaccharide A, which induces IL-10-secreting Treg cells and suppress the T-helper (Th)-17 subpopulation [22,23]. Moreover, when fecal samples from MS patients were transferred to germ-free mice, genetically susceptible to EAE, the mice developed the disease and significantly produced less IL-10 than mice colonized with feces from healthy subjects [24]. These data suggest that the gut microbiota is linked to disease severity and immune response during MS development [10].

In humans, the gut microbiota from untreated RRMS patients, from different populations (China, Japan, Germany, USA), differs from that of healthy controls, and patients with active disease present decreased microbiota diversity. Intestinal dysbiosis in MS was predominantly characterized by decreased Firmicutes, Clostridia clusters XIVa and IV, *Faecalibacterium*, *Butyricimonas*, *Prevotella*, and *Lactobacillus* species, and increased abundance of *Pseudomonas*, *Mycoplasma*, *Haemophilus*, *Streptococcus*,*Akkermansia muciniphila*, and *Methanobrevibacter smithii* [24–33]. In addition, MS patients with increased peripheral Th17 lymphocytes and higher disease activity presented an increased Firmicutes/Bacteroidetes ratio, *Streptococcus* amounts, and decreased relative abundance of *Prevotella* species [34]. Interestingly, the taxonomic composition during remission showed richness and evenness similar to those of healthy individuals, and even the frequency of relapses seemed to be influenced by the intestinal microbiota [29,35].

There are few studies evaluating the effect of disease-modifying therapies (DMTs), used to treat MS patients on intestinal microbiota composition. Some studies suggest that these therapies are capable of reversing dysbiosis and restore a "healthy" gut microbiota, similar to that of control subjects [19]. Patients on IFN-β or glatiramer acetate treatment showed increased abundance of *Prevotella*, *Sutterella*, and *Prevotella copri* and decreased *Sarcina* species and gut microbiota richness [29,36,37]. Besides that, evidence from animal models and human studies demonstrated that gut microbes and their metabolites can influence drug bioavailability, pharmacokinetics, clinical response, as well as adverse events, supporting the importance of studies on the interaction of the gut microbiota with DMTs [38,39]. The future goal is to predict therapeutic responses based on microbiome analyses and propose diet interventions and the use of probiotics or other microbiota modulators as adjuvant therapy to enhance the therapeutic efficacy of DMTs [40,41].

On the basis of this background and the fact that there are no studies evaluating the gut microbiota in Brazilian MS patients, the aim of the present study was to evaluate the gut microbiota in RRMS patients receiving DMTs and correlate these data with dietary habits, clinical parameters, cytokines, and zonulin concentrations.

2. Materials and Methods

2.1. Selection of Relapsing–Remitting MS Patients and Controls

Relapsing–remitting multiple sclerosis (RRMS) patients, diagnosed according to the Poser and colleagues criteria [42], were selected by the Neurologist from the School of Health Sciences Dr. Paulo Prata, Barretos, Sao Paulo, Brazil. The Ethics Committee on Human Research from the Barretos Educational Foundation approved the present study (Process number 1522.762/2016), and all subjects signed the informed consent in accordance with the Declaration of Helsinki.

A total of 18 RRMS patients, 16 females and 2 males (mean age − standard deviation (SD) = 46.06 − 11.83 years), were included in this study. Eighteen control subjects, age- and-sex-matched, were included as a control group (mean age − SD = 45.50 − 11.03 years). After the consent, all of subjects answered a food frequency questionnaire (FFQ) that was designed by specialized nutritionists. The FFQ included questions concerning dietary habits, such as consumption of vegetables, fruits, carbohydrates, animal-derived proteins, saturated and trans fats, dairy products, and canned products. The options for frequency of consumption in the FFQ was classified as (1) Never consumes; (2) Less than once a month; (3) One to three times a month; (4) Once or twice a week; (5) Three to five times a week; (6) Six to seven times a week. Data were expressed in percentages based on the responses of patients and controls. Thereafter, peripheral blood (8 mL) was collected, and stool samples were requested and delivered within five days.

At enrollment, exclusion criteria for patients and controls included use of antibiotics and laxatives and vaccination in the last 60 days. Chronic diarrhea and gastrointestinal surgeries, such as bariatric, cholecystectomy, and appendectomy, were also considered as exclusion criteria for both groups.

Clinical data from MS patients, such as body mass index (BMI), disease duration, Expanded Disability Status Score (EDSS), presence/absence of gadolinium (Gd)-enhanced brain magnetic resonance imaging (MRI) lesions, and disease-modifying therapies (DMTs) were recorded. The mean body mass index of the MS patients was 26. Three patients reported having systemic arterial hypertension, and two patients reported taking vitamin D. All other patients included in this study reported no other comorbidity. Demographic characteristics and clinical data from RRMS patients are summarized in Table 1.

2.2. Bacterial DNA Extraction, Real-Time PCR, and 16S Sequencing

DNA was extracted from 200 mg of stool samples by using QIAamp DNA Stool Mini Kit (QIAGEN, Hilden, Germany), according to the manufacturer's instructions. DNA was quantified by Nanodrop and adjusted to 5 ng/mL. Primers were specific for *Bacteroides*, *Bifidobacterium*, *Lactobacillus*, *Prevotella*, and *Roseburia* species [43]. Reactions were performed by using Power SYBR Green PCR Master Mix (Applied Biosystems, Life Technologies, Carlsbad, CA, USA), 2 uM of forward/reverse primers, and 5 ng of DNA. For relative quantification, DNA copy numbers from target primers were normalized for the copy numbers of universal primer. The relative abundance was calculated by using the cycle-threshold (Ct) values and was expressed by the relative expression units method (REU) [44], per 200 mg of stool.

Table 1. Demographic and clinical data of the relapsing–remitting multiple sclerosis patients.

Patients	Gender/Age	BMI	Ethnicity	Disease Duration	EDSS	MRI	DMT
MS01	F/59	23.11	Caucasian	21 years	5.0	Gd-	IFN-β-1b
MS02	F/62	19.65	Asiatic	22 years	ND	ND	IFN-β-1b
MS03	F/50	23.33	Afrodescendent	26 years	ND	ND	AZA
MS04	F/26	24.44	Caucasian	3.2 years	4.5	Gd+	GA
MS05	F/69	23.42	Caucasian	7 years	3.0	Gd-	GA
MS06	F/45	34.41	Caucasian	9 years	3.0	Gd+	TER
MS07	F/37	26.67	Caucasian	7 years	4.0	Gd-	IFN-β-1b
MS08	F/33	34.42	Caucasian	10 years	3.0	ND	GA
MS09	F/30	22.98	Caucasian	6 years	3.0	Gd+	FTY720
MS10	F/57	25.39	Caucasian	15 years	ND	ND	FTY720
MS11	M/44	28.40	Caucasian	18 years	4.5	Gd-	IFN-β-1a
MS12	F/37	23.05	Caucasian	13 years	ND	ND	GA
MS13	F/50	23.22	Caucasian	7 years	3.5	Gd+	IFN-β-1a
MS14	F/33	28.00	Caucasian	3 years	4.0	Gd+	IFN-β-1a
MS15	F/47	27.05	Caucasian	7 months	2.5	Gd+	IFN-β-1b
MS16	F/49	23.82	Caucasian	2 years	4.0	Gd+	NAT
MS17	F/56	29.41	Caucasian	12 years	ND	ND	FTY720
MS18	M/45	29.66	Caucasian	7 years	3.0	Gd-	IFN-β-1b

F: Female; M: Male; BMI: Body Mass Index; EDSS: Expanded Disability Status Score; MRI: Magnetic resonance imaging; Gd+: Presence of gadolinium-enhanced brain lesions; ND: not determined; Gd-: Absence of inflammatory active lesions; DMT: Disease-modifying therapy; IFN-β-1b: Interferon-β-1b; AZA: Azathioprine; GA: Glatiramer acetate; TER: Teriflunomide; FTY720: Fingolimod; NAT: Natalizumab.

For bacterial 16S sequencing, DNA was quantified by Quantus fluorometer and adjusted to 5 ng/mL using Tris buffer (10 mM, pH 8.5). V3 and V4 regions of the bacterial 16S [45] were amplified by using bacterial DNA, V3/V4 primers, and the 2X KAPA HiFi HotStart Ready Mix (Kapa Biosystems, MA, USA). PCR purification was performed using AMPure XP Beads Kit (BD Biosciences, San Jose, CA, USA). DNA libraries were constructed according to the Illumina protocols, and sequencing was conducted by an Illumina MiSeq platform system.

2.3. Cytokine Determination by Cytometric Bead Array

After peripheral blood collection (8 mL) in gel tubes with clot activator, samples were incubated for 50 min and then centrifuged at 1372 g for 5 min, 25 °C. Isolated serum samples were stored until cytokine determination. Cytokine detection was performed by using a cytometric bead array (Human Th1/Th2/Th17 Cytokine Kit, BD Biosciences, Franklin Lakes, NJ, USA). Serum levels of IL-2, IL-4, IL-6, IL-10, IL-17A, tumor necrosis factor (TNF), and IFN-γ were determined by flow cytometer FACSCanto™ II (BD Biosciences). Analyses were performed by BDFCAP array™ software, and data were expressed in pg/mL.

2.4. Zonulin Serum Quantification by Sandwich ELISA

Serum samples were isolated from peripheral blood collected in gel tubes with clot activator. After collection, samples were incubated for 50 min, centrifuged at 1372 g for 5 min, and stored until zonulin determination. A human Zonulin ELISA Kit (Elabscience,

MD, USA) was used to quantify zonulin concentrations. Plates were pre-coated with antibodies to human zonulin, and serum samples and standards were incubated for 1 h, 37 °C. Then, incubation with biotinylated detection antibodies and avidin–horseradish peroxidase conjugate was performed for 30 min. Three washing steps followed to remove unbound and free molecules. The substrate solution was added to each well and incubated for 15 min. The enzyme–substrate reaction was blocked by a stop solution, and the color turned yellow. The optical density was measured in a spectrophotometer at 450 nm. A standard curve was constructed, and zonulin concentrations were calculated by converting the obtained optical density in ng/mL.

2.5. Statistical Analyses

Data extracted from the FFQ were analyzed by Pearson's chi-square. Comparisons between relative expression units and cytokines' concentrations in MS patients and controls were performed by a nonparametric Mann–Whitney U test. Zonulin concentrations were analyzed by unpaired t test with Welch's correction, since the data presented < Gaussian distribution. Correlations among the read percentages of the gut microbiota, cytokines, and zonulin concentrations were performed by Spearman's correlation.

We performed analyses of variance and obtained rarefaction curves and diversity indexes by using annotated operational taxonomic units (OTUs). Alpha diversity summarizes the microbial diversity within each sample, and beta diversity measures differences between samples. Sequencing analysis of bacterial 16S was conducted as described in a previous study [46]. p values less than 0.05 were considered statistically significant.

3. Results

3.1. Dietary Habits and Correlations with the Gut Microbiota in RRMS Patients

Since diet plays a significant role in gut microbiota composition, we used an FFQ in order to detect differences in dietary habits between RRMS patients and healthy controls. The interviewees reported daily consumption of vegetables (patients (Pt) = 77.8%; controls (Ct) = 61.1%), fruits (Pt = 44.4%; Ct = 27.8%), carbohydrates (Pt = 61.1%; Ct = 61.1%), animal-derived proteins (Pt = 50.0%; Ct = 27.8%), saturated/trans fats (Pt = 5.5%; Ct = 16.7%), dairy products (Pt = 55.6%; Ct = 72.2%), and canned products (Pt = 0.0%; Ct = 5.5%). We observed significant differences ($p < 0.05$) among intake of vegetables, fruits, carbohydrates, animal-derived proteins, and dairy products when we compared patients and controls. Table 2 summarizes the data obtained from the FFQ, with the frequencies of food consumption per patient and controls and the p values.

To find correlations between dietary habits and gut microbiota composition in RRMS patients, we used the consumption frequencies and the reads percentages detected in stool samples from RRMS patients. We detected significant moderate/strong correlation between vegetables consumption by patients and relative abundance of *Roseburia* ($p = 0.010$; $r = -0.60$). We also found negative correlations between animal-derived protein intake and relative abundance of Verrucomicrobiae/Verrucomicrobiales ($p = 0.041$; $r = -0.50$) and *Bacteroides vulgatus* ($p = 0.014$; $r = -0.58$).

3.2. Detection of Intestinal Dysbiosis and Prevalence of Gram-Negative Bacteria in RRMS Patients

For the purpose to detect intestinal dysbiosis in RRMS patients receiving DMTs, we sequenced the V3/V4 regions from bacterial 16S and determined the alpha and beta diversities by using the annotated operational taxonomic units (OTUs). According to the rarefaction curves, we observed no significant differences ($p = 0.38$) in richness and evenness between samples obtained from RRMS patients and controls (Figure 1A,B). However, when we used the unweighted UniFrac metric with Bonferroni correction, we detected a significant difference ($p = 0.01$) between microbial communities found in RRMS patients and controls (Figure 1D). Figure 1C shows the PcoA plot regarding the weighted UniFrac metric with Bonferroni correction.

Table 2. Description of the dietary habits of multiple sclerosis patients and controls.

Consumption Frequency	N	RRMS (%)	N	Controls (%)	p Value
Vegetables					
Once or twice a week	2	11.1%	2	11.1%	
Three to five days a week	2	11.1%	5	27.8%	$p < 0.001$
Six to seven days a week	14	77.8%	11	61.1%	
Fruits					
One to three times a month	0	0	4	22.2%	
Once or twice a week	0	0	5	27.8%	
Three to five days a week	10	55.6%	4	22.2%	$p = 0.047$
Six to seven days a week	8	44.4%	5	27.8%	
Carbohydrates					
Never consumes	1	5.55%	0	0	
Less than once a month	2	11.1%	0	0	
One to three times a month	0	0	1	5.5%	
Once or twice a week	1	5.5%	3	16.7%	$p < 0.001$
Three to five days a week	3	16.7%	3	16.7%	
Six to seven days a week	11	61.1%	11	61.1%	
Animal-derived proteins					
Never consumes	0	0	1	5.5%	
One to three times a month	1	5.5%	0	0	
Once or twice a week	6	33.4%	8	44.5%	$p < 0.001$
Three to five days a week	2	11.1%	4	22.2%	
Six to seven days a week	9	50.0%	5	27.8%	
Saturated/trans fats					
Never consumes	6	33.4%	2	11.1%	
Less than once a month	2	11.1%	6	33.4%	
One to three times a month	3	16.7%	1	5.5%	
Once or twice a week	4	22.2%	5	27.8%	$p = 0.444$
Three to five days a week	2	11.1%	1	5.5%	
Six to seven days a week	1	5.5%	3	16.7%	
Dairy products					
Never consumes	3	16.7%	1	5.5%	
Once or twice a week	1	5.5%	2	11.1%	
Three to five days a week	4	22.2%	2	11.1%	$p < 0.001$
Six to seven days a week	10	55.6%	13	72.2%	
Canned products					
Never consumes	7	38.9%	3	16.7%	
Less than once a month	5	27.7%	3	16.7%	
One to three times a month	3	16.7%	4	22.2%	$p = 0.083$
Once or twice a week	3	16.7%	7	38.9%	
Six to seven days a week	0	0	1	5.5%	

The consumption of dairy products by patients correlated with the presence of the Bacteroidetes phylum ($p = 0.015$; $r = -0.58$), Bacteroidia/Bacteroidales ($p = 0.011$; $r = -0.60$), Bacteroidaceae/*Bacteroides* ($p = 0.016$; $r = -0.57$), *Bacteroides rodentium* ($p = 0.044$; $r = -0.49$), and *Bacteroides uniformis* ($p = 0.049$; $r = -0.48$). Furthermore, we reported a positive correlation between saturated/trans fat consumption and the abundance of Firmicutes ($p = 0.044$; $r = 0.49$), Clostridia ($p = 0.039$; $r = 0.50$), and Clostridiales ($p = 0.035$; $r = 0.51$).

To compare the microbiota composition in treated RRMS patients and controls, we sequenced the bacterial 16S in stool samples and analyzed specific bacterial groups by real-time PCR. The prevalent phyla in RRMS patients were Firmicutes (patient reads (Pr) = 43.78%; control reads (Cr) = 50.12%) and Bacteroidetes (Pr = 30.52%; Cr = 14.47%), and the prevalent classes were Clostridia (Pr = 39.29%; Cr = 41.15%) e Bacteroidia (Pr = 25.96%; Cr = 11.99%) (Figure 2A,B). The prevalent orders were Clostridiales (Pr = 35.80%; Cr = 37.16%) and Bacteroidales (Pr = 25.96%; Cr = 11.99%), and the prevalent families were Bacteroidaceae

(Pr = 18.86%; Cr = 9.25%), Ruminococcaceae (Pr = 11.35%; Cr = 16.74%), and Lachnospiraceae (Pr = 10.19%; Cr = 6.24%) (Figure 2C,D). The prevalent genera in RRMS patients were *Bacteroides* (Pr = 18.86%; Cr = 9.25%), *Akkermansia* (Pr = 7.35%; Cr = 6.95%), *Blautia* (Pr = 5.18%; Cr = 2.16%), and *Faecalibacterium* (Pr = 4.31%; Cr = 9.91%). The prevalent species in stool samples from RRMS patients were *Akkermansia muciniphila* (Pr = 7.35%; Cr=7.27%), *Bacteroides vulgatus* (Pr = 4.68%; Cr = 1.07%), *Methanobrevibacter smithii* (Pr = 2.99%; Cr = 10.01%), *Bacteroides rodentium* (Pr = 1.95%; Cr = 3.43%), *Blautia coccoides* (Pr = 1.33%; Cr = 2.05%), and *Prevotella copri* (Pr = 1.28%; Cr = 1.09%) (Figure 2E,F). Additionally, we found significant differences ($p < 0.05$) in the relative abundances of Bacteroidetes and Actinobacteria phyla, Bacteroidia, Gammaproteobacteria and Actinobacteriia classes, Bacteroidales, Lactobacillales, and Bifidobacteriales orders, Bacteroidaceae, Ruminococcaceae, Flavobacteriaceae, Porphyromonadaceae, and Bifidobacteriaceae families, *Bacteroides, Flavobacterium, Parabacteroides, Streptococcus, Bifidobacterium* genera, *Bacteroides vulgatus* and *Bifidobacterium stercoris* between samples derived from patients and controls (Figure 2). Interestingly, the *Parabacteroides* genus (Pr = 1.31%; Cr = 0%) was detected only in stool samples from RRMS patients, and the *Bifidobacterium* (Pr = 0%; Cr = 4.59%) and *Enterobacter* (Pr = 0%; Cr = 1.12%) genera were found exclusively in stool samples from controls (Figure 2E).

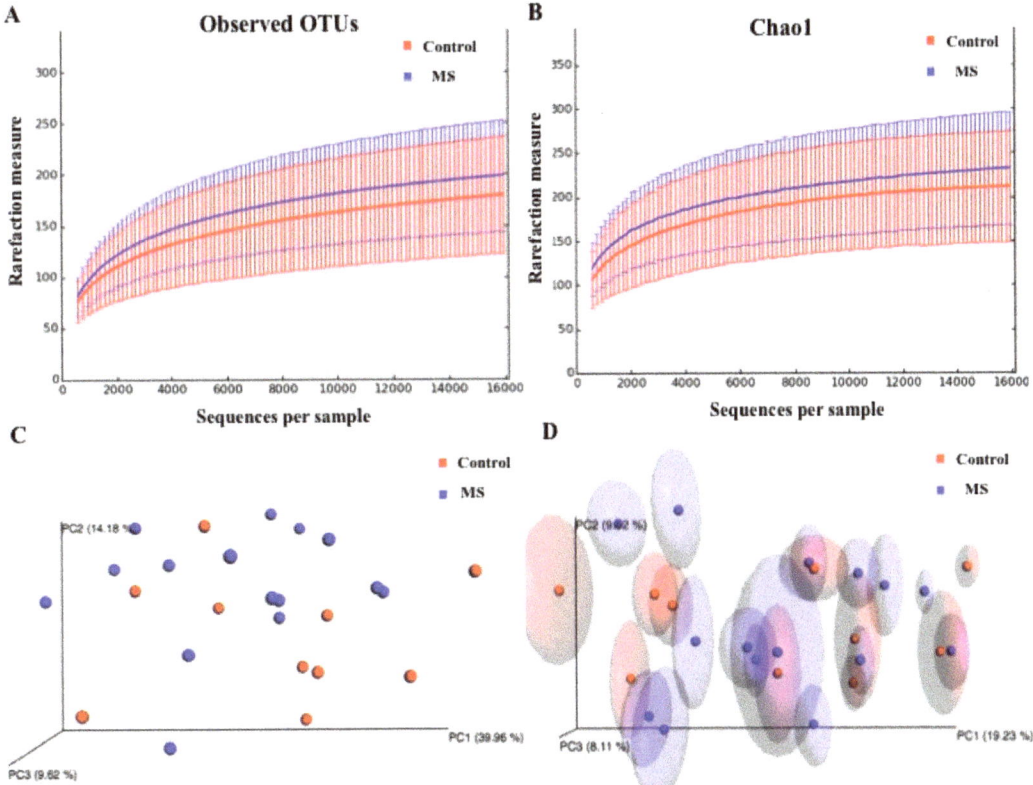

Figure 1. Alpha and beta diversity in the gut microbiota of RRMS patients receiving DMTs and that of healthy controls. Rarefaction curves are a representation of species richness for a given number of individual samples: (**A**) Observed and (**B**) Chao 1-estimated OTUs. Principal component analysis (PcoA) is a transformation of weighted or unweighted Unifrac distance, a pair-wise distance between samples based on the calculation of the shared branches of the phylogenetic tree of the representative rRNA genes from OTUs present in at least one sample: (**C**) PcoA plot with weighted and (**D**) unweighted UniFrac metric with Bonferroni's correction.

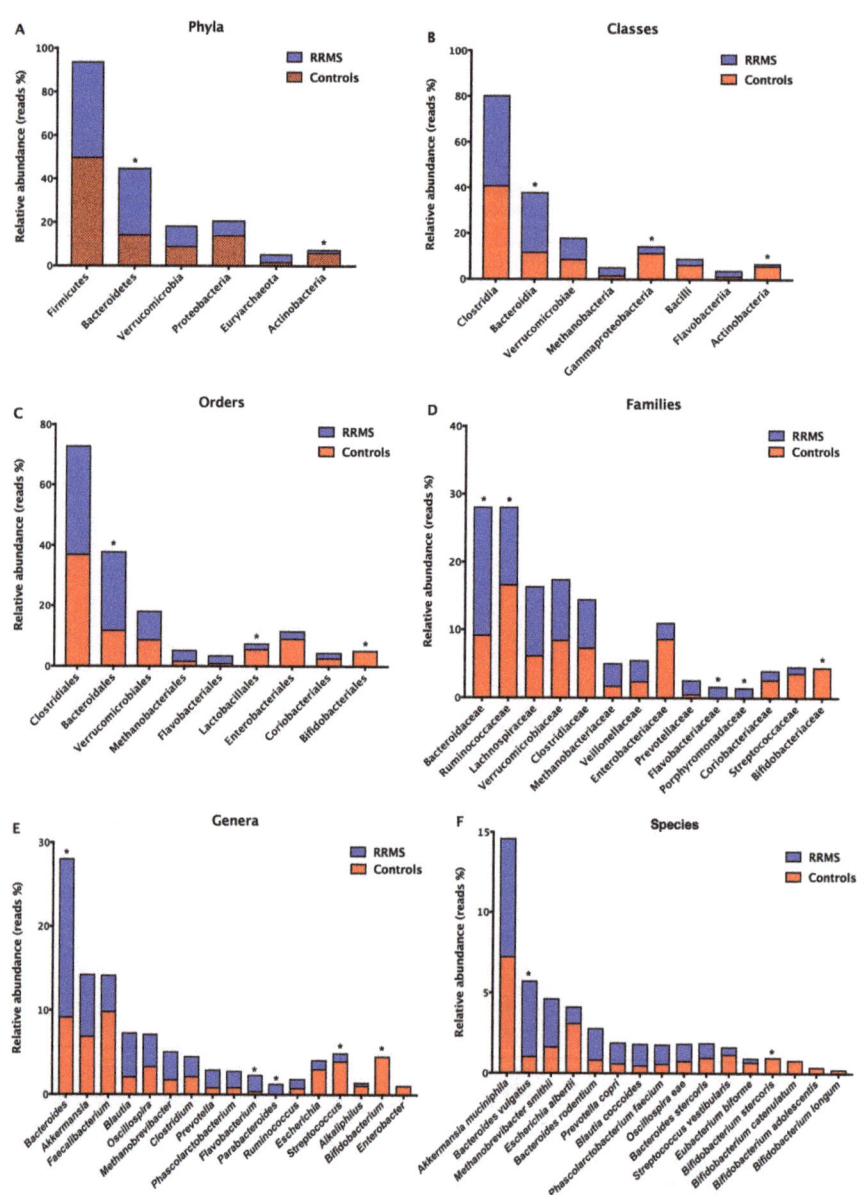

Figure 2. Relative abundances of bacterial taxa in stool samples from RRMS patients and controls. Predominant phyla (**A**), classes (**B**), orders (**C**), families (**D**), genera (**E**), and species (**F**). Bars represent the reads percentages found in metagenomics analyses. * $p < 0.05$.

Regarding the characterization of the gut microbiota by real-time PCR, we observed similar relative expression units ($p > 0.05$) of *Bacteroides*, *Lactobacillus*, *Prevotella*, and *Roseburia* species when we compared patients' and controls' samples (Figure 3). In contrast, we found a significant decrease ($p = 0.036$) in relative expression units of *Bifidobacterium* species detected in stool samples derived from RRMS patients (median = 239.7) compared to controls (median = 7791) (Figure 3B). Moreover, when we classified MS patients based on different DMTs, there were no significant differences ($p > 0.05$) in relative expression units of *Bacteroides*, *Bifidobacterium*, *Clostridium coccoides*, *Clostridium coccoides-Eubacterium rectale*, *Clostridium leptum*, *Lactobacillus*, *Prevotella*, and *Roseburia* in stool samples from MS patients.

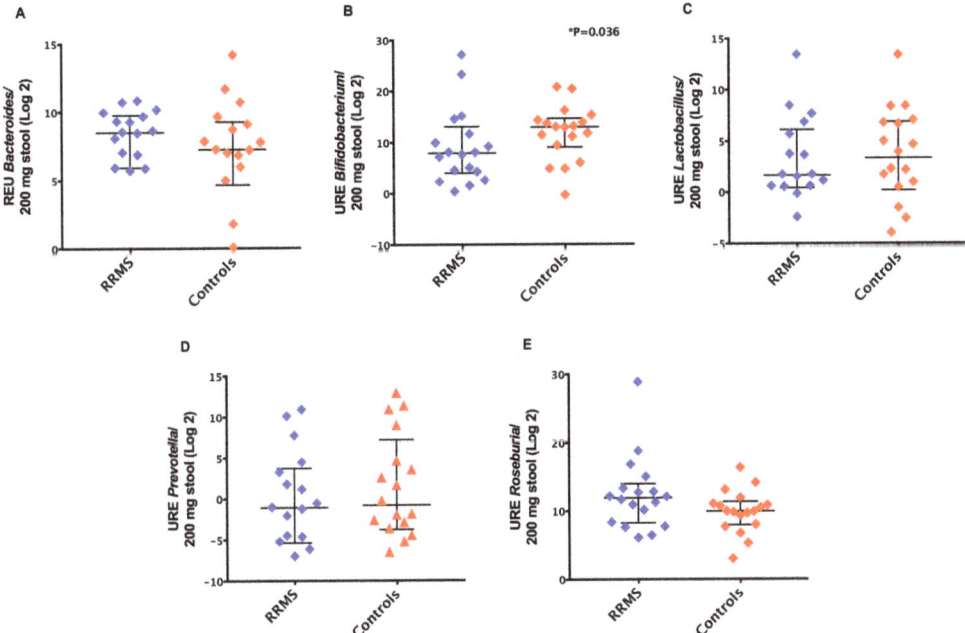

Figure 3. Relative abundance of bacterial community in stool samples from RRMS patients and controls. (**A**) *Bacteroides* species, (**B**) *Bifidobacterium* species, (**C**) *Lactobacillus* species, (**D**) *Prevotella* species, and (**E**) *Roseburia* species. Bars represent the median with interquartile range of relative expression units (REU) per 200 mg of stool.

3.3. Detection of Decreased Pro-Inflammatory IL-6 Cytokine in MS Patients

To determine the serum concentrations of anti- and pro-inflammatory cytokines in RRMS patients, we quantified IL-2, IL-4, IL-6, IL-10, IL-17A, IFN-gamma, and TNF by cytometric bead array. There were no significant differences ($p < 0.05$) in the concentrations of IL-2, IL-4, IL-10, IL-17A, TNF in patients' serum (mean ± standard error IL-2: 0.1867 ± 0.0687 pg/mL; IL-4: 0.3239 ± 0.0743 pg/mL; IL-10: 0.265 ± 0.0429 pg/mL; IL-17A: 2.708 ± 0.8544 pg/mL; TNF: 1.138 ± 0.1372 pg/mL; IFN-gamma: 0.4222 ± 0.1076 pg/mL) when compared with control group (IL-2: 0.4294 ± 0.4051 pg/mL; 233IL-4: 0.2839 ± 0.2244 pg/mL; IL-10: 0.2422 ± 0.18 pg/mL; IL-17A: 4.796 ± 1.43 pg/mL; TNF: 0.7572 ± 0.4383 pg/mL; IFN-gamma: 0.5028 ± 0.158 pg/mL) (Figure 4A–G). IL-6 serum concentrations were decreased ($p = 0.003$) in RRMS patients (0.7261 ± 0.1244 pg/mL) when compared with controls (1.242 ± 0.1601 pg/mL) (Figure 4C). In addition, IL-6 concentrations inversely correlated with Clostridiaceae family members ($p = 0.001$; $r = -0.70$), and TNF levels correlated with Actinobacteria ($p = 0.025$; $r = 0.48$) and *Bacteroides vulgatus* ($p = 0.001$; $r = -0.70$) (Figure 5A–C).

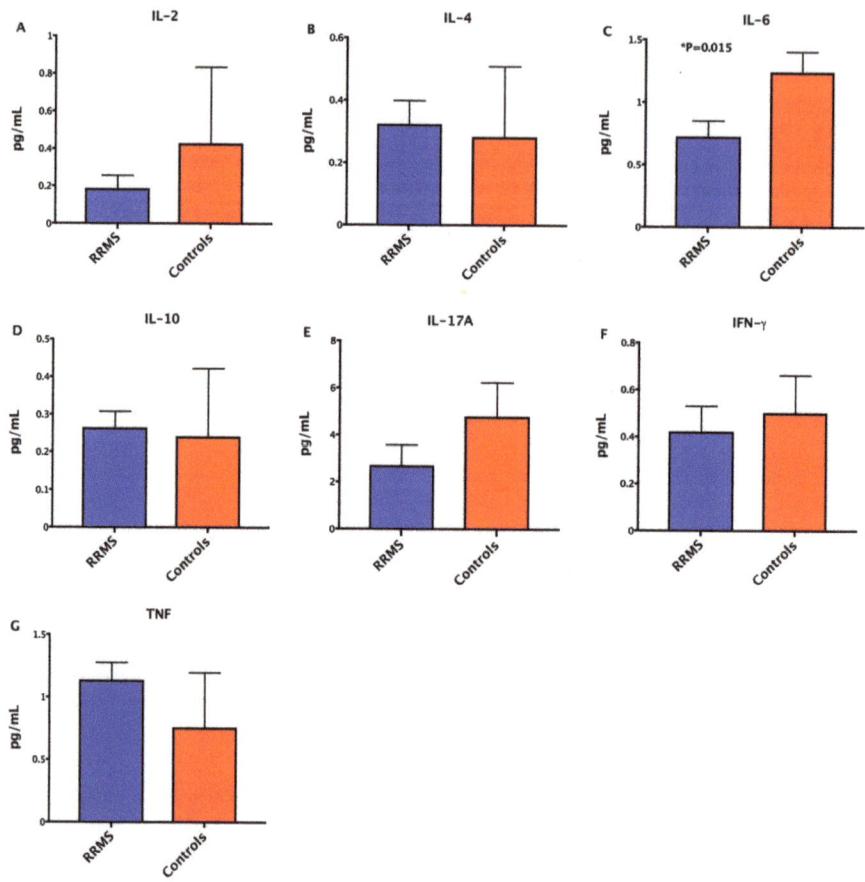

Figure 4. Cytokine profile in treated RRMS patients and control subjects. Serum concentrations of (**A**) IL-2, (**B**) IL-4, (**C**) IL-6, (**D**) IL-10, (**E**) IL-17A, (**F**) IFN-gamma, and (**G**) TNF. Statistical analyses were performed by the Mann–Whitney test. Significance was set at $p < 0.05$.

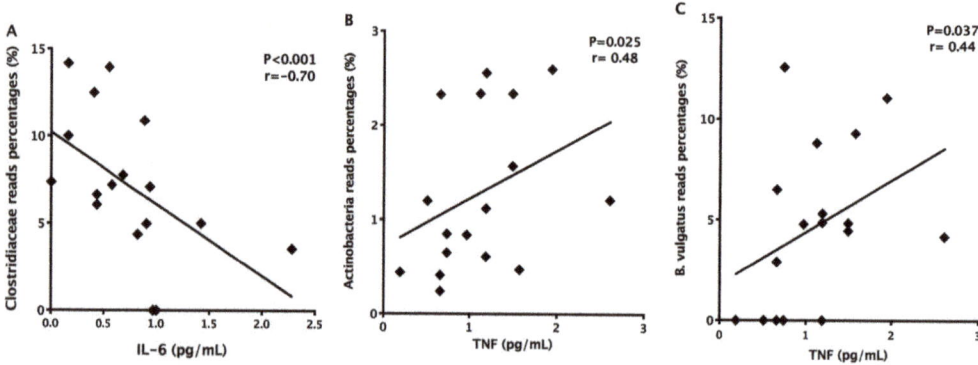

Figure 5. Correlations among relative abundances of bacterial taxa and serum concentrations of inflammatory cytokines. (**A**) Negative correlation between relative abundance of Clostridiaceae and IL-6 concentrations in RRMS patients; (**B**) Positive correlation between relative abundance of Actinobacteria and TNF concentrations; (**C**) Positive correlation between *Bacteroides vulgatus* and TNF concentrations. Statistical analyses were performed by Spearman's test. Significance was set at $p < 0.05$.

3.4. Detection of Increased Intestinal Permeability in RRMS Patients

In order to find whether RRMS patients presented increased intestinal permeability, since alterations in the gut microbiota were detected, we evaluated the serum concentrations of zonulin. Zonulin levels were significantly increased ($p = 0.017$) in MS patients' samples (mean ± standard error: 27.13 ± 2.08 ng/mL) when compared with controls' (mean ± standard error: 19.01 ± 2.98 pg/mL) (Figure 6A). Besides that, zonulin concentrations positively correlated with disease duration ($p = 0.025$; $r = 0.55$; Figure 6B) and with the relative abundance of Bacilli class members ($p = 0.045$; $r = 0.49$; Figure 6C) in MS patients.

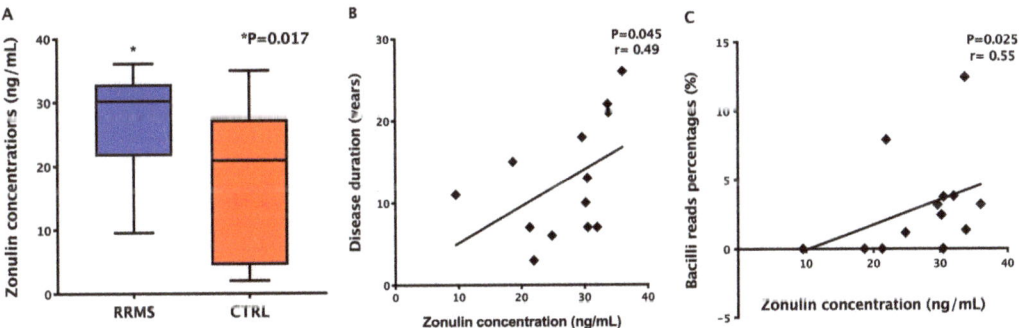

Figure 6. Zonulin concentrations and correlations with clinical data and gut microbiota. (**A**) Serum zonulin concentrations in RRMS patients and controls (CTRL); (**B**) Positive correlation between zonulin concentrations and disease duration; (**C**) Positive correlation between zonulin concentrations and relative abundance of Bacilli class members.

4. Discussion

The dietary habits in industrialized societies have considerable changed in the last years, and concomitant to this changes, the frequency of autoimmune diseases has increased [47]. Western diets include low fiber and high fat consumption, which alters the gut microbiota diversity and function, affecting the mucosal immune system and influencing the development of autoimmune diseases [48]. Berer and colleagues (2018) demonstrated that the supplementation of non-fermentable fiber to transgenic mice of the spontaneous EAE model (opticospinal encephalomyelitis mice) impacted gut microbiota and metabolic profile, increased long-chain fatty acids production, induced polarization to Th2 immune responses, and prevented autoimmune diseases [49]. Furthermore, exercise practice and low-calorie diets based on the consumption of vegetables, fruits, fish, prebiotics, and probiotics induced a decrease in inflammatory mediators and reestablished eubiosis by acting via nuclear receptors [50]. Additionally, Wu and colleagues (2011) showed the influence of diet on the gut microbiota and the prevalence of *Bacteroides* species when animal proteins and saturated fats were consumed, while the presence of *Prevotella* species was associated with carbohydrates and simple sugar intake [51]. In our study, we detected significant differences in the consumption of vegetables, fruits, carbohydrates, animal-derived proteins, and dairy products between patients and controls and, in contrast to Wu et al., we detected an inverse correlation between increased animal-derived protein intake by patients (50% vs. 27.8% in controls) and relative abundance of *Bacteroides vulgatus*. There are no studies evaluating the intestinal microbiota of the Brazilian population as a whole, and it should be noted that the human intestinal microbiota is considered to be variable between individuals and presents geographic variation [52].

Several clinical trials are underway to test the effects of dietary interventions on inflammatory diseases, such as MS (NCT03539094, NCT02580435, NCT04574024, NCT04042415, NCT03451955). So far, protective effects have been proposed for a Mediterranean diet enriched in fibers, vegetables, polyunsaturated fatty acids, and low levels of proteins [51,53]. On the other hand, the consumption of large amounts of milk and derivatives, meat, or animal fats correlates with an increasing prevalence of MS [54]. We detected differences in dairy products consumption between patients and controls, and inverse correlations with Bacteroidetes members, carbohydrate-degrading, Gram negatives bacteria, including *Bacteroides uniformis* [55]. In MS patients, it has been suggested that dysbiosis caused by an inadequate diet may indirectly influence Tregs/Th17 cell balance in the gut mucosa and activate inflammatory pathways, contributing to intestinal and systemic inflammation and MS pathogenesis [56]. Although we detected differences in diet and alterations in the gut microbiota, the levels of inflammatory IL-17 and IFN-γ cytokines, which are involved in MS pathogenesis [57], were similar in patients and controls. However, we detected a significant decrease in IL-6 levels, which are probably associated with DMTs, which impacts the immune response in relapsing–remitting patients [58].

The gut microbiota and the CNS are connected in a bidirectional manner, including neural, endocrine, and immunological interactions [59]. Commensal microbes can interfere with the secretion of neurotransmitters by intestinal cells, stimulate the vagus nerve thus affecting the brain and behavior, produce neuroactive molecules, and modulate mucosal immune cells and systemic populations that can cross the blood–brain barrier (BBB) into the CNS [60]. In turn, the CNS modulates the microbiota by adrenergic signaling and impacts intestinal motility and neurotransmitters actions in immunological cells that shape the gut microbiota composition [60]. Interestingly, a small fraction of metabolites generated by the gut microbiota in response to diet can reach the systemic circulation, cross the blood BBB through vascular epithelial receptors, and modulate CNS inflammation [10,61–63]. Besides that, these metabolites can indirectly act through SCFA receptors in MS patients and through aryl hydrocarbon receptors that influence microglia activation and gene transcription in astrocytes [53,63,64]. In animal models, previous studies showed that germ-free mice with a breakdown of tight-junctions at the BBB had defective permeability, restored when these mice were colonized with conventional microbiota [65]. Therefore, a disbiotic microbiota secretes metabolites that enter the blood stream and impact the development of local and systemic diseases [49]. Moreover, these microbes may influence therapeutic responses by activating or inhibiting exogenous molecules [60].

In the present study, we detected intestinal dysbiosis in RRMS patients receiving DMTs, and our results present some similarities with previous studies in non-treated patients [24–33]. Some of these similarities include decreased *Lactobacillus* spp. (Lactobacillales) and predominance of *Akkermansia muciniphila* and *Methanobrevibacter smithii*, chemilitotrophic specie. *Methanobrevibacter* is involved in inflammatory conditions by recruiting macrophages and activating dendritic cells [66]. *Akkermansia* have immunoregulatory effects by converting mucin into SCFAs [54]; however, they play a role in the degradation of the mucus layer and can promote intestinal inflammation [56]. In addition, we detected a reduced relative abundance of *Bifidobacterium* spp. and Ruminocaceae members including *Faecalibacterium* spp. and *Ruminococcus* spp. *Bifidobacterium* represents one of the first colonizers of the human gut and exerts health-promoting effects [67]. *Faecalibacterium* spp. are butyrate-producing bacteria in the human colon, a bioindicator of human health, and are reduced in inflammatory conditions [68]. *Ruminococcus* spp. re part of the healthy gut microbiota in humans, and some mucus-degrading species are increased in inflammatory diseases [69].

There are few studies evaluating the effect of DMTs on gut microbiota composition, and previous works suggest that these therapies are able to reestablish the gut ecosystem towards a eubiosis condition [19]. Patients on IFN-β or glatiramer acetate treatment showed increased abundance of *Prevotella*, *Sutterella*, and *Prevotella copri* and decreased *Sarcina* species [29,36,37]. In our MS patients, we also observed an increase in *Prevotella* spp. (Bacteroidales) in treated RRMS patients. The *Prevotella* genus is associated with a high-fiber diet and has regulatory roles via butyrate generation [28]. Butyrate has anti-inflammatory effects, induces Tregs in the gut mucosa, and maintains the epithelial barrier [70]. It is important to note that metabolites produced by the gut microbiota are capable of influencing drug bioavailability, pharmacokinetics, and clinical response, which supports the importance of studies on the interaction of the gut microbiota with DMTs [38,39]. In our work, the treated RRMS patients had a different microbiota profile when compared with healthy controls, suggesting that the disbiotic microbiota could interfere with the therapeutic response and with intestinal permeability, which was significantly increased in our patients.

In addition to changes in the gut microbiota, recent studies have associated small intestine rupture with the development of MS, and, based on this, Rahman and colleagues hypothesized that a leaky gut is mechanistically linked to BBB disruption through receptors for zonulin [71]. One of the predictors of intestinal permeability in humans is the serum zonulin level. Zonulin is a physiological modulator of tight junctions involved in the traffic of macromolecules and in the maintenance of epithelial barrier integrity and immune tolerance in the gut mucosa. [72]. A leaky gut in mice induces inflammatory cytokines release that promote an increased permeability, establishing a vicious circle favoring the entry of antigens derived from diet and gut microbes, inducing a tolerance breakdown and the activation of immune cells in the gastrointestinal mucosa [73,74]. The activated immune cells can remain in the gut or migrate to distant organs, including the brain [73–75].

Intestinal dysbiosis can activate the zonulin pathway and stimulate cytokines release allowing the leakage of luminal contents through the epithelial barrier [73]. A study from Camara-Lemarroy and colleagues detected an increase in serum zonulin concentrations in RRMS patients, which positively correlated with BBB disruption, confirmed by positive gadolinium images in MRI [76]. In the present study, we detected a significant increase in serum zonulin concentrations in treated RRMS patients, suggesting that increased gut permeability could be a consequence of the intestinal dysbiosis detected in treated RRMS patients.

5. Conclusions

We conclude that diet plays an important role in the composition of the intestinal microbiota in MS patients and controls. In addition, intestinal dysbiosis, detected in RRMS patients receiving DMTs, could be involved in increased intestinal permeability and affect clinical response, future relapses, and disease progression in MS patients. Additional studies in patients with different forms of MS, using DMTs, in different populations are needed, and the future goal is to predict therapeutic responses based on individual microbiome analyses (personalized medicine) and propose dietary interventions and the use of probiotics or other microbiota modulators as adjuvant therapy to enhance the therapeutic efficacy of DMTs.

Author Contributions: Conceptualization, G.L.V.d.O.; data curation, F.P.P., A.Z.L., N.d.C.R., M.J.U., M.I.G., N.N.C.T., V.S.M., W.P.O., D.G.P., and G.L.V.d.O.; formal analysis, F.P.P., A.Z.L., V.S.M. and G.L.V.d.O.; funding acquisition, N.d.C.R., E.M.J. and G.L.V.d.O.; investigation, F.P.P., A.Z.L., N.d.C.R., M.J.U., M.I.G., V.S.M., and G.L.V.d.O.; methodology, F.P.P., A.Z.L., N.d.C.R., M.I.G., N.N.C.T., V.S.M., W.P.O., D.G.P., and V.S.M.; project administration, E.G. and G.L.V.d.O.; resources, E.G. and G.L.V.d.O.; supervision, D.G.P., E.M.J., E.G. and G.L.V.d.O.; validation, D.G.P., E.G., G.L.V.d.O.; visualization, G.L.V.d.O.; writing—original draft, F.P.P., A.Z.L., and G.L.V.d.O.; writing—review and editing, E.G. and G.L.V.d.O. All authors have read and agreed to the published version of the manuscript.

Funding: This research was funded by the Brazilian governmental agency, Fundação de Amparo à Pesquisa do Estado de São Paulo (FAPESP), grant numbers #2016/50204-0, #2016/05062-2, #2017/04508-0, #2021/03866-5.

Institutional Review Board Statement: The study was conducted according to the guidelines of the Declaration of Helsinki, and approved by the Ethics Committee on Human Research from the Barretos Educational Foundation (protocol code 1522.762/2016; 29 April 2016).

Informed Consent Statement: Informed consent was obtained from all subjects involved in the study.

Conflicts of Interest: The authors declare no conflict of interest.

Abbreviations

Abbreviations

MS: multiple sclerosis; RRMS: relapsing-remitting MS; CNS: central nervous system; MRI: magnetic resonance imaging; PPMS: primary progressive MS; SPMS: secondary progressive MS; HLA: human leucocyte antigens; SCFAs, short-chain fatty acids; EAE: experimental autoimmune encephalomyelitis; IFN: interferon; IL: interleukin; Treg: regulatory T cells; Th: T helper; DMTs: disease modifying therapies; SD: standard deviation; FFQ: food frequency questionnaire; F: female; M: male; BMI: body mass index; EDSS: expanded disability status score; Gd+: presence of gadolinium-enhancement brain lesions; ND: not determined; Gd-: Absence of inflammatory active lesions; AZA: Azathioprine; GA: Glatiramer acetate; TER: Teriflunomide; FTY720: Fingolimod; NAT: Natalizumab; REU: relative expression units; Ct: cycle threshold; TNF: tumor necrosis factor; OTUs: operational taxonomic units; PcoA: principal component analysis; BBB: blood-brain barrier.

References

1. Filippi, M.; Bar-Or, A.; Piehl, F.; Preziosa, P.; Solari, A.; Vukusic, S.; Rocca, M.A. Multiple sclerosis. *Nat. Rev. Dis. Primers* **2018**, *4*, 43. [CrossRef] [PubMed]
2. Dobson, R.; Giovannoni, G. Multiple sclerosis—A review. *Eur. J. Neurol.* **2019**, *26*, 27–40. [CrossRef] [PubMed]
3. McGinley, M.P.; Goldschmidt, C.H.; Rae-Grant, A.D. Diagnosis and Treatment of Multiple Sclerosis: A Review. *JAMA* **2021**, *325*, 765–779. [CrossRef] [PubMed]
4. Hauser, S.L.; Cree, B.A.C. Treatment of Multiple Sclerosis: A Review. *Am. J. Med.* **2020**, *133*, 1380–1390. [CrossRef]
5. Thompson, A.J.; Baranzini, S.E.; Geurts, J.; Hemmer, B.; Ciccarelli, O. Multiple sclerosis. *Lancet* **2018**, *391*, 1622–1636. [CrossRef]
6. Shahi, S.K.; Freedman, S.N.; Mangalam, A.K. Gut microbiome in multiple sclerosis: The players involved and the roles they play. *Gut Microbes* **2017**, *8*, 607–615. [CrossRef]
7. Sassone-Corsi, M.; Raffatellu, M. No Vacancy: How Beneficial Microbes Cooperate with Immunity To Provide Colonization Resistance to Pathogens. *J. Immunol.* **2015**, *194*, 4081–4087. [CrossRef]
8. Chung, H.; Pamp, S.J.; Hill, J.A.; Surana, N.K.; Edelman, S.M.; Troy, E.B.; Reading, N.N.; Villablanca, E.J.; Wang, S.; Mora, J.R.; et al. Gut Immune Maturation Depends on Colonization with a Host-Specific Microbiota. *Cell* **2012**, *149*, 1578–1593. [CrossRef] [PubMed]
9. Hansen, N.W.; Sams, A. The Microbiotic Highway to Health—New Perspective on Food Structure, Gut Microbiota, and Host Inflammation. *Nutrients* **2018**, *10*, 1590. [CrossRef] [PubMed]
10. Rutsch, A.; Kantsjö, J.B.; Ronchi, F. The Gut-Brain Axis: How Microbiota and Host Inflammasome Influence Brain Physiology and Pathology. *Front. Immunol.* **2020**, *11*, 604179. [CrossRef] [PubMed]
11. Burberry, A.; Wells, M.F.; Limone, F.; Couto, A.; Smith, K.S.; Keaney, J.; Gillet, G.; van Gastel, N.; Wang, J.-Y.; Pietilainen, O. C9orf72 suppresses systemic and neural inflammation induced by gut bacteria. *Nature* **2020**, *582*, 89–94. [CrossRef] [PubMed]
12. Blacher, E.; Bashiardes, S.; Shapiro, H.; Rothschild, D.; Mor, U.; Dori-Bachash, M.; Kleimeyer, C.; Moresi, C.; Harnik, Y.; Zur, M. Potential roles of gut microbiome and metabolites in modulating ALS in mice. *Nature* **2019**, *572*, 474–480. [CrossRef]
13. Kuwahara, A.; Matsuda, K.; Kuwahara, Y.; Asano, S.; Inui, T.; Marunaka, Y. Microbiota-gut-brain axis: Enteroendocrine cells and the enteric nervous system form an interface between the microbiota and the central nervous system. *Biomed. Res.* **2020**, *41*, 199–216. [CrossRef] [PubMed]
14. Mittal, R.; Debs, L.H.; Patel, A.P.; Nguyen, D.; Patel, K.; O'Connor, G.; Grati, M.; Mittal, J.; Yan, D.; Eshraghi, A.A. Neurotransmitters: The Critical Modulators Regulating Gut-Brain Axis. *J. Cell Physiol.* **2017**, *232*, 2359–2372. [CrossRef] [PubMed]
15. Dalile, B.; Van Oudenhove, L.; Vervliet, B.; Verbeke, K. The role of short-chain fatty acids in microbiota-gut-brain communication. *Nat. Rev. Gastroenterol. Hepatol.* **2019**, *16*, 461–478. [CrossRef]
16. Camara-Lemarroy, C.R.; Metz, L.M.; Yong, V.W. Focus on the gut-brain axis: Multiple sclerosis, the intestinal barrier and the microbiome. *World J. Gastroenterol.* **2018**, *24*, 4217–4223. [CrossRef] [PubMed]
17. Buscarinu, M.C.; Fornasiero, A.; Romano, S.; Ferraldeschi, M.; Mechelli, R.; Reniè, R.; Morena, E.; Romano, C.; Pellicciari, G.; Landi, A.C. The Contribution of Gut Barrier Changes to Multiple Sclerosis Pathophysiology. *Front. Immunol.* **2019**, *10*, 1916. [CrossRef] [PubMed]
18. Grigg, J.B.; Sonnenberg, G.F. Host-Microbiota Interactions Shape Local and Systemic Inflammatory Diseases. *J. Immunol.* **2017**, *198*, 564–571. [CrossRef] [PubMed]
19. Brown, J.; Quattrochi, B.; Everett, C.; Hong, B.-Y.; Cervantes, J. Gut commensals, dysbiosis, and immune response imbalance in the pathogenesis of multiple sclerosis. *Mult. Scler.* **2020**, *8*, 1–5. [CrossRef] [PubMed]
20. Lee, Y.K.; Menezes, J.S.; Umesaki, Y.; Mazmanian, S.K. Proinflammatory T-cell responses to gut microbiota promote experimental autoimmune encephalomyelitis. *Proc. Natl. Acad. Sci. USA* **2011**, *108* (Suppl. 1), 4615–4622. [CrossRef]
21. Chu, F.; Shi, M.; Lang, Y.; Shen, D.; Jin, T.; Zhu, J.; Chui, L. Gut Microbiota in Multiple Sclerosis and Experimental Autoimmune Encephalomyelitis: Current Applications and Future Perspectives. *Mediat. Inflamm.* **2018**, *2018*, 8168717. [CrossRef] [PubMed]

22. Takata, K.; Kinoshita, M.; Okuno, T.; Moriya, M.; Kohda, T.; Honorat, J.A.; Sugimoto, T.; Kumanogoh, A.; Kayama, H.; Takeda, K. The lactic acid bacterium Pediococcus acidilactici suppresses autoimmune encephalomyelitis by inducing IL-10-producing regulatory T cells. *PLoS ONE* **2011**, *6*, e27644. [CrossRef]
23. Arpaia, N.; Campbell, C.; Fan, X.; Dikiy, S.; van der Veeken, J.; deRoos, P.; Liu, H.; Cross, J.R.; Pfeffer, K.; Coffer, P.J. Metabolites produced by commensal bacteria promote peripheral regulatory T-cell generation. *Nature* **2013**, *504*, 451–455. [CrossRef] [PubMed]
24. Berer, K.; Gerdes, L.A.; Cekanaviciute, E.; Jia, X.; Xiao, L.; Xia, Z.; Liu, C.; Klotz, L.; Stauffer, U.; Baranzini, S.E. Gut microbiota from multiple sclerosis patients enables spontaneous autoimmune encephalomyelitis in mice. *Proc. Natl. Acad. Sci. USA* **2017**, *114*, 10719–10724. [CrossRef] [PubMed]
25. Bhargava, P.; Mowry, E.M. Gut microbiome and multiple sclerosis. *Curr. Neurol. Neurosci. Rep.* **2014**, *14*, 492. [CrossRef] [PubMed]
26. Miyake, S.; Kim, S.; Suda, W.; Oshima, K.; Nakamura, M.; Matsuoka, T.; Chihara, N.; Tomita, A.; Sato, W.; Kim, S.-W. Dysbiosis in the Gut Microbiota of Patients with Multiple Sclerosis, with a Striking Depletion of Species Belonging to Clostridia XIVa and IV Clusters. *PLoS ONE* **2015**, *10*, e0137429. [CrossRef]
27. Cantarel, B.L.; Waubant, E.; Chehoud, C.; Kuczynski, J.; DeSantis, T.Z.; Warrington, J.; Venkatesan, A.; Fraser, C.M.; Mowry, E.M. Gut microbiota in multiple sclerosis: Possible influence of immunomodulators. *J. Investig. Med.* **2015**, *63*, 729–734. [CrossRef] [PubMed]
28. Chen, J.; Chia, N.; Kalari, K.R.; Yao, J.Z.; Novotna, M.; Paz Soldan, M.M.; Luckey, D.H.; Marietta, E.V.; Jeraldo, P.R.; Chen, X. Multiple sclerosis patients have a distinct gut microbiota compared to healthy controls. *Sci. Rep.* **2016**, *6*, 28484. [CrossRef]
29. Jangi, S.; Gandhi, R.; Cox, L.M.; Li, N.; von Glehn, F.; Yan, R.; Patel, B.; Mazzola, M.A.; Liu, S.; Glanz, B.L. Alterations of the human gut microbiome in multiple sclerosis. *Nat. Commun.* **2016**, *7*, 12015. [CrossRef]
30. Cekanaviciute, E.; Pröbstel, A.-K.; Thomann, A.; Runia, T.F.; Casaccia, P.; Katz Sand, I.; Crabtree, E.; Singh, S.; Morrissey, J.; Barba, P. Multiple Sclerosis-Associated Changes in the Composition and Immune Functions of Spore-Forming Bacteria. *mSystems* **2018**, *3*, e00083–18. [CrossRef]
31. Ling, Z.; Cheng, Y.; Yan, X.; Shao, L.; Liu, X.; Zhou, D.; Zhang, L.; Yu, K.; Zhao, L. Alterations of the Fecal Microbiota in Chinese Patients with Multiple Sclerosis. *Front. Immunol.* **2020**, *11*, 590783. [CrossRef] [PubMed]
32. Takewaki, D.; Suda, W.; Sato, W.; Takayasu, L.; Kumar, N.; Kimura, K.; Kaga, N.; Mizuno, T.; Miyake, S.; Hattori, M. Alterations of the gut ecological and functional microenvironment in different stages of multiple sclerosis. *Proc. Natl. Acad. Sci. USA* **2020**, *117*, 22402–12. [CrossRef]
33. Zeng, Q.; Gong, J.; Liu, X.; Chen, C.; Sun, X.; Li, H.; Zhou, Y.; Cui, C.; Wang, Y.; Yang, Y. Gut dysbiosis and lack of short chain fatty acids in a Chinese cohort of patients with multiple sclerosis. *Neurochem. Int.* **2019**, *129*, 104468. [CrossRef]
34. Cosorich, I.; Dalla-Costa, G.; Sorini, C.; Ferrarese, R.; Messina, M.J.; Dolpady, J.; Radice, E.; Mariani, A.; Testoni, P.A.; Canducci, F. High frequency of intestinal TH17 cells correlates with microbiota alterations and disease activity in multiple sclerosis. *Sci. Adv.* **2017**, *3*, e1700492. [CrossRef] [PubMed]
35. Tremlett, H.; Fadrosh, D.W.; Faruqi, A.A.; Hart, J.; Roalstad, S.; Graves, J.; Lynch, S.; Waubant, E.; US Network of Pediatric MS Centers. Gut microbiota composition and relapse risk in pediatric MS: A pilot study. *J. Neurol. Sci.* **2016**, *363*, 153–157. [CrossRef] [PubMed]
36. Castillo-Álvarez, F.; Pérez-Matute, P.; Oteo, J.A.; Marzo-Sola, M.E. The influence of interferon β-1b on gut microbiota composition in patients with multiple sclerosis. *Neurologia* **2018**, S0213-4853, 30158. [CrossRef]
37. Reynders, T.; Devolder, L.; Valles-Colomer, M.; Van Remoortel, A.; Joossens, M.; De Keyser, J.; Nagels, G.; D'hooghe, M.; Raes, J. Gut microbiome variation is associated to Multiple Sclerosis phenotypic subtypes. *Ann. Clin. Transl. Neurol.* **2020**, *7*, 406–419. [CrossRef] [PubMed]
38. Maini Rekdal, V.; Bess, E.N.; Bisanz, J.E.; Turnbaugh, P.J.; Balskus, E.P. Discovery and inhibition of an interspecies gut bacterial pathway for Levodopa metabolism. *Science* **2019**, *364*, eaau6323. [CrossRef]
39. Scher, J.U.; Nayak, R.R.; Ubeda, C.; Turnbaugh, P.J.; Abramson, S.B. Pharmacomicrobiomics in inflammatory arthritis: Gut microbiome as modulator of therapeutic response. *Nat. Rev. Rheumatol.* **2020**, *16*, 282–292. [CrossRef]
40. Weersma, R.K.; Zhernakova, A.; Fu, J. Interaction between drugs and the gut microbiome. *Gut* **2020**, *69*, 1510–1519. [CrossRef] [PubMed]
41. Spanogiannopoulos, P.; Bess, E.N.; Carmody, R.N.; Turnbaugh, P.J. The microbial pharmacists within us: A metagenomic view of xenobiotic metabolism. *Nat. Rev. Microbiol.* **2016**, *14*, 273–287. [CrossRef] [PubMed]
42. Poser, C.M.; Paty, D.W.; Scheinberg, L.; McDonald, W.I.; Davis, F.A.; Ebers, G.C.; Johnson, K.P.; Sibley, W.A.; Silberberg, D.H.; Tourtellotte, W.W. New diagnostic criteria for multiple sclerosis: Guidelines for research protocols. *Ann. Neurol.* **1983**, *13*, 227–231. [CrossRef] [PubMed]
43. Larsen, N.; Vogensen, F.K.; van den Berg, F.W.J.; Nielsen, D.S.; Andreasen, A.S.; Pedersen, B.K.; Al-Soud, W.A.; Sorensen, S.J.; Hansen, L.H.; Jakobsen, M. Gut microbiota in human adults with type 2 diabetes differs from non-diabetic adults. *PLoS ONE* **2010**, *5*, e9085. [CrossRef] [PubMed]
44. Albesiano, E.; Messmer, B.T.; Damle, R.N.; Allen, S.L.; Rai, K.R.; Chiorazzi, N. Activation-induced cytidine deaminase in chronic lymphocytic leukemia B cells: Expression as multiple forms in a dynamic, variably sized fraction of the clone. *Blood* **2003**, *102*, 3333–3339. [CrossRef]
45. Klindworth, A.; Pruesse, E.; Schweer, T.; Peplies, J.; Quast, C.; Horn, M.; Glockner, F.O. Evaluation of general 16S ribosomal RNA gene PCR primers for classical and next-generation sequencing-based diversity studies. *Nucleic Acids Res.* **2013**, *41*, e1. [CrossRef]

46. Leite, A.Z.; de Campos Rodrigues, N.; Gonzaga, M.I.; Paiolo, J.C.C.; de Souza, C.A.; Stefanutto, N.A.V.; Omori, W.P.; Pinheiro, D.G.; Brisotti, J.L.; Matheucci Junior, E. Detection of Increased Plasma Interleukin-6 Levels and Prevalence of Prevotella copri and Bacteroides vulgatus in the Feces of Type 2 Diabetes Patients. *Front. Immunol.* **2017**, *8*, 1107. [CrossRef]
47. Bach, J.-F. The hygiene hypothesis in autoimmunity: The role of pathogens and commensals. *Nat. Rev. Immunol.* **2018**, *18*, 105–20. [CrossRef] [PubMed]
48. Maslowski, K.M.; Mackay, C.R. Diet, gut microbiota and immune responses. *Nat. Immunol.* **2011**, *12*, 5–9. [CrossRef] [PubMed]
49. Berer, K.; Mues, M.; Koutrolos, M.; Rasbi, Z.A.; Boziki, M.; Johner, C.; Wekerle, H.; Krishnamoorthy, G. Commensal microbiota and myelin autoantigen cooperate to trigger autoimmune demyelination. *Nature* **2011**, *479*, 538–541. [CrossRef] [PubMed]
50. Riccio, P.; Rossano, R. Nutrition facts in multiple sclerosis. *ASN Neuro* **2015**, *7*, 1759091414568185. [CrossRef]
51. Wu, G.D.; Chen, J.; Hoffmann, C.; Bittinger, K.; Chen, Y.-Y.; Keilbaugh, S.A.; Bewtra, M.; Knights, D.; Walters, W.A.; Knight, R. Linking long-term dietary patterns with gut microbial enterotypes. *Science* **2011**, *334*, 105–108. [CrossRef] [PubMed]
52. Gupta, V.K.; Paul, S.; Dutta, C. Geography, Ethnicity or Subsistence-Specific Variations in Human Microbiome Composition and Diversity. *Front. Microbiol.* **2017**, *8*, 1162. [CrossRef] [PubMed]
53. Saresella, M.; Marventano, I.; Barone, M.; La Rosa, F.; Piancone, F.; Mendozzi, L.; d'Arma, A.; Rossi, V.; Pugnetti, L.; Roda, G. Alterations in Circulating Fatty Acid Are Associated With Gut Microbiota Dysbiosis and Inflammation in Multiple Sclerosis. *Front. Immunol.* **2020**, *11*, 1390. [CrossRef] [PubMed]
54. Haghikia, A.; Jörg, S.; Duscha, A.; Berg, J.; Manzel, A.; Waschbisch, A.; Hammer, A.; Lee, D.-H.; May, C.; Wilck, N. Dietary Fatty Acids Directly Impact Central Nervous System Autoimmunity via the Small Intestine. *Immunity* **2016**, *44*, 951–953. [CrossRef] [PubMed]
55. Lapébie, P.; Lombard, V.; Drula, E.; Terrapon, N.; Henrissat, B. Bacteroidetes use thousands of enzyme combinations to break down glycans. *Nat. Commun.* **2019**, *10*, 2043. [CrossRef] [PubMed]
56. Esposito, S.; Bonavita, S.; Sparaco, M.; Gallo, A.; Tedeschi, G. The role of diet in multiple sclerosis: A review. *Nutr. Neurosci.* **2018**, *21*, 377–390. [CrossRef] [PubMed]
57. Dendrou, C.A.; Fugger, L.; Friese, M.A. Immunopathology of multiple sclerosis. *Nat. Rev. Immunol.* **2015**, *15*, 545–58. [CrossRef] [PubMed]
58. Vargas, D.L.; Tyor, W.R. Update on disease-modifying therapies for multiple sclerosis. *J. Investig. Med.* **2017**, *65*, 883–91. [CrossRef]
59. Collins, S.M.; Surette, M.; Bercik, P. The interplay between the intestinal microbiota and the brain. *Nat. Rev. Microbiol.* **2012**, *10*, 735–742. [CrossRef]
60. Cox, L.M.; Weiner, H.L. Microbiota Signaling Pathways that Influence Neurologic Disease. *Neurother. J. Am. Soc. Exp. Neurother.* **2018**, *15*, 135–45. [CrossRef]
61. Oldendorf, W.H. Blood brain barrier permeability to lactate. *Eur. Neurol.* **1971**, *6*, 49–55. [CrossRef] [PubMed]
62. Oldendorf, W.H. Carrier-mediated blood-brain barrier transport of short-chain monocarboxylic organic acids. *Am. J. Physiol.* **1973**, *224*, 1450–1453. [CrossRef] [PubMed]
63. Silva, Y.P.; Bernardi, A.; Frozza, R.L. The Role of Short-Chain Fatty Acids From Gut Microbiota in Gut-Brain Communication. *Front. Endocrinol.* **2020**, *11*, 25. [CrossRef] [PubMed]
64. Rothhammer, V.; Borucki, D.M.; Tjon, E.C.; Takenaka, M.C.; Chao, C.-C.; Ardura-Fabregat, A.; Lima, K.A.; Gutiérrez-Vásquez, C.; Hewson, P.; Staszewski, O. Microglial control of astrocytes in response to microbial metabolites. *Nature* **2018**, *557*, 724–728. [CrossRef] [PubMed]
65. Braniste, V.; Al-Asmakh, M.; Kowal, C.; Anuar, F.; Abbaspour, A.; Tóth, M.; Korecka, A.; Bakocevic, N.; Ng, L.G.; Kundu, P. The gut microbiota influences blood-brain barrier permeability in mice. *Sci. Transl. Med.* **2014**, *6*, 263ra158. [CrossRef] [PubMed]
66. Grine, G.; Boualam, M.A.; Drancourt, M. Methanobrevibacter smithii, a methanogen consistently colonising the newborn stomach. *Eur. J. Clin. Microbiol. Infect. Dis.* **2017**, *36*, 2449–2455. [CrossRef] [PubMed]
67. Hidalgo-Cantabrana, C.; Delgado, S.; Ruiz, L.; Ruas-Madiedo, P.; Sánchez, B.; Margolles, A. Bifidobacteria and Their Health-Promoting Effects. *Microbiol. Spectr.* **2017**, *5*, 3.
68. Ferreira-Halder, C.V.; de Sousa Faria, A.V.; Andrade, S.S. Action and function of Faecalibacterium prausnitzii in health and disease. *Best Pract. Res. Clin. Gastroenterol.* **2017**, *31*, 643–648. [CrossRef]
69. Bell, A.; Brunt, J.; Crost, E.; Vaux, L.; Nepravishta, R.; Owen, C.D.; Latousakis, D.; Xiao, A.; Li, W.; Chen, X. Elucidation of a sialic acid metabolism pathway in mucus-foraging Ruminococcus gnavus unravels mechanisms of bacterial adaptation to the gut. *Nat. Microbiol.* **2019**, *4*, 2393–2404. [CrossRef] [PubMed]
70. Furusawa, Y.; Obata, Y.; Fukuda, S.; Endo, T.A.; Nakato, G.; Takahashi, D.; Nakanishi, Y.; Uetake, C.; Kato, K.; Kato, T. Commensal microbe-derived butyrate induces the differentiation of colonic regulatory T cells. *Nature* **2013**, *504*, 446–450. [CrossRef] [PubMed]
71. Rahman, M.T.; Ghosh, C.; Hossain, M.; Linfield, D.; Rezaee, F.; Janigro, D.; Marchi, N.; van Boxel-Dezaire, A.H.H. IFN-γ, IL-17A, or zonulin rapidly increase the permeability of the blood-brain and small intestinal epithelial barriers: Relevance for neuro-inflammatory diseases. *Biochem. Biophys. Res. Commun.* **2018**, *507*, 274–279. [CrossRef] [PubMed]
72. Fasano, A. Zonulin and its regulation of intestinal barrier function: The biological door to inflammation, autoimmunity, and cancer. *Physiol. Rev.* **2011**, *91*, 151–75. [CrossRef] [PubMed]
73. Fasano, A. All disease begins in the (leaky) gut: Role of zonulin-mediated gut permeability in the pathogenesis of some chronic inflammatory diseases. *F1000Research* **2020**, *9*, 9. [CrossRef]

74. El Asmar, R.; Panigrahi, P.; Bamford, P.; Berti, I.; Not, T.; Coppa, G.V.; Catassi, C.; Fasano, A. Host-dependent zonulin secretion causes the impairment of the small intestine barrier function after bacterial exposure. *Gastroenterology* **2002**, *123*, 1607–1615. [CrossRef]
75. Drago, S.; El Asmar, R.; Di Pierro, M.; Grazia Clemente, M.; Tripathi, A.; Sapone, A.; Thakar, M.; Iacono, G.; Carroccio, A.; D'Agate, C. Gliadin, zonulin and gut permeability: Effects on celiac and non-celiac intestinal mucosa and intestinal cell lines. *Scand. J. Gastroenterol.* **2006**, *41*, 408–419. [CrossRef] [PubMed]
76. Olsson, A.; Gustavsen, S.; Hasselbalch, I.C.; Langkilde, A.R.; Sellebjerg, F.; Oturai, A.B.; Sondergaard, H.B. Biomarkers of inflammation and epithelial barrier function in multiple sclerosis. *Mult. Scler. Relat. Disord.* **2020**, *46*, 102520. [CrossRef] [PubMed]

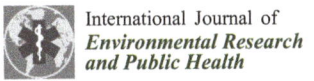

Review

Impact of Food Additive Titanium Dioxide on Gut Microbiota Composition, Microbiota-Associated Functions, and Gut Barrier: A Systematic Review of In Vivo Animal Studies

Emanuele Rinninella [1,*], Marco Cintoni [2], Pauline Raoul [3], Vincenzina Mora [4], Antonio Gasbarrini [3,4] and Maria Cristina Mele [3,5]

1. UOC di Nutrizione Clinica, Dipartimento di Scienze Mediche e Chirurgiche, Fondazione Policlinico Universitario A. Gemelli IRCCS, Largo A. Gemelli 8, 00168 Rome, Italy
2. Scuola di Specializzazione in Scienza dell'Alimentazione, Università di Roma Tor Vergata, Via Montpellier 1, 00133 Rome, Italy; marco.cintoni@gmail.com
3. Dipartimento di Medicina e Chirurgia Traslazionale, Università Cattolica Del Sacro Cuore, Largo F. Vito 1, 00168 Rome, Italy; pauline.raoul1@gmail.com (P.R.); antonio.gasbarrini@unicatt.it (A.G.); mariacristina.mele@unicatt.it (M.C.M.)
4. UOC di Medicina Interna e Gastroenterologia, Dipartimento di Scienze Mediche e Chirurgiche, Fondazione Policlinico Universitario A. Gemelli IRCCS, Largo A. Gemelli 8, 00168 Rome, Italy; vincenzina.mora@policlinicogemelli.it
5. UOSD di Nutrizione Avanzata in Oncologia, Dipartimento di Scienze Mediche e Chirurgiche, Fondazione Policlinico Universitario A. Gemelli IRCCS, Largo A. Gemelli 8, 00168 Rome, Italy
* Correspondence: emanuele.rinninella@unicatt.it; Tel.: +39-06-3015-5579

Abstract: Background: Titanium dioxide (TiO_2) is used as a food additive in pastries, sweets, and sauces. It is recognized as safe by food safety authorities, but in recent years, governments and scientists have raised concerns about its genotoxicity. This systematic review aims to assess the potential associations between food TiO_2 exposure and microbiota composition and functions. Methods: A systematic literature search was performed up to December 2020 in PubMed, Web of Science, and Scopus databases. The PRISMA guidelines followed. The risk of bias was assessed from ARRIVE and SYRCLE tools. Results: A total of 18 animal studies were included (n = 10 mice, n = 5 rats, n = 2 fruit flies, n = 1 silkworm). Studies varied significantly in protocols and outcomes assessment. TiO_2 exposure might cause variations in abundance in specific bacterial species and lead to gut dysfunctions such as a reduction in SCFAs levels, goblet cells and crypts, mucus production, and increased biomarkers of intestinal inflammation. Conclusions: Although the extrapolation of these results from animals to humans remains difficult, this review highlights the key role of gut microbiota in gut nanotoxicology and stimulates discussions on the safe TiO_2 use in food and dietary supplements. This systematic review was registered at PROSPERO as CRD42020223968.

Keywords: dioxide titanium; TiO_2; E171; CI 77891; food additive; gut microbiota; gut barrier; immunity; toxicity; diet

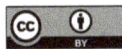

1. Introduction

Titanium dioxide (TiO_2) is one of the main food additives used for its coloring and opacifying properties to improve the appearance and taste of processed foods. Food-grade TiO_2 is found in over 900 food products such as pastries, sauces, ice-creams, candies, chocolates, and chewing gum. In foods, TiO_2 is commonly reported as E171. It is also referred to as CI 77891 when used in cosmetics and toothpaste as a white colorant [1]. E171 consists of a wide range of particle TiO_2 sizes and can contain up to 36% nanosized TiO_2 particles, i.e., less than 100 nm in diameter [2,3]. Compared with their macroscopic counterparts, nanoparticles (NPs) can easier pass through the body's cells and then into the bloodstream and internal organs such as liver, kidney, and lung tissues. Daily, the human dietary exposure dose of TiO_2 NPs can reach one to four micrograms per kilogram body weight per day (μg per kg bw per day) [3]. In 1966, the Food and Drug Administration (FDA) approved the use of food-grade TiO_2 referred to as INS171, specifying that the quantity of TiO_2 must not exceed one percent by weight of the food [4]. In Europe, in 2006, the European Food Safety Authority (EFSA) authorized the use of E171 in food concluding that E171 is safe for consumers, having margins of safety (MoS) of 2.25 mg per kg bw per day [5,6]. However, TiO_2 NPs raise health concerns among the scientific community and governments given their potential to cross the gut barrier and distribute to other organs eliciting immunological response. In June 2018, the EFSA evaluated four new in vivo and in vitro studies [7–10] assessing potential toxicities and reaffirmed the safety of E171 [11]. In April 2019, the French Agency for Food, Environmental and Occupational Health and Safety (ANSES) published a review suggesting a genotoxic and carcinogenic potential even if further in vivo mammalian studies are warranted to confirm or rule out these hypotheses [12]. As requested by the European Commission, EFSA provided urgent scientific and technical review regarding the opinion issued by ANSES [13]. The EFSA concluded that the latest ANSES opinion does not identify any major new findings that would overrule the conclusions made in the previous two scientific opinions in 2016 and 2018. The latest ANSES opinion reiterated the previously identified uncertainties and emphasized that there was still not enough data available to carry out a proper assessment of the risks associated with the food use of E171. EFSA considered this recommendation should be revisited once the ongoing work on the physicochemical characterization of E171 will be completed. In January 2020, France has adopted a decree to ban the use of E171 in foods as a precautionary measure to protect consumers' health.

In a scientific context of "microbiota revolution", potential health risks of TiO_2 NPs and their impact on the intestinal tract and the gut microbiota are increasingly being studied. Gut microbiota is composed of millions of bacterial species that bi-directionally interact with the host in the intestinal tract, regulating the development of immune cells. Alterations in the abundance and composition of intestinal microbiota, known as dysbiosis, are associated with host health such as brain function, lipid metabolism, immune responses, and development of diseases [14]. Recent studies reported adverse effects of in vitro exposure of intestinal epithelial cells to E171 [9,15,16]. Indeed, TiO_2 NPs could damage microvilli structure and alter epithelial integrity [17,18]. TiO_2 NPs can be internalized and can cross the epithelial barrier to enter the bloodstream and potentially affect the function of distant organs, such as the liver [19]. Moreover, in vitro, NPs have the potential to negatively affect intestinal functions and gut homeostasis associated with gut microbiota [20]. New evidence from numerous recent animal studies has emerged highlighting the effects of various physiological doses of TiO_2 NPs on gut microbiota composition and gut homeostasis. Such evidence has not yet been systematically reviewed. Hence, we sought to systematically review current evidence from in vivo animal models to disentangle the TiO_2 effects on the gut microbiome composition and functions.

2. Methods

This systematic review is structured following the general principles published in the Preferred Reporting Items for Systematic Reviews and Meta-Analyses (PRISMA) guidelines [21]. The PRISMA checklist was detailed in Table S1. Full details of the search strategies were specified and documented in a protocol that was registered at PROSPERO (https://www.crd.york.ac.uk/PROSPERO; accessed on 24 December 2020) as CRD42020223968.

2.1. Eligibility Criteria

The eligibility criteria are outlined using the PICOS format (Table 1).

Table 1. PICOS criteria for inclusion of studies.

Criteria	Definition
Participants	Adult animals
Exposure	TiO_2 NPs (rutile or anastase forms, with any size of nanoparticles)
Comparator	Any comparator
Outcomes	Primary outcomes - Between-group differences in α diversity of fecal microbiota at the end of the intervention: total number of observed operational taxonomic units (OTUs); Chao1 index; Shannon diversity index; Simpson diversity index; - Between-group differences in abundances of bacterial groups such as *Bifidobacterium* spp.; *Lactobacillus* spp.; *Akkermansia muciniphila*; *Faecalibacterium prausnitzii*; and *Ruminococcus bromii*. Secondary outcomes - Between-group differences in fecal SCFAs, Muc-2 gene expression, fasting blood glucose levels, lipid metabolism (such as LPS, HDL, LDL, and cholesterol levels); - Between-group differences in the inflammatory response (such as TNFα, IL-1α, IL-6, IL-10 levels, CD8+ T cells, CD4 + T cells, reg T cells production)
Study design	Peer-reviewed original animal experimental studies

The exclusion criteria were the following: (1) Non-English articles; (2) in vitro models; (3) review articles; (4) not fulfilling the inclusion criteria.

2.2. Data Sources and Search Strategy

The search was carried out on 1 December 2020 using three electronic databases, MEDLINE (via PubMed), ISI Web of Science, and Scopus. Multiple search terms are used including the microbiome, microflora, intestinal microbiota, gut microbiota, titanium dioxide, TiO_2, and E171. The search string for each database is described in Table S2. Hand searching of eligible studies was done to find studies that may not have been found in the databases.

2.3. Study Selection

The study selection process was independently carried out by two reviewers (P.R.; E.R.). All articles generated from the electronic search were imported into Mendeley© (Elsevier, Amsterdam, The Netherlands), a references management software, and duplicates were removed. Titles and abstracts were screened for eligibility based on inclusion criteria. All titles assessed as ineligible were excluded. Differences in judgment during the selection process between the two reviewers were settled by discussion and consensus.

2.4. Data Extraction and Reporting

After full-text analysis, the following information was extracted from the included articles: title, author information, year of publication, type of study performed, assessed outcome/s, the animal model used, animal gender, age, and weight at baseline, administered dose, length of study, administration route, and main conclusions.

Data was reported using an Excel© (Microsoft Office, Redmond, WA, USA) spreadsheet specifically developed for this study. Each full-text article was retrieved, and any ineligible articles were excluded from the reasoning reported. Differences in judgment between two reviewers (P.R.; E.R.) were settled by discussion and consensus.

2.5. Quality Assessment

The quality of the included studies was assessed following the Animal Research Reporting of In Vivo Experiments (ARRIVE) guidelines [22]. These guidelines consist of the minimum information that animal research studies should include such as the number and specific characteristics of animals, details of housing and husbandry, experimental and statistical methods, reporting and interpretation of the results.

Moreover, SYRCLE's risk of bias tool [23] was used to assess the risk of bias of animal studies. SYRCLE's tool is an adapted version of the Risk of Bias tool provided by the Cochrane Collaboration. It consists of ten entries associated with selection bias, performance bias, detection bias, attrition bias, reporting bias, and other biases. Quality assessment was independently performed by two reviewers (P.R. and E.R.) and a consensus should be reached for discrepancies.

3. Results

3.1. Study Selection

The flow diagram in Figure 1 displays the results of the literature search and study selection process. A total of 6254 studies were initially identified. After duplicate removal, 4915 studies remained for titles and abstracts screening. Thirteen studies were excluded for the following reasons: in vitro studies (n = 8) [9,19,24–29], no assessment outcomes of interest (n = 1) [30], microbiota of mussel hemolymph (n = 1) [31], review (n = 1) [32], Chinese language (n = 1) [33], TiO_2 and bisphenol A co-exposure (n = 1) [34]. Eighteen studies [8,35–51] were identified for inclusion in the systematic review.

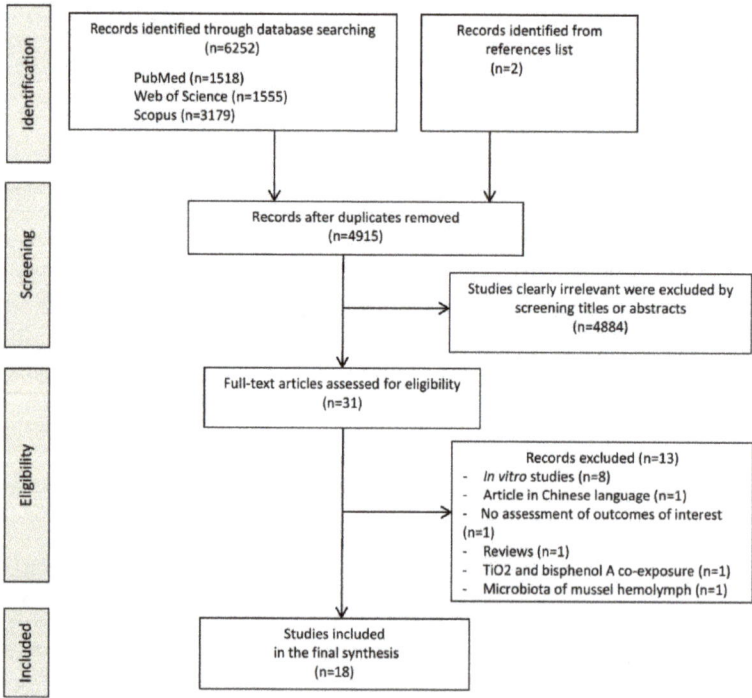

Figure 1. Preferred reporting items for systematic reviews and meta-analyses (PRISMA) flow diagram.

3.2. Study Characteristics

Included studies used different animal models: C57BL/6J mice (n = 5) [44,45,47,50,51], Sprague-Dawley rats (n = 3) [36,37,43], C57BL/6 (n = 3) [35,39,40], Wistar rats (n = 2) [8,48], Drosophila Melanogaster (n = 2) [42,46], CD-1 mice (n = 1) [38], ICR mice (n = 1) [49], and *Bombyx mori* (n = 1) [41]. Sample size ranged from 8 [43] to 80 animals [38]. Dose exposure ranged from 2 mg/day/kg body weight of TiO_2 NPs [36,37,42,45] to 1 g/day/kg body weight of TiO_2 NPs [39] and exposure period ranged from 24 h [39] to 100 days [8]. The characteristics of each included study are detailed in Table 2.

Table 2. Characteristics of included animal studies (listed by animal type).

Animal Species	First Author, Year	Sex	Age *	Weight *	Sample Size	TiO$_2$ Particules Type and Size	Dose Exposure and Administration Route	Duration of Exposure	Significant Compositional Changes of Gut Microbiota (Compared with the Control Group)	Significant Effects on Microbiota-Associated Functions (Compared with the Control Group)
Mice Obese and non-obese C57BL/6	Cao, 2020 [45]	M	6 weeks	n.r.	N = 20 • low-fat diet (control) n = 5 • high fat diet n = 5 • high-fat diet + E171 n = 5 • high-fat diet + TiO$_2$ NPs n = 5	E171, 112 nm TiO$_2$ NPs, 33 nm	0.1 weight percent	8 weeks	In mice treated with TiO$_2$ NPs + high-fat diet: • ↑ Firmicutes • ↓ Actinobacteria and Bacteroidetes • ↓ Bifidobacterium, Allobaculum, Lactobacillus • ↑ Oscillospira	In mice treated with TiO$_2$ NPs + high-fat diet: • ↓ SCFAs production • Loss of goblet cells and crypts • ↑ IL-12 • ↑ IL-17
Mice CD-1 (ICR)	Duan, 2010 [38]	F	n.r.	22 ± 2 g	N = 80 • control group (n = 20) • 62.5 mg/kg bw TiO$_2$ (n = 20) • 125 mg/kg bw TiO$_2$ (n = 20) • 250 mg/kg bw TiO$_2$ (n = 20)	Anatase TiO$_2$ NPs 5 nm	62.5, 125, 250 mg/kg bw/day TiO$_2$ NPs via intragastric administration	30 days		• ↑ IL-2 activity in the exposed groups in a dose-dependent manner • ↓ CD3, CD4, and CD8 in the group treated with 250 mg/kg bw TiO$_2$ • ↓ B cells and NK cells in all exposure groups
Mice C57/BL/6	Kurtz, 2020 [39]	F	7–8 weeks	n.r.	N = 48 • control group (n = 16) • TiO$_2$ NPs (n = 32)	TiO$_2$ NPs with irregular shapes	1 g/kg bw TiO$_2$ NPs by oral gavage	24 h, 48 h, 7 days, and 14 days	• ↑ Firmicutes in the ileum at 14 days post-exposure • ↓ Lactobacillus spp. at 24 h	• ↑ SCFAs production in stools • Higher body weight • ↑ mucus production from 48 h post gavage to 7 days • ↑ IL-4 levels at 24 h
Mice C57BL/6	Li, 2018 [40]	M	8 weeks	22–26 g	N = 30 • control group (n = 10) • rutile TiO$_2$ NPs (n = 10) • anatase TiO$_2$ NPs (n = 10)	Anatase NPs in water 20.13 ± 0.18 nm Rutile NPs in water 15.91 ± 0.05 nm	100 mg/kg bw/day by oral gavage	28 days	• No decrease in overall microbiota diversity (Chao1 index, Shannon index, Simpson diversity index) • Shift of microbiota composition in a time-dependent manner • ↑ Proteobacteria by rutile TiO$_2$ NPs but not by anatase TiO$_2$ NPs • ↑ Prevotella by both TiO$_2$ NPs • ↑ Rikukococcus, Escherichia-Shigella by rutile TiO$_2$ NPs • ↑ Bacteroides, Akkermansia by anatase TiO$_2$ NPs	In rutile TiO$_2$ NPs-exposed mice: • Longer intestinal villi • Irregular arrangement of villus epithelial cells.
Mice C57BL/6J	Mu, 2019 [44]	F	3 weeks	n.r.	N = 20 • control group (n = 5) • NP10 (n = 5) • NP50 (n = 5) • NP100 (n = 5)	TiO$_2$ NPs were added to the diet as an ingredient in the feed preparation process NP10: anatase; 10 nm NP50: anastase 50 nm NP100: anatase 100 nm	Diet containing 0.1% TiO$_2$ NPs	3 months	• No significant bacterial diversity changes • ↑ Bacteroidetes in NP10 and NP50 treatment groups • ↑ Actinobacteria in NP10 and NP50 treated groups • ↓ Lactobacillus and Bifidobacterium in NP10 and NP50 treatment groups	• Lower body weight in mice fed with NP10 and NP50 for 3 months • ↑ LCN2 levels in stools (a marker for intestinal inflammation) in NP10 and NP50-treated groups • Aggravation of DSS-induced chronic colitis • Aggravation of immune response • CD4 + T cells, regulatory T cells, and macrophages

Table 2. Cont.

Animal Species	First Author, Year	Sex	Age *	Weight *	Sample Size	TiO$_2$ Particles Type and Size	Dose Exposure and Administration Route	Duration of Exposure	Significant Compositional Changes of Gut Microbiota (Compared with the Control Group)	Significant Effects on Microbiota-Associated Functions (Compared with the Control Group)
Mice C57BL/6Jausb	Pinget, 2019 [45]	M	5–6 weeks	n.r.	N = 24 • control group (n = 6) • 2 mg TiO$_2$/kg bw/day (n = 6) • 10 mg TiO$_2$/kg bw/day (n = 6) • 50 mg TiO$_2$/kg bw/day (n = 6)	TiO$_2$ NPs, 28 to 1158 nm	2, 10, 50 mg TiO$_2$/kg bw/day orally administrated via drinking water	3 weeks	• Limited variations of bacterial diversity (Simpson, Shannon analyses), bacterial richness, and evenness in all exposed groups (although these trended toward a decrease with increasing dose of TiO$_2$) • ↑ *Parabacteroides* in TiO$_2$-treated mice, at a dose of 50 mg TiO$_2$/kg bw/day • ↑ *Lactobacillus* and *Allobaculum* in all exposed groups • ↓ *Adlercreutzia* and unclassified *Desulfovibrio* in mice treated with TiO$_2$ at the doses of 10 and 50 mg TiO$_2$/kg bw/day	In mice treated with 50 mg TiO$_2$/kg bw/day: • ↓ SCFAs • ↓ TMA • ↓ crypt length In mice treated with 10 and 50 mg TiO$_2$/kg bw/day: • ↓ MUC2 gene expression • ↑ expression of the β defensin gene • infiltration of CD8+ T cells • ↑ production of macrophages (CD45 + F4/80 + CD8 - Ly6 g - lab +CD11b+ CD1f0-) • ↑inflammatory cytokines (IL-6, TNF-α and IL-10)
Mice Wild-type (C57BL/6) and NLRP3-deficient	Ruiz, 2016 [47]	F	12–14 weeks	n.r.	N = 56 WT mice (n = 36) • water (n = 12) • 50 mg/day/kg body weight of TiO$_2$ NPs (n = 12) • 500 mg/day/kg body weight of TiO$_2$ NPs (n = 12) NLRP3-deficient mice (n = 20) • water (n = 10) • 500 mg/day/kg body weight of TiO$_2$ NPs (n = 10)	Suspension of TiO$_2$, rutile NPs, 30–50 nm	50 and 500 mg/day/kg bw of rutile TiO$_2$ NPs by oral gavage	8 days		• TiO$_2$ NPs enhance intestinal inflammation in the DSS mouse model of colitis. • TiO$_2$ proinflammatory effects required NLRP3 inflammasome activation when comparing WT with NLRP3-deficient mice
Mice ICR	Yan, 2020 [46]	M	Adult	18–20 g	N = 28 • control group (n = 7) • 10 mg/kg bw/day TiO$_2$ NPs (n = 7) • 40 mg/kg bw/day TiO$_2$ NPs (n = 7) • 160 mg/kg bw/day TiO$_2$ NPs (n = 7)	Anatase TiO$_2$ NPs, 20 nm	10, 40, 160 mg/kg bw/day by oral gavage	28 days	• ↑ Firmicutes in all exposed groups • ↓ Verrucomicrobia in all exposed groups • ↓ Bacteroidetes at 160 mg/kg bw/day TiO$_2$ • ↓ *Barnesiella* in all exposed groups in a dose-dependent manner • ↓ *Akkermansia* genus and *Porphyromonadaceae* family	• ↑ TG and glucose levels in the exposed group with 160 mg/kg bw/day TiO$_2$ • ↑ LPS levels in all exposed groups • ↑ IL-1α levels in the exposed group with 160 mg/kg bw/day TiO$_2$ • ↑ IL-6 levels in all exposed groups • ↑ TNF-α levels in the exposed groups treated with 40 and 160 mg/kg/day TiO$_2$ • ↑ PKC protein at 40 mg/kg • Elevated TLR4 protein levels in the 40 and 160 mg/kg groups and P-P65 in all exposed groups • ↓ MUC2 expression at 160 mg/kg • ↓ intestinal mucus thickness in all exposed groups
Mice C57BL/6J	Zhang, 2020 [50]	M	7 weeks	20–24 g	N = 30 • control group (n = 15) • TiO$_2$ NPs (n = 15)	TiO$_2$ NPs, 21 nm	150 mg/kg bw/day by intragastric administration	30 days	- ↓ Richness and evenness of gut microbiota (decreased Shannon's diversity, Chao, observed species and elevated Simpson's diversity) • ↑ Proteobacteria	• No changes in body weight • Abnormal excitement on the enteric neurons • ↑ expression of TuJ1 (a neuronal marker of the peripheral nervous system) • No changes of IL-6 and IL-1β in the gut tissues

Table 2. Cont.

Animal Species	First Author, Year	Sex	Age	Weight	Sample Size	TiO$_2$ Particles Type and Size	Dose Exposure and Administration Route	Duration of Exposure	Significant Compositional Changes of Gut Microbiota (Compared with the Control Group)	Significant Effects on Microbiota-Associated Functions (Compared with the Control Group)
Mice C57BL/6J	Zhu, 2020 [55]	F	4–5 weeks	n.r.	N = 24 • control fed with CHOW diet (n = 6) • TiO$_2$ NPs fed with CHOW diet (n = 6) • control fed with HFD (n = 6) • TiO$_2$ NPs fed with HFD (n = 6)	TiO$_2$ NPs, 30 ± 7 nm	10 μL/g bw/day via oral gavage	8 weeks	• ↑ Firmicutes to Bacteroidetes ratio in TiO$_2$ NPs treated mice fed with HFD compared with both CHOW group and controls • ↑ Desulfovibrionaceae in TiO$_2$ NPs treated mice fed with CHOW or HFD compared with controls • ↑ Ruminococcaceae in TiO$_2$ NPs treated mice fed with CHOW diet or HFD compared with controls • ↑ Lachnospiraceae in TiO$_2$ NPs treated mice fed with CHOW controls	• ↓ crypt length in TiO$_2$ groups compared with controls • ↑ muc2 expression in TiO$_2$ groups compared with controls • ↓ MUC2 proteins levels in TiO$_2$ groups compared with controls • ↑ LPS levels in TiO$_2$ groups compared with controls with a significant increase in TiO$_2$ mice fed HFD compared with TiO$_2$ mice fed CHOW. • ↑ IL-1β, IL-6, and TNFα in TiO$_2$ groups compared with controls with a significant increase in TiO$_2$ mice fed HFD compared with TiO$_2$ mice fed CHOW
Rats Wistar	Bettini, 2017 [6]	M	adult	175–200 g	First series of experiments N = 30 • control group (n = 10) • food-grade E171 (n = 10) • NM-105 (n = 10) Second series of experiments N = 34 • water (n = 11) treated with DMH • food-grade E171 (n = 11) treated with DMH • control (n = 12) water only	NM-105: TiO$_2$ NPs, 105 nm	10 mg/kg bw/day by intragastric gavage 10 mg/kg bw/day TiO$_2$ NPs through drinking water	7 days 100 days		• No changes in epithelium permeability • Accumulation of dendritic cells in the immune cells of Peyer's patches regardless of the TiO$_2$ treatment • ↓ regulatory T cells • ↑ IL8, IL10, TNFα in food-grade E171 group after 100 days • At 7 days, no intestinal inflammation in E171 and NM-105 groups • Initiation of colon inflammation and pre-neoplastic lesions in the 100-day E171 group.
Rats Sprague-Dawley	Chen, 2019 [56]	M	3 weeks	n.r.	N = 12 • control group (n = 6) • TiO$_2$ NPs (n = 6)	Anatase TiO$_2$ NPs, 29 ± 9 nm	2, 10, 50 mg/kg bw/day TiO$_2$ NPs via oral gavage	30 days	• ↑ L. gasseri in the high-dose group • ↑ Turicibacter in the low-dose group • ↑ L. NK4A136_group in the medium-dose group • ↓ Veillonella in all exposure groups	• Increase of N-acetylhistamine, caprolactam, and glycerophosphocholine • ↓ 4-methyl-5-thiazoleethanol, L-histidine, and L-ornithine • No significant changes in SCFAs levels • ↑ LPS production • ↑ IL-6 in the high-dose group • ↑ intestinal oxidative stress and inflammatory response
Rats Sprague-Dawley	Chen, 2020 [57]	M	3 weeks	n.r.	N = 12 • control group (n = 6) • TiO$_2$ NPs (n = 6)	Anatase TiO$_2$ NPs, 29 ± 9 nm	2, 10, 50 mg/kg bw/day TiO$_2$ NPs via oral gavage	90 days		• No significant changes in SCFAs levels • ↓ TG levels in medium and high-dose groups • Significant serum lipophilic metabolites changes in the high-dose group with ↑ phosphatidylcholines and ↓ lysophosphatidylcholine and glycerophosphocholine levels • ↓ activity of the antioxidant enzyme SOD

Table 2. Cont.

Animal Species	First Author, Year	Sex	Age *	Weight *	Sample Size	TiO$_2$ Particles Type and Size	Dose Exposure and Administration Route	Duration of Exposure	Significant Compositional Changes of Gut Microbiota (Compared with the Control Group)	Significant Effects on Microbiota-Associated Functions (Compared with the Control Group)
Rats Pregnant Sprague-Dawley	Mao, 2019 [42]	F	12 weeks	n.r.	N = 8 • control group (n = 4) • TiO$_2$ NPs (n = 4)	TiO$_2$ NPs, 21 nm	5 mg/kg bw/day of TiO$_2$ NPs	from the 5th to 18th day after pregnancy	• No significant changes of alpha-diversity (although the increasing trend in Shannon, and a significant change in Simpson index but no difference in Chao1) • ↓ *Ellin60*7 at GD 10 and GD 17 • Increase of *Clostridiales* at GD 10 • ↓ *Debalobacteriaceae* at GD 17	• ↑ fasting blood glucose levels at GD 10 and GD 17 after exposure. • Strengthened genes about type 2 diabetes mellitus related function and lipid biosynthesis in the exposure group • Weakened taurine and hypotaurine metabolism in the exposure group
Rats Wistar	Talbot, 2018 [43]	M	Adult	175–200 g	First series of experiments N = 24 • control group (n = 8) • food-grade E171 (n = 8) • NM-105 (n = 8) Second series of experiments N = 30 • water (n = 10) • food-grade E171 (n = 10) • NM-105 (n = 10)	Food-grade E171, TiO$_2$, 364 nm NM-105: TiO$_2$ NPs, 105 nm	0.1 mg/kg bw./day intragastric ga-vage 10 mg/kg bw/day through the drinking water	7 days 60 days		• No impact on the overall caecal composition of SCFAs (irrespectively of TiO$_2$) • No effect on mucin O-glycosylation (irrespectively of TiO$_2$) • Absence of mucus barrier impairment irrespectively of TiO$_2$)
Fruit flies *Drosophila*	Liu, 2016 [44]	F	n.r.	n.r.	N = 45	10, 50, and 100 nm TiO$_2$ NPs	1, 2 mg/mL and 200 mg/mL dietary TiO$_2$ NPs of 3 different sizes	5 days	• No inhibition of the growth of symbiotic bacteria in the gut of *Drosophila* larva or adults	• No alteration of pupation cycle • No alteration of weight and lipid levels
Fruit flies *Drosophila Melanogaster*	Richter, 2018 [45]	n.r.	2 to 6 days	n.r.	N = 24 • control group (n = 6) • 5 ppM TiO$_2$ NPs (n = 6) • 50 ppM TiO$_2$ NPs (n = 6) • 500 ppM TiO$_2$ NPs (n = 6)	TiO$_2$ NPs, 30 nm	5 ppm, 50 ppm, 500 ppm of TiO$_2$ NPs suspended in the food during cooking	From first instar larvae to adulthood		• Alterations of metabolic gut homeostasis with significant changes in pupation, time to pupation, time to emergence, body size, and glucose content.
Larvae of *Bombyx mori*	Li, 2020 [46]	n.r.	n.r.	n.r.	N = 16 • control group (n = 8) • TiO$_2$ NPs (n = 8)	TiO$_2$ NPs, 6–10 nm	Mulberry leaves soaked in 5 mg/L TiO$_2$ NPs and naturally dried	From the 3rd day of fifth-instar larvae until morning	↑ *Staphylococcus*, *Lachnospiraceae*, *Pseudomonas*, *Sphingomonas*, *Kineococcus*, *Norank_f_bacteroidales*, ↓ *Methylobacterium* and *Serratia*	

Abbreviations: ↓, decrease; ↑, increase; bw, body weight; DMH, dimethylhydrazine; F, female; GD, gestational day; HFD, high-fat diet; IFN, interferon; IL, interleukin; LPS, lipopolysaccharide; M, male; MUC2, oligomeric mucin-gel forming; NP, nano-particles; n.r, not reported; ppm, parts per million; SCFA, short chain fatty acid; SOD, superoxide dismutase; spp, species; TG, triglyceride; TLR4, toll-like receptor 4; TMA, trimethylamine. * Age at the start of the study.

3.3. Quality Assessment

The detailed results of quality assessment are presented in Tables S3 and S4. First, the quality of the eighteen included animal studies was assessed through the ARRIVE guidelines. As a result, the included animal articles adequately provide an accurate title and abstract, a structured and thorough introduction, an ethical statement only for mammalian studies, and an adequate study design except for two studies [44,45] which are unclear. None of them justified the sample size, and consequently, the use of a too small number of animals may lead to a lack of experimental statistical significance given the use of too many animals may lead to unnecessary wastage of resources and ethical issues. Only one study did not clearly describe statistical methods [42]. Baseline characteristics (body weight, age, and gender) before treatment are reported in five of the total of studies [8,40,48–50]. For twelve studies [35–37,39,41–47,51], body weight was not specified, and for three studies [38,41,42], age was not reported. All studies adequately reported and interpreted their results in terms of numbers analyzed, outcomes, adverse events, interpretation, and generalizability.

Secondly, the risk of bias of the included animal studies was assessed using SYRCLE's tool. In regards to sequence generation, in twelve out of eighteen studies, the allocation sequence was randomly generated and applied. However, in eleven out of 12 studies, the investigators did not describe the sequence generation process such as the use of a random number table or a computer random number generation. Only in the study of Zhang et al. [50], mice were randomly allocated into the control group and the TiO_2 NPs' group using a web-based randomization service. For all studies, it is not clear how animals were allocated to different groups. In addition, for all studies, all groups had similar characteristics at baseline. Regarding allocation concealment, the concealment was not clear for all studies. Indeed, no studies have explicated the concealed procedure when the investigators have allocated the animals to different groups. Moreover, all included studies have a high risk of performance bias. Indeed, the animals did not randomly house during the experiment and it is not clear whether the investigators did not blind from knowledge which intervention each animal received during the experiment. Additionally, overall, it is not specified whether the investigators did not select animals at random for outcome assessment. However, the outcome assessment methods are the same in both groups for all studies. In regards to attrition and reporting bias, the risk is low for all studies since the outcome data reported in each study was completed for each outcome. All primary outcomes have been reported. Finally, the studies did not report other problems that could result in a high risk of bias. As a conclusion, according to SYRCLE's risk of bias tool, the quality of each study is debatable due to an inadequate or unclear randomization of allocation, housing and outcome assessment, and a lack of blinding. However, the studied population has similar characteristics at baseline making the sample homogenous and avoiding confounding bias. Moreover, in regards to the reporting of outcomes (complete outcome data reporting, adequate outcome reporting), the risk of bias is low.

3.4. Results

3.4.1. TiO_2 and gut Microbial Diversity

Alpha-diversity variations were measured in five studies [40,43–45,50]. Chao1—an estimate of species richness based on a vector or matrix of abundance data—did not significantly vary between exposed groups and controls groups in mice exposed to 100 mg/kg bw/day of TiO_2 NPs for eight weeks [40], in pregnant rats exposed to 5 mg/kg bw/day of TiO_2 NPs for 12 weeks [43], but decreased in mice exposed to 150 mg/kg bw/day of TiO_2 NPs for 30 days (p = 0.0052) [50]. In regards to Shannon's diversity—another index accounting for both abundance and evenness of the species with equal weighting given to abundant and rare species—no significant variations were observed between groups in mice exposed to 100 mg/kg bw/day of TiO_2 NPs for eight weeks [40], in mice exposed to a diet containing 0.1% TiO_2 NPs for three months [44], in mice exposed to 2, 10, 50 mg/kg bw/day of TiO_2 NPs for three weeks [45], and in pregnant rats exposed to 5 mg/kg bw/day of TiO$_2$ NPs for 13 days [43]. However, in the study of Zhang et al. [50], Shannon's diversity decreased in mice exposed to 150 mg/kg bw/day of TiO$_2$ NPs for 30 days (p = 0.0036) [50]. Finally, applying Simpson's diversity index—another diversity index measuring richness and evenness in which more weighting is given to abundant species—in four out of the same studies [43–45,50], no significant variations were found except for the study of Zhang et al. [50] showing a significant increase after TiO$_2$ NPs exposure (p = 0.0180).

3.4.2. TiO$_2$ and Abundance of Individual Microbial Species

In rodents, four studies showed an increase in Firmicutes abundance after TiO$_2$ exposure compared with controls [35,39,49,51]. *Lactobacillus* was the most studied genus and significantly decreased in four studies [35,36,39,44] but increased in one study [45] after TiO$_2$ NPs exposure compared with controls. Moreover, an increase in *Allobaculum* abundance was reported in one study [45] while a decrease was observed in another mice model [35]. Other variations in genera and family abundance after TiO$_2$ exposure compared with controls are observed such as an increase in *Oscillospira* [35,51], *Turicibacter* [36], and Clostridiales [43], and a decrease in *Veillonella* [36], *Prevotella* [40,51], and *Dehalobacteriaceae* [43].

Bacteroidetes abundance could also be influenced by TiO$_2$ exposure in rodent models. Three studies showed a decrease in Bacteroidetes levels [35,49,51] while one study reported an increase in Bacteroidetes levels [44]. Especially, TiO$_2$ exposure could lead to an increase in *Bacteroides* [40], *Parabacteroides* [45], and a decrease in *Barnesiella* [19].

Actinobacteria phylum could decrease in abundance [35] after TiO$_2$ exposure with a decrease in *Bifidobacterium spp* reported in two rodent studies [35,44]. Moreover, an increase in *Rhodococcus* abundance [40] and a decrease in *Adlercreutzia* levels [45] were observed.

In regards to other phyla, Proteobacteria could increase after TiO$_2$ exposure, as reported in three studies [40,50,51], and Desulfovibrionaceae [51] and Verrucomicrobia could decrease, in particular in the *Akkermansia* genus [51].

All these findings observed in rodent models showed that TiO$_2$ exposure could impact gut microbiota composition, although the variations in specific phyla and genera abundances remain to be elucidated with large sample size animal studies using the same dose and duration of TiO$_2$ exposure.

In regards to animal models other than rodents, a model organism *Drosophila melanogaster* [42] showed that the exposure of 1, 2, and 200 mg/mL dietary of three different sizes of TiO$_2$ NPs for five days did not inhibit the growth of gut bacteria in *Drosophila* larva or adults. On the other hand, a silkworm model [41] showed different gut microbiota compositional variations after intake of mulberry leaves soaked in 5 mg/L TiO$_2$ NPs and naturally dried from the third day of fifth instar larvae until morning.

3.4.3. TiO$_2$ and SCFAs Levels

A total of six rodent studies reported between-group differences in fecal SCFA concentrations after different TiO$_2$ NPs dose exposure and length of exposure. Three studies showed no significant variations in SCFAs levels [36,37,48] while two studies observed a decrease in SCFAs levels in mice treated with 0.1 weight percent of TiO$_2$ NPs for eight weeks [35] and in mice treated with 50 mg TiO$_2$/kg bw/day for three weeks [45]. Interestingly, one study [39] reported an increase of SCFAs in stools in mice exposed to 1 g/kg bw TiO$_2$ for 14 days. This can be explained by an increase in SCFAs production or a decrease in absorption.

3.4.4. TiO$_2$ and Metabolism

A total of seven studies [36,37,39,42,43,49,50] showed significant metabolic variations in TiO$_2$ exposed animals compared with controls. Lipopolysaccharides (LPS) proportionally increased in mice exposed to 2, 10, and 50 mg/kg bw/day of TiO$_2$ for 30 days [36], in mice exposed to 10, 40, and 160 mg/kg bw/day of TiO$_2$ for 28 days [49], and in mice exposed to 10 µL/g bw/day for eight weeks [51]. Interestingly, in TiO$_2$-treated mice fed with a high-fat diet (HFD), LPS significantly increased compared with TiO$_2$-treated mice fed with a high fiber diet (CHOW diet) [51]. Triglycerides levels (TG) levels increased in mice after exposure to 160 mg/kg bw/day of TiO$_2$ for 28 days, while TG levels reduced in rats exposed to 10 and 50 mg/kg bw/day of TiO$_2$ for 90 days. Moreover, glucose levels could increase after TiO$_2$ exposure, as reported in two rodent model studies [43,49]. Interestingly, in Sprague-Dawley pregnant rats, exposure of 5 mg/kg/day of TiO$_2$ NPs for 12 weeks could strengthen genes about type 2 diabetes mellitus related to function and lipid biosynthesis, compared with controls [43].

The two *Drosophila* model studies [42,46] reported contradictory results. One study showed no alterations of pupation cycle, weight, and lipid levels after 1, 2, and 200 mg/mL dietary TiO$_2$ NPs of different sizes for five days while Richter and colleagues [46] demonstrated alterations of metabolic gut homeostasis with significant changes in pupation, time to pupation, reduction of body size, and glucose levels.

3.4.5. TiO$_2$ and Gut Barrier Permeability

Bettini et al. observed no significant changes in epithelial paracellular permeability in the E171 group in comparison to the controls [8]. Additionally, a previous study [48] found no effect compared with controls on mucin O-glycosylation in the small intestine of the rats following 7- or 60-day TiO$_2$ exposure, regardless of TiO$_2$ type (E171 and NM-105) or E171 dose tested (0.1 mg/kg bw/day and 10 mg/kg bw/day). Another study [39] showed that at 24 h post-gavage, MUC2 gene expression was lower in TiO$_2$ NP-treated mice (1 g/kg bw/day) compared with controls but this trend was reversed from 48 h post-gavage to seven days with an elevated expression of mucin-2 for the rest of the study.

On the other hand, in mice exposed to 0.1 weight percent of TiO$_2$, goblet cells and crypts significantly decreased compared to controls. Furthermore, three studies [45,49,51] reported a decrease in MUC2 gene expression in mice treated with TiO$_2$ NPs. Yan et al. [49] also reported a reduction of mucus thickness in all exposed mice compared with controls. Interestingly, MUC2 gene expression and crypt length significantly decreased in TiO$_2$-treated mice fed with HFD compared with TiO$_2$-treated mice fed with CHOW diet [51].

3.4.6. TiO$_2$ and Inflammatory Responses

A total of ten studies have assessed levels of different gut microbiota associated biomarkers of mucosal immunity and intestinal inflammation such as interleukins (IL) levels, number of T reg cells, macrophages, and T helper cells. A reduction of T reg cells numbers was found in food-grade E171 treated mice after 100 days [8] and in mice exposed to a diet containing 0.1% TiO$_2$ NPs for three months [44]. Inflammatory cytokines levels increased in exposed rodents compared with controls in the majority of studies: IL1 [49,51], IL2 [38], IL6 [8,36,45,49,51], IL10 [45], IL12 [35], IL17 [8,35], IL18 [8], as well as TNFα levels [45,49,51]. The production of macrophages and the expression of β defensin gene are also stimulated [45]. Interestingly, TiO$_2$ NPs decreased the CD4+ T cells, T regs, and macrophages in the mesenteric lymph nodes and increased neutrophil gelatinase-associated lipocalin (LCN2) levels in mice aggravating the DSS-induced chronic colitis [44]. Moreover, IL-1 levels, IL-6 levels, TNFα levels increased in TiO$_2$-treated mice fed with HFD compared with TiO$_2$-treated mice fed CHOW diet [51]. All these results showed the potential involvement of TiO$_2$ in the imbalances in intestinal and systemic immune responses.

4. Discussion

This systematic review of animal studies found that TiO$_2$ dietary exposure might increase or decrease abundance in specific bacterial species, even if an overall impact on bacterial α-diversity has not been clearly demonstrated. Moreover, this review highlights that TiO$_2$ exposure could lead to perturbations in intestinal metabolism, gut barrier integrity, and gut immunity.

The limited effect of TiO$_2$ exposure on α-diversity of the gut microbiota was found in the majority of included studies. This could be explained by the short duration of the interventions, not exceeding three months. The lack of effects of different dietary interventions on gut microbiota diversity has been shown in previous systematic reviews investigating the effects of dietary patterns or dietary interventions—such as dietary fiber interventions or probiotics interventions—on gut microbiota [52]. Long-term studies are required to assess this hypothesis. In regards to bacterial abundances, in various included studies [35,39,44,49], significant compositional changes are reported after TiO$_2$ exposure compared with controls. TiO$_2$ exposure could lead to an alteration of the Firmicutes/Bacteroides ratio, a depletion of *Lactobacillus*, and enrichment of Proteobacteria [40,50]. Interestingly, these microbial variations are also found in studies investigating the effect of other food nanoparticles such as nano-Ag, ZnO, and SiO$_2$ exposure [53]. *Lactobacillus* is a genus well-known to produce SCFAs, metabolites involved in host metabolism, while Proteobacteria might be overrepresented in inflammatory intestinal and extra intestinal diseases. Indeed, this observed dysbiosis is also a hallmark of inflammatory bowel disease, colorectal cancer, or chronic metabolic disorders such as obesity [54].

The intestinal microbiota plays a key role in gastrointestinal functions such as the digestion and fermentation of indigestible polysaccharides, differentiation of the intestinal epithelium, and the maintenance of mucosal barrier integrity, including mucus characteristics. Mucus is a viscoelastic gel that separates the intestinal epithelium from the gut lumen. It consists of water and mucins, lipids, as well as epithelial and globets cells. Goblet cells are localized in the intestinal crypts and secrete proteins such as muc-2 (encoded by MUC2 gene). Intestinal bacteria influence the shaping of the mucus regulating LPS and SCFAs. Indeed, SCFAs—mainly butyrate—stimulate muc-2 protein production and influence mucus quality. Numerous studies [55–57] demonstrated that germ-free mice, comparing with conventionalized mice, were provided with an underdeveloped intestinal epithelium with decreased mucus production, intestinal epithelial cell differentiation, and villus thickness. These alterations could lead to an increased permeability allowing the passage of harmful intraluminal microorganisms and microbial toxins. These bidirectional interactions between gut microbiota composition and gut barrier functions could be impaired with TiO$_2$ exposure. Indeed, in some included studies [35,45,49], TiO$_2$ exposure could be associated with a reduction of SCFAs, a decrease of goblet cells and crypts, a reduction of mucus production with a lower MUC2 expression. These in vivo findings confirmed the results of in vitro studies demonstrating that TiO$_2$ NPs could alter microvilli structure and epithelial integrity [19,24]. Particularly, in vivo and ex vivo, TiO$_2$ NPs can cross the regular ileum and follicle-associated epithelium and alter the paracellular permeability of the ileum and colon epithelia, which is a sign of integrity alteration [58]. However, three studies [8,37,48] did not show significant changes in terms of epithelium permeability, SCFAs levels, and mucus barrier impairment. Considering the TiO$_2$ dose exposure of the studies, we can hypothesize that these discrepancies could be due to dose exposure and healthy conditions of the animals at baseline.

TiO$_2$ NPs also could interact with gut immunity. Indeed, a majority of included studies have assessed associations between TiO$_2$ exposure and increased biomarkers of intestinal inflammation such as increased interleukins levels. Recent in vitro studies [19,27] found that TiO$_2$ NPs could stimulate the production of pro-inflammatory cytokines. Moreover, in vivo, the number of T reg cells decreased after 100 days of TiO$_2$ exposure [8]. T reg cells are well-known to limit gut inflammatory responses and prevent food allergy development [59]. Thus, long-term TiO$_2$ exposure could have an immunosuppressive role by limiting the production of T reg cells. Interestingly, there are significant changes in terms of IL production, significantly aggravated in obese mice treated with TiO$_2$ compared with non-obese mice [35,51]. This shows that TiO$_2$ could exacerbate intestinal inflammation in mice affected by metabolic diseases such as obesity. Mu et al. [44] analyzed the effect of TiO$_2$ NPs on DSS-induced chronic colitis in mice showing that DSS-induced chronic colitis worsened by chronic TiO$_2$ NPs exposure with a reduction of immune cells such as CD4 + T cells and Tregs. Further studies are required to deepen the effects of TiO$_2$ NPs on immunity responses, and specifically on the gut microbiota immune axis.

Overall, TiO$_2$ exposure can raise concerns if we consider the cocktail effects of daily consumption of the different food additives. Indeed, other NPs present in food, emulsifiers, and artificial sweeteners have also dysbiotic effects on gut microbiota [60]. This cocktail effect raises particular concerns since the quantity of food additives is not detailed in the ingredient list, making impossible the calculation of the daily quantity of food additives. For example, chewing one piece of chewing gum can result in an intake of 1.5–5.1 mg of TiO$_2$ NPs [61]. These concerns are even more important in children. Indeed, candies, gums, desserts, and beverages—products containing the highest levels of TiO$_2$ NPs—are consumed two to four times higher for children than for adults [3]. A Dutch survey estimated a mean TiO$_2$ NPs intake of 2.16 (2.13–2.26) mg/kg bw per day among children aged two to six years old, and a mean of 0.55 (0.52–0.58) among people aged 7–69 years old, with toothpaste, candy, coffee creamer, fine bakery wares, and sauces mostly contributing to the TiO$_2$ daily intake [62]. Childhood is a key development time for the shape of the microbiota that can have considerable consequences in later life [63]. Although TiO$_2$ consumption has considerably increased in the last few decades in Western countries and despite dietary composition having an impact on gut and overall health [64], the possible impacts of long term effects of TiO$_2$ are still poorly understood.

This systematic review has some limitations. Although the majority of included studies have used rodent models, the methods of administration (gastric gavage, addition to drinking water, addition to food), TiO$_2$ doses, and exposure durations differ between studies and do not allow pooling results. Thus, since some studies detect only a limited impact on the microbiota, others reporting various significant changes, it remains difficult to reach firm conclusions. Another limitation are the very high doses used in animal studies compared to the estimated daily intake in humans. Indeed, the amount of TiO$_2$ consumed is estimated to 1 mg of TiO$_2$/kg bw/day in adults in the United Kingdom and Germany, while the ingested quantity can exceed 3 mg of TiO$_2$/kg bw/day in children [3,65]. Thus, the results from animal studies cannot be directly extrapolated to humans. Furthermore, only 15% of the 16S rRNA sequence dataset for the mouse microbiota are shared with humans [66]. Since randomized controlled studies are unethical, the use of germ-free mice inoculated with the human microbiota could be feasible to elucidate the impact of TiO$_2$ NPs on gut bacteria that colonize the human intestine. Moreover, different dietary patterns such as HFD or high fiber diet should be evaluated to compare the impact on TiO$_2$ NPs in healthy individuals with those in poor health.

5. Conclusions

In conclusion, in vivo consumption of TiO$_2$ could alter the composition and the activity of intestinal bacteria, promoting an inflammatory environment in the gut and aggravating gut barrier impairment and immune responses in animals already affected by diseases such as colitis or obesity. Therefore, although these findings did not allow us to reach firm conclusions in humans, this systematic review highlights the key role of gut microbiota in nanotoxicology in the gut and stimulates discussions on the safe TiO$_2$ use in food and dietary supplements.

Supplementary Materials: The following are available online at https://www.mdpi.com/1660-4601/18/4/2008/s1, Table S1. PRISMA checklist; Table S2. Search strategy; Table S3. Reporting of in vivo experiments (ARRIVE) guideline assessment for the included animal studies; Table S4. SCYRCLE's tool for assessing the risk of bias in animal studies.

Author Contributions: Conceptualization, E.R. and P.R.; methodology, P.R.; validation, M.C.M. and A.G.; investigation, M.C.; resources, V.M.; writing—original draft preparation, P.R.; writing—review and editing, E.R.; visualization, A.G.; supervision, M.C.M. All authors have read and agreed to the published version of the manuscript.

Funding: This research received no external funding.

Institutional Review Board Statement: Not applicable.

Informed Consent Statement: Not applicable.

Data Availability Statement: Not applicable.

Conflicts of Interest: The authors declare no conflict of interest.

References

1. Martirosyan, A.; Schneider, Y.-J. Engineered nanomaterials in food: Implications for food safety and consumer health. *Int. J. Environ. Res. Public Health* **2014**, *11*, 5720–5750. [CrossRef]
2. Yang, Y.; Doudrick, K.; Bi, X.; Hristovski, K.; Herckes, P.; Westerhoff, P.; Kaegi, R. Characterization of food-grade titanium dioxide: The presence of nanosized particles. *Environ. Sci. Technol.* **2014**, *48*, 6391–6400. [CrossRef] [PubMed]
3. Weir, A.; Westerhoff, P.; Fabricius, L.; Hristovski, K.; Von Goetz, N. Titanium dioxide nanoparticles in food and personal care products. *Environ. Sci. Technol.* **2012**, *46*, 2242–2250. [CrossRef] [PubMed]
4. U.S. Food and Drug Administration. CFR—Code of Federal Regulations Title 21. Available online: https://www.accessdata.fda.gov/scripts/cdrh/cfdocs/cfCFR/CFRSearch.cfm?fr=73.575 (accessed on 15 December 2020).
5. EFSA ANS Panel (EFSA Panel on Food Additives and Nutrient Sources Added to Food). Scientific opinion on the re-evaluation of titanium dioxide (E 171) as a food additive. *EFSA J.* **2016**, *14*, 4545.
6. NTP (National Toxicology Program). *Bioassay of Titanium Dioxide for Possible Carcinogenicity*; U.S. Department of Health, Education, and Welfare: Rockville, MD, USA, 1979.
7. Heringa, M.B.; Geraets, L.; van Eijkeren, J.C.H.; Vandebriel, R.J.; deJong, W.; Oomen, A.G. Risk assessment of titanium dioxide nanoparticles via oral exposure, including toxicokinetic considerations. *Nanotoxicology* **2016**, *10*, 1515–1525. [CrossRef]
8. Bettini, S.; Boutet-Robinet, E.; Cartier, C.; Coméra, C.; Gaultier, E.; Dupuy, J.; Naud, N.; Taché, S.; Grysan, P.; Reguer, S.; et al. Food-grade TiO_2 impairs intestinal and systemic immune homeostasis, initiates preneoplastic lesions and promotes aberrant crypt development in the rat colon. *Sci. Rep.* **2017**, *7*, srep40373. [CrossRef] [PubMed]
9. Guo, Z.; Martucci, N.J.; Moreno-Olivas, F.; Tako, E.; Mahler, G.J. Titanium dioxide nanoparticle ingestion alters nutrient absorption in an in vitro model of the small intestine. *NanoImpact* **2017**, *5*, 70–82. [CrossRef]
10. Proquin, H.; Rodríguez-Ibarra, C.; Moonen, C.G.J.; Urrutia Ortega, I.M.; Briedé, J.J.; De Kok, T.M.; Van Loveren, H.; Chirino, Y.I. Titanium dioxide food additive (E171) induces ROS formation and genotoxicity: Contribution of micro and nano-sized fractions. *Mutagenesis* **2017**, *32*, 139–149. [CrossRef] [PubMed]
11. EFSA Panel on Food Additives and Nutrient Sources added to Food (ANS); Younes, M.; Aggett, P.; Aguilar, F.; Crebelli, R.; Dusemund, B.; Filipič, M.; Frutos, M.J.; Galtier, P.; Gott, D.; et al. Evaluation of four new studies on the potential toxicity of titanium dioxide used as a food additive (E 171). *EFSA J.* **2018**, *16*, e05366. [CrossRef]
12. ANSES. Avis de l'Agence Nationale de Securit e Sanitaire de l'Alimentation, de l'environnement et du Travail Relatif au Risques Lies a la Ingestion de l'Additif Alimentaire E 171. Available online: https://www.anses.fr/fr/system/files/ERCA2019SA0036.pdf (accessed on 20 December 2020).
13. EFSA (European Food Safety Authority). EFSA statement on the review of the risks related to the exposure to the food additive titanium dioxide (E 171) performed by the French Agency for Food, Environmental and Occupational Health and Safety (ANSES). *EFSA J.* **2019**, *17*, e05714. [CrossRef]
14. Rinninella, E.; Raoul, P.; Cintoni, M.; Franceschi, F.; Miggiano, G.A.D.; Gasbarrini, A.; Mele, M.C. What is the healthy gut microbiota composition? a changing ecosystem across age, environment, diet, and diseases. *Microorganisms* **2019**, *7*, 14. [CrossRef]
15. Dorier, M.; Béal, D.; Marie-Desvergne, C.; Dubosson, M.; Barreau, F.; Houdeau, E.; Herlin-Boime, N.; Carriere, M. Continuous in vitro exposure of intestinal epithelial cells to E171 food additive causes oxidative stress, inducing oxidation of DNA bases but no endoplasmic reticulum stress. *Nanotoxicology* **2017**, *11*, 751–761. [CrossRef]
16. Dorier, M.; Brun, E.; Veronesi, G.; Barreau, F.; Pernet-Gallay, K.; Desvergne, C.; Rabilloud, T.; Carapito, C.; Herlin-Boime, N.; Carrière, M. Impact of anatase and rutile titanium dioxide nanoparticles on uptake carriers and efflux pumps in Caco-2 gut epithelial cells. *Nanoscale* **2015**, *7*, 7352–7360. [CrossRef] [PubMed]
17. Faust, J.J.; Masserano, B.M.; Mielke, A.H.; Abraham, A.; Capco, D.G. Engineered nanoparticles induced brush border disruption in a human model of the intestinal epithelium. *Adv. Exp. Med. Biol.* **2014**, *811*, 55–72. [PubMed]
18. Song, B.; Liu, J.; Feng, X.; Wei, L.; Shao, L. A review on potential neurotoxicity of titanium dioxide nanoparticles. *Nanoscale Res. Lett.* **2015**, *10*, 342. [CrossRef] [PubMed]
19. Pedata, P.; Ricci, G.; Malorni, L.; Venezia, A.; Cammarota, M.; Volpe, N.; Iannaccone, N.; Guida, V.; Schiraldi, C.; Romano, M.; et al. In vitro intestinal epithelium responses to titanium dioxide nanoparticles. *Food Res. Int.* **2019**, *119*, 634–642. [CrossRef]
20. Kolba, N.; Guo, Z.; Olivas, F.M.; Mahler, G.J.; Tako, E. Intra-amniotic administration (*Gallus gallus*) of TiO_2, SiO_2, and ZnO nanoparticles affect brush border membrane functionality and alters gut microflora populations. *Food Chem. Toxicol.* **2020**, *135*, 110896. [CrossRef]
21. Moher, D.; Liberati, A.; Tetzlaff, J.; Altman, D.G.; PRISMA Group. Preferred reporting items for systematic reviews and me-ta-analyses: The PRISMA statement. *PLoS Med.* **2009**, *6*, e1000097. [CrossRef]
22. Kilkenny, C.; Browne, W.J.; Cuthill, I.C.; Emerson, M.; Altman, D.G. Improving bioscience research reporting: The ARRIVE guidelines for reporting animal research. *PLoS Biol.* **2010**, *8*, e1000412. [CrossRef]

23. Hooijmans, C.R.; Rovers, M.M.; De Vries, R.B.M.; Leenaars, M.; Ritskes-Hoitinga, M.; Langendam, M.W. SYRCLE's risk of bias tool for animal studies. *BMC Med. Res. Methodol.* **2014**, *14*, 43. [CrossRef] [PubMed]
24. Limage, R.; Tako, E.; Kolba, N.; Guo, Z.; García-Rodríguez, A.; Marques, C.N.H.; Mahler, G.J. TiO$_2$ nanoparticles and com-mensal bacteria alter mucus layer thickness and composition in a gastrointestinal tract model. *Small* **2020**, *16*, e2000601. [CrossRef]
25. Dudefoi, W.; Moniz, K.; Allen-Vercoe, E.; Ropers, M.H.; Walker, V.K. Impact of food-grade and nano-TiO$_2$ particles on a human intestinal community. *Food Chem. Toxicol.* **2017**, *106*, 242–249. [CrossRef]
26. Agans, R.T.; Gordon, A.; Hussain, S.; Paliy, O. Titanium dioxide nanoparticles elicit lower direct inhibitory effect on human gut microbiota than silver nanoparticles. *Toxicol. Sci.* **2019**, *172*, 411–416. [CrossRef]
27. Dorier, M.; Béal, D.; Tisseyre, C.; Marie-Desvergne, C.; Dubosson, M.; Barreau, F.; Houdeau, E.; Herlin-Boime, N.; Rabilloud, T.; Carriere, M. The food additive E171 and titanium dioxide nanoparticles indirectly alter the homeostasis of human intestinal epithelial cells in vitro. *Environ. Sci. Nano* **2019**, *6*, 1549–1561. [CrossRef]
28. Taylor, A.A.; Marcus, I.M.; Guysi, R.L.; Walker, S.L. metal oxide nanoparticles induce minimal phenotypic changes in a model colon gut microbiota. *Environ. Eng. Sci.* **2015**, *32*, 602–612. [CrossRef]
29. Waller, T.; Chen, C.; Walker, S.L. Food and industrial grade titanium dioxide impacts gut microbiota. *Environ. Eng. Sci.* **2017**, *34*, 537–550. [CrossRef]
30. Hong, F.; Zhou, Y.; Zhao, X.; Sheng, L.; Wang, L. Maternal exposure to nanosized titanium dioxide suppresses embryonic development in mice. *Int. J. Nanomed.* **2017**, *12*, 6197–6204. [CrossRef] [PubMed]
31. Auguste, M.; Lasa, A.; Pallavicini, A.; Gualdi, S.; Vezzulli, L.; Canesi, L. Exposure to TiO$_2$ nanoparticles induces shifts in the microbiota composition of Mytilus galloprovincialis hemolymph. *Sci. Total. Environ.* **2019**, *670*, 129–137. [CrossRef]
32. Mercier-Bonin, M.; Despax, B.; Raynaud, P.; Houdeau, E.; Thomas, M. Mucus and microbiota as emerging players in gut nanotoxicology: The example of dietary silver and titanium dioxide nanoparticles. *Crit. Rev. Food Sci. Nutr.* **2018**, *58*, 1023–1032. [CrossRef]
33. Han, S.; Chen, Z.; Zhou, D.; Zheng, P.; Zhang, J.; Jia, G. Effects of titanium dioxide nanoparticles on fecal metabolome in rats after oral administration for 90 days. *J. Peking Univ.* **2020**, *52*, 457–463.
34. Chen, L.; Guo, Y.; Hu, C.; Lam, P.K.; Lam, J.C.; Zhou, B. Dysbiosis of gut microbiota by chronic coexposure to titanium dioxide nanoparticles and bisphenol A: Implications for host health in zebrafish. *Environ. Pollut.* **2018**, *234*, 307–317. [CrossRef]
35. Cao, X.; Han, Y.; Gu, M.; Du, H.; Song, M.; Zhu, X.; Ma, G.; Pan, C.; Wang, W.; Zhao, E.; et al. Foodborne titanium dioxide nanoparticles induce stronger adverse effects in obese mice than non-obese mice: Gut microbiota dysbiosis, colonic inflammation, and proteome alterations. *Small* **2020**, *16*, e2001858. [CrossRef]
36. Chen, Z.; Han, S.; Zhou, D.; Zhou, S.; Jia, G. Effects of oral exposure to titanium dioxide nanoparticles on gut microbiota and gut-associated metabolism in vivo. *Nanoscale* **2019**, *11*, 22398–22412. [CrossRef]
37. Chen, Z.; Han, S.; Zheng, P.; Zhou, D.; Zhou, S.; Jia, G. Effect of oral exposure to titanium dioxide nanoparticles on lipid me-tabolism in Sprague-Dawley rats. *Nanoscale* **2020**, *12*, 5973–5986. [CrossRef]
38. Duan, Y.; Liu, J.; Ma, L.; Li, N.; Liu, H.; Wang, J.; Zheng, L.; Liu, C.; Wang, X.; Zhao, X.; et al. Toxicological characteristics of nanoparticulate anatase titanium dioxide in mice. *Biomaterials* **2010**, *31*, 894–899. [CrossRef]
39. Kurtz, C.C.; Mitchell, S.; Nielsen, K.; Crawford, K.D.; Mueller-Spitz, S.R. Acute high-dose titanium dioxide nanoparticle ex-posure alters gastrointestinal homeostasis in mice. *J. Appl. Toxicol.* **2020**, *40*, 1384–1395. [CrossRef] [PubMed]
40. Li, J.; Yang, S.; Lei, R.; Gu, W.; Qin, Y.; Ma, S.; Chen, K.; Chang, Y.; Bai, X.; Xia, S.; et al. Oral administration of rutile and anatase TiO$_2$ nanoparticles shifts mouse gut microbiota structure. *Nanoscale* **2018**, *10*, 7736–7745. [CrossRef] [PubMed]
41. Li, M.; Li, F.; Lu, Z.; Fang, Y.; Qu, J.; Mao, T.; Wang, H.; Chen, J.; Li, B. Effects of TiO$_2$ nanoparticles on intestinal microbial composition of silkworm, Bombyx mori. *Sci. Total. Environ.* **2020**, *704*, 135273. [CrossRef]
42. Liu, L.-Y.; Sun, L.; Zhong, Z.-T.; Zhu, J.; Song, H.-Y. Effects of titanium dioxide nanoparticles on intestinal commensal bacteria. *Nucl. Sci. Tech.* **2016**, *27*, 1–5. [CrossRef]
43. Mao, Z.; Li, Y.; Dong, T.; Zhang, L.; Zhang, Y.; Li, S.; Hu, H.; Sun, C.; Xia, Y. Exposure to titanium dioxide nanoparticles during pregnancy changed maternal gut microbiota and increased blood glucose of rat. *Nanoscale Res. Lett.* **2019**, *14*, 26. [CrossRef]
44. Mu, W.; Wang, Y.; Huang, C.; Fu, Y.; Li, J.; Wang, H.; Jia, X.; Ba, Q. Effect of Long-Term Intake of Dietary Titanium Dioxide Nanoparticles on Intestine Inflammation in Mice. *J. Agric. Food Chem.* **2019**, *67*, 9382–9389. [CrossRef] [PubMed]
45. Pinget, G.; Tan, J.; Janac, B.; Kaakoush, N.O.; Angelatos, A.S.; O'Sullivan, J.; Koay, Y.C.; Sierro, F.; Davis, J.; Divakarla, S.K.; et al. Impact of the food additive titanium dioxide (E171) on gut microbiota-host interaction. *Front. Nutr.* **2019**, *6*, 57. [CrossRef] [PubMed]
46. Richter, J.W.; Shull, G.M.; Fountain, J.H.; Guo, Z.; Musselman, L.P.; Fiumera, A.C.; Mahler, G.J. Titanium dioxide nanoparti-cle exposure alters metabolic homeostasis in a cell culture model of the intestinal epithelium and Drosophila melanogaster. *Nanotoxicology* **2018**, *12*, 390–406. [CrossRef] [PubMed]
47. Ruiz, P.A.; Morón, B.; Becker, H.M.; Lang, S.; Atrott, K.; Spalinger, M.R.; Scharl, M.; Wojtal, K.A.; Fischbeck-Terhalle, A.; Frey-Wagner, I.; et al. Titanium dioxide nanoparticles exacerbate DSS-induced colitis: Role of the NLRP3 inflammasome. *Gut* **2017**, *66*, 1216–1224. [CrossRef]
48. Talbot, P.; Radziwill-Bienkowska, J.M.; Kamphuis, J.B.J.; Steenkeste, K.; Bettini, S.; Robert, V.; Noordine, M.-L.; Mayeur, C.; Gaultier, E.; Langella, P.; et al. Food-grade TiO$_2$ is trapped by intestinal mucus in vitro but does not impair mucin O-glycosylation and short-chain fatty acid synthesis in vivo: Implications for gut barrier protection. *J. Nanobiotechnol.* **2018**, *16*, 1–14. [CrossRef]

49. Yan, J.; Wang, D.; Li, K.; Chen, Q.; Lai, W.; Tian, L.; Lin, B.; Tan, Y.; Liu, X.; Xi, Z. Toxic effects of the food additives titanium dioxide and silica on the murine intestinal tract: Mechanisms related to intestinal barrier dysfunction involved by gut micro-biota. *Environ. Toxicol. Pharmacol.* **2020**, *80*, 103485. [CrossRef]
50. Zhang, S.; Jiang, X.; Cheng, S.; Fan, J.; Qin, X.; Wang, T.; Zhang, Y.; Zhang, J.; Qiu, Y.; Qiu, J.; et al. Titanium dioxide nanoparticles via oral exposure leads to adverse disturbance of gut microecology and locomotor activity in adult mice. *Arch. Toxicol.* **2020**, *94*, 1173–1190. [CrossRef]
51. Zhu, X.; Zhao, L.; Liu, Z.; Zhou, Q.; Zhu, Y.; Zhao, Y.; Yang, X. Long-term exposure to titanium dioxide nanoparticles promotes diet-induced obesity through exacerbating intestinal mucus layer damage and microbiota dysbiosis. *Nano Res.* **2020**, 1–11. [CrossRef]
52. Leeming, E.R.; Johnson, A.J.; Spector, T.D.; Le Roy, C.I. Effect of diet on the gut microbiota: Rethinking intervention duration. *Nutrients* **2019**, *11*, 2862. [CrossRef]
53. Lamas, B.; Martins Breyner, N.; Houdeau, E. Impacts of foodborne inorganic nanoparticles on the gut microbiota-immune axis: Potential consequences for host health. *Part. Fibre Toxicol.* **2020**, *17*, 1–22. [CrossRef] [PubMed]
54. Carding, S.; Verbeke, K.; Vipond, D.T.; Corfe, B.M.; Owen, L.J. Dysbiosis of the gut microbiota in disease. *Microb. Ecol. Health Dis.* **2015**, *26*, 26191. [CrossRef]
55. Jakobsson, H.E.; Rodríguez-Piñeiro, A.M.; Schütte, A.; Ermund, A.; Boysen, P.; Bemark, M.; Sommer, F.; Bäckhed, F.; Hansson, G.C.; Johansson, M.E.V. The composition of the gut microbiota shapes the colon mucus barrier. *EMBO Rep.* **2015**, *16*, 164–177. [CrossRef] [PubMed]
56. Johansson, M.E.; Jakobsson, H.E.; Holmén-Larsson, J.; Schütte, A.; Ermund, A.; Rodríguez-Piñeiro, A.M.; Arike, L.; Wising, C.; Svensson, F.; Bäckhed, F.; et al. Normalization of host intestinal mucus layers requires long-term microbial colonization. *Cell Host Microbe* **2015**, *18*, 582–592. [CrossRef]
57. Becker, S.; Oelschlaeger, T.A.; Wullaert, A.; Vlantis, K.; Pasparakis, M.; Wehkamp, J.; Stange, E.F.; Gersemann, M. Bacteria regulate intestinal epithelial cell differentiation factors both in vitro and in vivo. *PLoS ONE* **2013**, *8*, e55620.
58. Brun, E.; Barreau, F.; Veronesi, G.; Fayard, B.; Sorieul, S.; Chanéac, C.; Carapito, C.; Rabilloud, T.; Mabondzo, A.; Herlin-Boime, N.; et al. Titanium dioxide nanoparticle impact and translocation through ex vivo, in vivo and in vitro gut epithelia. *Part. Fibre Toxicol.* **2014**, *11*, 13. [CrossRef]
59. Coombes, J.L.; Maloy, K.J. Control of intestinal homeostasis by regulatory T cells and dendritic cells. *Semin. Immunol.* **2007**, *19*, 116–126. [CrossRef]
60. Rinninella, E.; Cintoni, M.; Raoul, P.; Gasbarrini, A.; Mele, M.C. Food additives, gut microbiota, and irritable Bowel syndrome: A hidden track. *Int. J. Environ. Res. Public Heal.* **2020**, *17*, 8816. [CrossRef] [PubMed]
61. Chen, X.-X.; Cheng, B.; Yang, Y.-X.; Cao, A.; Liu, J.-H.; Du, L.-J.; Liu, Y.; Zhao, Y.; Wang, H. Characterization and preliminary toxicity assay of nano-titanium dioxide additive in sugar-coated chewing gum. *Small* **2013**, *9*, 1765–1774. [CrossRef]
62. Rompelberg, C.; Heringa, M.B.; Van Donkersgoed, G.; Drijvers, J.; Roos, A.; Westenbrink, S.; Peters, R.; Van Bemmel, G.; Brand, W.; Oomen, A.G. Oral intake of added titanium dioxide and its nanofraction from food products, food supplements and toothpaste by the Dutch population. *Nanotoxicology* **2016**, *10*, 1404–1414. [CrossRef] [PubMed]
63. Derrien, M.; Alvarez, A.-S.; De Vos, W.M. The gut microbiota in the first decade of life. *Trends Microbiol.* **2019**, *27*, 997–1010. [CrossRef]
64. Rinninella, E.; Cintoni, M.; Raoul, P.; Lopetuso, L.R.; Scaldaferri, F.; Pulcini, G.; Miggiano, G.A.D.; Gasbarrini, A.; Mele, M.C. Food components and dietary habits: Keys for a healthy gut microbiota composition. *Nutrients* **2019**, *11*, 2393. [CrossRef] [PubMed]
65. Bachler, G.; Von Goetz, N.; Hungerbuhler, K. Using physiologically based pharmacokinetic (PBPK) modeling for dietary risk assessment of titanium dioxide (TiO_2) nanoparticles. *Nanotoxicology* **2014**, *9*, 373–380. [CrossRef] [PubMed]
66. Ley, R.E.; Bäckhed, F.; Turnbaugh, P.; Lozupone, C.A.; Knight, R.D.; Gordon, J.I. Obesity alters gut microbial ecology. *Proc. Natl. Acad. Sci. USA* **2005**, *102*, 11070–11075. [CrossRef] [PubMed]

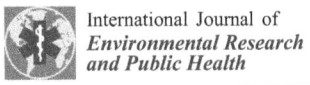

Article

Casomorphins and Gliadorphins Have Diverse Systemic Effects Spanning Gut, Brain and Internal Organs

Keith Bernard Woodford

Agri-Food Systems, Lincoln University, Lincoln 7674, New Zealand; keith.woodford@lincoln.ac.nz

Abstract: Food-derived opioid peptides include digestive products derived from cereal and dairy diets. If these opioid peptides breach the intestinal barrier, typically linked to permeability and constrained biosynthesis of dipeptidyl peptidase-4 (DPP4), they can attach to opioid receptors. The widespread presence of opioid receptors spanning gut, brain, and internal organs is fundamental to the diverse and systemic effects of food-derived opioids, with effects being evidential across many health conditions. However, manifestation delays following low-intensity long-term exposure create major challenges for clinical trials. Accordingly, it has been easiest to demonstrate causal relationships in digestion-based research where some impacts occur rapidly. Within this environment, the role of the microbiome is evidential but challenging to further elucidate, with microbiome effects ranging across gut-condition indicators and modulators, and potentially as systemic causal factors. Elucidation requires a systemic framework that acknowledges that public-health effects of food-derived opioids are complex with varying genetic susceptibility and confounding factors, together with system-wide interactions and feedbacks. The specific role of the microbiome within this puzzle remains a medical frontier. The easiest albeit challenging nutritional strategy to modify risk is reduced intake of foods containing embedded opioids. In future, constituent modification within specific foods to reduce embedded opioids may become feasible.

Keywords: food-derived opioids; casomorphin; gliadorphin; opioid receptors; A1 beta-casein; beta-casomorphin-7; gut-to-brain; microbiome; DPP4

1. Introduction

This paper reviews and integrates evidence relating to food-derived opioid peptides in public health, focusing on casomorphins from dairy and gliadorphin peptides from cereals. The systemic nature of the evidence, which spans the gut, brain, and many internal organs, arises as a direct consequence of the widespread presence of opioid receptors throughout the human body. Influencing factors beyond diet itself include human genetic variability, specific microbiota, and aspects of health that mediate absorption of the peptides from the gut into the circulatory system. Some of these same factors then impact on inflammatory and autoimmune responses. The role of the gut and associated microbiome is clearly important within the system but much remains to be elucidated [1].

One of the challenges of investigating and documenting the wide-ranging effects of food-derived opioids is that dietary exposure is long-term, with effects often due to chronic rather than short-term high-intensity exposure, and therefore difficult to investigate within clinical trials. A further investigational challenge is that the multiple influencing factors, including genetic factors and other disease factors, in combination with the diverse locations of opioid receptors within human tissues, can lead to great effect-diversity between individuals.

The specific focus of this paper on casomorphin and gliadin peptides reflects that these are the most researched of the food-derived opioids based on the prevalence of dairy and wheat within human diets, together with evidence that they are the peptide groupings most clearly implicated in food-derived opioid health issues. However, they are not the only opioid peptides in either gluten or dairy. For example, there are opioid peptide sequences within glutenin, the alcohol-insoluble proteins that along with the alcohol-soluble gliadins comprise the overarching gluten grouping. Additionally, opioid peptides can be released from other food products. For example, barley and rye have homologous proteins to the gluten proteins found in wheat. These barley and rye proteins release opioid hordein peptides and opioid secalin peptides, respectively [2]. Indeed, there is diversity of practice within the literature as to whether the term 'gluten' encompasses all of the prolamin (high proline) proteins derived from species of the Triticeae, thereby including the various wheat species plus barley, rye, and triticale, or whether it should be reserved as a term for prolamin proteins from wheat. In this paper, wherever the terms 'gluten' and 'gliadin' are used, it is as encompassing terms that include relevant prolamin proteins within all of the Triticeae, but recognizing that there will be differences between species and even between strains and varieties of a species in terms of both gluten and gliadin intensity plus specific opioid structure [3]. A notable feature of gluten proteins is the variety and complexity of structure [4].

Non-homologous opioid peptides can also be released from soy as soymorphins [5] and from spinach as rubiscolins [6]. Those issues lie specifically beyond the scope of this paper.

Both dairy casomorphins and gluten peptides are largely specific to modern diets. This is because neither dairy nor cereals were of dietary importance prior to the gradual emergence of agricultural and animal domestication activities. This began to occur approximately 10,000 years ago within Neolithic communities in the Fertile Crescent of West Asia. In many parts of the world, dairy plus wheat and other gluten-producing cereals from the Triticeae have only become important dietary components in the most recent centuries. Further, there is evidence of considerably lower levels of gluten peptides in early strains of wheat compared to modern wheat varieties [7] and also in durum varieties used in pasta compared to bread-making varieties [8].

The potential importance of casomorphin and gluten peptides in relation to human health remains an emergent field. For example, the presence of opioid casomorphins in dairy was not identified until 1979 [9], and the full extent of casomorphin-relevance to multiple issues of human health is far from resolved. In contrast, early insights that coeliac disease was protein-related and with particular relevance to wheat protein were known with clarity by 1950 and suspected much earlier [10]. However, the opioid connection appears to have not been explicitly identified until 1987 [11]. The broadening of the association between coeliac disease to other gluten-producing species within the Triticeae came considerably later [3]. In regard to non-celiac aspects of gluten science and pharmacology, there is still much to be elucidated.

Emergent evidence includes that not all effects of opioid peptides are necessarily dependent on attachment to opioid receptors. For example, there is compelling evidence as to the role of toll-like receptors, and in particular TLR4, in relation to both food-derived exorphins and pharmaceutical opioids [12,13]. There is also evidence that the casomorphins directly influence the serotonergic system independent of opioid receptors [14].

In this paper, evidence will be documented to show that casomorphins and specific gliadin peptides have structural elements in common and that they thereby have potential to 'hunt together' in terms of inflammatory and autoimmune effects. This is reflected in arguments in favor of diets that are free of both gluten and casein (GFCF). However, there are also obvious needs to consider gluten and casein separately, given both the known structural differences and the fact that they may favor different opioid receptors. With casomorphins, it is clear that they predominantly associate with mu-opioid (MOP) receptors, whereas with gluten peptides, there is evidence that there can also be close associations with delta-opioid (DOP) receptors [15].

The key amino acid sequence at the N-terminus that is common to casomorphins and gliadorphins, and which is fundamental to the opioid characteristics, is tyrosine–proline. However, despite the widespread presence of this sequence in relation to opioid structure, together with its relevance to particular opioid characteristics, it is not a necessary structure for all food opioids [16]. The other key characteristic of casomorphins and gliadiorphins is that they are proline-rich, thereby creating resistance to peptidase enzymes.

2. Methodology

This is a perspectives paper that draws together and thereby integrates evidence relating to systemic effects of casomorphins and gliadorphins, spanning gut, brain, and internal organs. Accordingly, the literature was searched via Google Scholar and PubMed using various combinations of the following keywords: food-derived opioids, beta-casein, casomorphin, gliadorphin, microbiome, microbiota, opioid receptors, beta-casomorphin-7, BCM7, beta-casomorphin-9, gut-to-brain, and various specific internal organs. This literature was then filtered by the author based on manuscript focus. Some background industry information was drawn from the author's professional involvement in agrifood systems spanning farming practices through to human nutrition.

3. The Role of Opioid Receptors

The widespread presence of opioid receptors spanning gut, brain, internal, and peripheral organs provides a theoretical framework to explain the current evidence and associated postulates laid out in this paper relating to diverse and systemic effects of food-derived opioids. The presence of opioid receptors in the gut and brain became well established in the 1970s [17]. It was also well understood by 1980 that opioid receptors are a key component of internal messaging systems involving endorphins and enkephalins [18]. However, identification of the widespread presence of these receptors in other organs of the body came later [19] and has been an emerging field, linked primarily to identifying and explaining the effects of opioid drugs. There is also now a substantial literature on specific molecular functional mechanisms of the opioid system [20]. This overarching suite of opioid knowledge has been central to understanding the effects that opioid drugs have on a range of internal biological processes, with opioid drugs having potential to not only exhibit inflammatory effects on specific tissues but to also disrupt internal messaging systems. This system disruption then lays a theoretical foundation for immune and auto-immune responses.

Casomorphins were first identified in the late 1970s as having opioid characteristics [9], and this is recognized with the 'morphin' nomenclature. Similarly, opioid peptides within gliadin were clearly identified in the 1980s [11]. However, no prior evidence has been found of extant literature on the presence of opioid receptors as a key element in identifying mechanisms whereby food-derived opioids might themselves have widespread systemic effects that extend well beyond the gut and brain. These concepts will be drawn upon in subsequent sections of the paper.

4. Casomorphins

By definition, casomorphins can be any opioid released from casein during digestion. In practice, the human-health interest relates to casomorphins released from beta-casein, and in particular the release of bovine beta-casomorphin-7 (bBCM7) from bovine milk. The longer chain beta-casomorphin-9 (bBCM9) is also of relevance. As background, beta-caseins are present in all mammalian milk, and in bovine milk they are the second most important of the casein proteins by volume, comprising about 35% of the casein proteins and approximately 28% of total protein [21].

The amino acid structure of bBCM7 is tyrosine–proline–phenylalaline–proline–glycine–proline–isoleucine. The first three amino acids confirm that it will be opioid in character, with the first two of fundamental importance. Additionally, the presence of the three proline amino acids in close proximity ensures that bBCM7 will be resistant to internal cleavage at the C-terminus by the peptidases [22]. Accordingly, bBCM7 is normally broken down from the N-terminus, with the key requirement being the enzyme dipeptidyl peptidase-4 (DPP4) [23]. Given the resistance to enzymatic degradation from the C-terminus, shorter-chain casomorphins are of limited practical importance within in vivo settings, despite in vitro investigations showing bBCM5 to be a stronger opioid than bBCM7 [24].

Bovine beta-casein is categorized into two broad types, these being A1 and A2, with the A1-type being fundamental to the release of bBCM7 (Figure 1). This bBCM7 peptide is located at positions 59–66 of the 209 amino acids contained within the bovine beta-casein protein [21]. In A1 beta-casein, the release of bBCM7 is facilitated by the presence of histidine at position 67, with the C-terminus bond between positions 66 and 67 being readily broken by carboxyl peptidases such as elastase [25]. In contrast, in A2 beta-casein, the amino acid at position 67 is another proline, leading to preferential cleavage of the longer peptide bBCM9 and creating a major constraint to formation of bBCM7 during in vivo digestion [21]. Although bBCM9 is itself also an opioid with consequent potential pharmacologic properties, these properties are fundamentally different, and bBCM9 is considered a potential beneficial bioactive carrying both antihypertensive properties [26] and antioxidant properties [27]. Additionally, in contrast to A1 beta-casein and bBCM7, no digestive differences have been recorded when A2 beta-casein digests containing bBCM9 are tested with and without naloxone [28]. Human-based in vivo data on beta-casein metabolism to casomorphins and intermediate peptides has been summarized within a systematic review of digestive effects undertaken by Brooke-Taylor and colleagues [22].

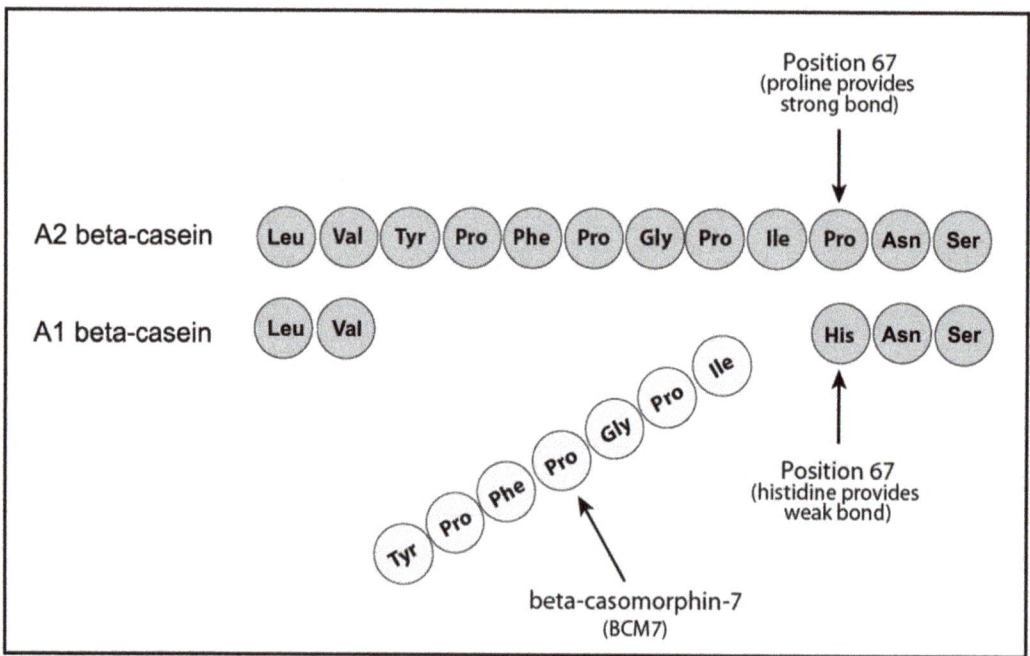

Figure 1. Preferential release of bovine beta-casomorphin-7 from A1 beta-casein.

Subsequent to the allocation of the beta-casein terminology, it has become evident from phylogenetic analyses that A2 is the original type with A1 beta-casein being the consequence of a mutation occurring in some European cattle approximately 5000 years ago, but with considerable uncertainty as to the precise time thereof [29]. The phylogenetic evidence is also clear that there have been subsequent mutations at other loci in the bovine beta-casein protein, but with these occurring at relatively lower levels, and these are generally considered as lying within the A1 and A2 families of bovine beta-casein [30]. Accordingly, the presence of any beta-casein of the A1-type in bovine milk is evidence of at least some European cow ancestry. In contrast, the beta-caseins of sheep, goats, horses, camels, yaks, buffalo, pure African cattle, pure Asian cattle, and even human milk are all classified as being exclusively of the A2 type, with no reliable evidence of exceptions even at low levels. However, some cattle classified as African or Asian types may have a small hidden proportion of European-breed ancestry due to crossbreeding within the last 200 years, leading to low levels of A1 beta-casein [31].

The proportion of A1 to A2 beta-casein within bovine herds will depend on the relative frequency of the A1 and A2 alleles of the beta-casein gene sited on the sixth-chromosome [31]. The two alleles are co-dominant, meaning that a cow carrying one copy of each of the A1 and A2 alleles produces A1 and A2 beta-casein in equal amounts and is commonly termed an 'A1A2' cow. The relative frequency of the alleles varies between countries and between breeds, but typically the ratio at a country level in modern industries based on European breeds is between 1:3 and 3:1. Specific herds may lie outside these ratios depending on historical bull choices. Additionally, there are European niche breeds such as Guernsey and Fleckvieh which tend to carry higher levels of the A2 allele. There is also a tendency for breeds with Northern European origins to carry higher A1 levels than breeds with Southern European origins [31], with this flowing through to national herd data and consequent between-country differences.

Given that some cows carry one copy of each allele with associated co-dominance, the proportion of cows producing only A2 beta casein and termed 'A2 cows' will be less than the proportion of the A2 beta-casein in bulk milk in all situations where some A1A2 cows are present. At the retail level, milk in which all of the beta-casein is A2 is called 'A2 milk'. In contrast, milk that contains some A1 beta-casein is commonly called 'A1 milk' despite typically also containing some A2 beta-casein.

There is also a human version of beta-casomorphin-7 with the structure tyrosine–proline–phenylalanine–valine–glutamine–proline–isoleucine, denoted here as hBCM7 (Figure 2). However, the human version of BCM7 is a much weaker opioid than the bovine form [32]. It is found mainly within colostrum and early lactation-stage milk [33] and it has been postulated to play a role in bonding of baby to mother. It is also much more susceptible than bBCM7 to internal cleavage by peptidases given the internal phenylalanine–valine–glutamine sequence. The specific mechanisms leading to hBCM7 in early-stage breast-milk remain to be fully elucidated. However, it is clear that hBCM7 is released in much smaller quantities than is the case with bBCM7 in most commercial milks, with this being entirely logical given that human beta-casein is of the A2 type.

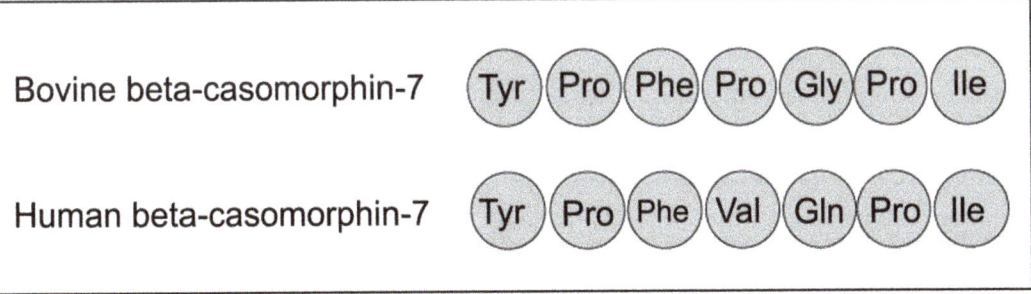

Figure 2. Comparing human and bovine beta-casomorphin-7.

In summary, it has become progressively evident over the last 40 years that the important casomorphin from a human-health perspective is bBCM7, with this peptide being preferentially released by cattle carrying beta-casein alleles belonging to the A1 family. Milk from cattle exclusively carrying double copies of the A2 allele, and also the milks from all other species of animal, are generally not considered to have casomorphin issues that are of public-health concern.

5. Casomorphin Effects on Human Health

5.1. Type 1 Diabetes

The initial evidence linking casomorphins to specific health issues was epidemiological with the investigational hypothesis deriving from clinical-practice insights. Between-country population studies identified remarkable associations between the intake of A1 beta-casein and the incidence of Type 1 diabetes in children with data from years 1990–1994 [34,35]. The hypothesis driving those investigations arose from empirical evidence that Polynesian children living in New Zealand had much higher levels of Type-1 diabetes than Polynesian children living in the Pacific Islands, with the key dietary difference being the much lower quantity of milk consumed in the Islands. The other evidence contributing to the initial hypothesis was that African children on very high-milk diets and in situations where the beta-casein was of the A2 type from indigenous African cattle were not susceptible to Type-1 diabetes [24,36]. The notion that milk might be a contributory causal factor for Type 1 diabetes was well established at that time [37–39] but the suggestion that the causal factor was a specific opioid-derived milk peptide was novel. Given the very high levels of statistical significance from the hypothesis-driven A1 versus A2 epidemiological investigations, the associations were unlikely to be random, and could not be argued to be a consequence of data-mining. However, a counter perspective was that between-country associations can never provide proof.

Given the widely accepted evidence that Type 1 diabetes is an auto-immune disease, then, if A1 beta-casein is a causal factor, it is logical that the antigen has to be the difference between the two beta-caseins in relation to the release of bBCM7. This logic is reinforced by evidence for a homologous peptide embedded within beta-cells within the pancreas that has the same sequence as the last four amino acids of bBCM7 [40]. Additionally, there is historical evidence from Germany that Type 1 diabetes sufferers have high levels of A1 beta-casein antibodies relative to those who do not have the disease [41]. However, at that time and ensuing times, there was no acknowledged mechanism by which bBCM7 was transported from the gut system to the pancreas. Accordingly, the mainstream medical perspective remained that bBCM7 would be broken down by the enzyme DPP4 before entering the circulatory system and was therefore unlikely to be relevant.

Subsequently, there has been a stream of work linking Type 1 diabetes to intestinal permeability and also to particular microbiota. Vaarala and colleagues in 2008 described the concept of a 'perfect storm' of aberrant intestinal microbiota, a leaky intestinal mucosal barrier, and altered intestinal immune responsiveness linking to other susceptibility factors [42]. Of relevance here is that the enzyme DPP4, which is the only peptidase enzyme known to break down bBCM7, is a brush-border enzyme, also present in serum, but human DPP4 does not circulate within the gut contents. Impaired brush border DPP4 production is clearly associated with intestinal permeability [43]. There is also a literature showing that specific microbiota themselves produce DPP4 and hence have the ability to degrade casomorphins and other food-derived opioids [44,45]. Additionally, there is a separate stream of work that now demonstrates that bBCM7 is present both in blood and urine [46,47]. Accordingly, some key elements of the initial skepticism have now been invalidated.

A more recent paper has developed a more sophisticated argument that A1 beta-casein and hence bBCM7 is a primary trigger for Type 1 diabetes while recognizing, consistent with the above knowledge, that there is a multiplicity of influencing factors that can enhance the opportunity for bBCM7 to act as the trigger [48]. There is also evidence of epigenetic effects [49]. It is also possible for bBCM7 to be a powerful mediating factor without necessarily being the final trigger. For example, the final trigger may include viruses, impacting via intestinal damage and decreased brush-border DPP4 biosynthesis [50]. Accordingly, it is not helpful to develop arguments based on single-factor causation expressed on an 'either/or' basis.

Within a broader framework, any factor that increases intestinal permeability by damaging the mucosal barrier is likely to increase susceptibility. It is notable that bBCM7 stimulates mucin biosynthesis [51–53], with this likely to be a protective response. It is also notable that although genetic susceptibility to Type 1 diabetes and the role of gut permeability are well established, direct linkage of Type 1 diabetes to specific microbiota and dysbiosis is relatively new and of increasing interest [54,55].

One issue that has not previously been integrated within the overall casomorphin and Type 1 diabetes synthesis is the role of opioid receptors within the pancreas and Islets of Langerhans where the insulin-producing beta cells are located. However, it has been known since the late 1970s that both mu-opioid and delta-opioid receptors are located there [56,57]. More recently, an extensive literature has been developing linking mu-opioids in the brain to insulin secretion [58,59]. This provides evidential logic as to why bBCM7 will be attracted to the pancreas and how it can therefore be expected to interfere with endorphin messaging. Given the homology of bBCM7 to sequences within the GLUT2 molecule, together with cross-reactivity of beta-casein T cell lines to human insulinoma extracts and GLUT2 peptide [60], there is a credible pathway as to how an autoimmune reaction then occurs, leading to auto-immune destruction.

5.2. Heart Disease

As with Type 1 diabetes, major differences in incidence between countries within the developed world correlate remarkably with A1 beta-casein intake [34,61]. Supporting evidence is provided by a causal relationship identified in rabbits having been exposed to A1 beta-casein intake versus A2 beta-casein intake, leading to increased deposits of arterial plaque with A1 beta-casein [62]. Additionally, formula-fed babies have been shown to have high antibodies to oxidized LDL [63], with this being associated with A1 beta-casein intake [64]. In piglets, a direct trial comparison between A1 beta-casein and A2 beta-casein intake has shown a statistically significant difference in relation to oxidized LDL antibodies, but it is only published in the Czech language [65]. It had previously been demonstrated that BCM7 has the ability to catalyze the oxidation of LDL [66]. In humans, it has long been recognized that high milk diets for stomach ulcer sufferers (a potential cause of stomach permeability) lead to high death rates from heart disease [67], and there is hypothesis potential for this linking to A1 beta-casein with release of bBCM7 within sera following the absorption of larger protein components.

The same logical pathway linking the passage of bBCM7 from the gut to the circulatory system occurs for heart disease as for Type 1 diabetes. There is also extensive evidence of the presence of mu, delta, and kappa opioid receptors within the cardiovascular system [68]. However, although the presence of opioids within heart muscles has been known for a considerable time [69], there is no evidence of this knowledge of opioids and opioid receptors being previously linked to risk issues associated with food-derived opioids. One difference between heart disease and Type 1 diabetes is that whereas Type 1 diabetes susceptibility is clearly associated with specific HLA haplotypes, any such links remain highly speculative in relation to heart disease apart from rheumatic fever, which is known to have genetic HLA factors [70].

5.3. Links to the Brain

There is extensive evidence that bBCM7 crosses the blood–brain barrier and affects behavior and physiology in multiple ways and that this is carrier-facilitated [71]. As one example, for more than 30 years bBCM7 has been suspected as a cause of sudden infant death syndrome (SIDS) following evidence that bBCM7 induced apnea and irregular breathing in both adult rats and newborn rabbits [72]. Subsequently, casomorphins were identified in the brainstems of children who have died from SIDS [73] but comparisons with normal children are obviously not possible. This evidence was subsequently integrated by Cade and colleagues in 2003 [71]. Thereafter, there was a research hiatus in relation to respiratory depression until evidence from Poland was published showing that babies who suffer acute life-threatening events (ALTE) through apnea are characterized by circulating levels of bovine BCM7 that are three times higher than in normal children [47]. These same ALTE children had DPP4 serum activity levels only 58 ± 3% of those in normal children.

Russian scientists have found that bovine BCM7 enters the blood of babies fed milk-formula diets [74]. Whereas some of these babies could quickly metabolize the BCM7, others were slow metabolizers. It was found that where bovine BCM7 levels in the blood stayed high between feeds, there was a high risk of delayed psychomotor development. The cause of slow metabolization was not explored or discussed within that specific research, but insufficient ability to upregulate DPP4 must be considered as a prime explanatory contributor.

Bovine BCM7 has long been considered a risk factor for autism, but the hypothesis remains controversial. Cade and his team integrated evidence linking autism and schizophrenia to casein and gliadin and characterized the conditions as intestinal disorders [75]. Trials with animals show that when bBCM7 crosses the blood–brain barrier, it leads to autistic type behavior [76]. Milk elimination trials in humans have produced positive results [77,78] but are often criticized for lack of double-blind protocols. Many autistic children suffer from digestive complaints, which may make them susceptible to bBCM7 absorption [75]. Recent research confirms bBCM7 in serum is associated with upregulation in serum of DPP4 [79]. It is also known that bBCM7 reaching the brain affects the serotonergic system [14] with potential implications for neurological development.

More recent research has extended neurological evidence in otherwise healthy people from behavior to cognition in adults [80] and children [81]. It has been found that the consumption of milk containing A1 beta-casein decreases both cognitive processing speed and accuracy. The key difference between behavior and cognition measures is that behavior is a response to stimuli, whereas cognition relates to information processing.

Trivedi and colleagues have demonstrated across a range of both in vitro [82–84] and in vivo investigations [27] that A1 beta-casein and bBCM7 are inflammatory, including decreased glutathione and cysteine expression in a range of epithelial and neuronal cells together with decreased DNA methylation in differentiating neural stem cells, with redox and epigenetic implications. They also report major divergence between bBCM7 and hBCM7 in redox status and neurogenesis, consistent with a hypothesis that hBCM7 plays a positive role in neurogenesis contrasting to the negative role of bBCM7. From these overall findings, they draw links to a body of evidence demonstrating that the same glutathione, methylation, redox, and inflammatory parameters are also associated with development of autistic conditions and Alzheimer's disease.

5.4. Gut Conditions

The evidence linking A1 beta-casein to specific digestive issues has developed almost exclusively since 2010. When the first edition of my book 'Devil in the Milk' was written in 2007 [36] covering various health conditions relating to A1 beta-casein, it was not possible to present any significant human or animal scientific evidence relating to digestive intolerances or gut inflammation that came from trials incorporating treatments plus comparative controls. Instead, the evidence was restricted to anecdotal case information. However, since then, an extensive literature has developed [22], initially with rodents and subsequently focusing on human trials. A paper published in 2013 found that consumption of A1 beta-casein by mice induced inflammatory responses in the gut by activating a Th2 pathway as compared to A2 beta-casein [12]. Significant differences included myeloperoxidase (MPO) activity, inflammatory cytokines, various antibodies including IgE and IgG, and mRNA expression for toll-like receptors (TL2 and TLR4). A paper published in 2014 found that consumption by Wistar rats of milks containing A1 beta-casein compared to A2 beta-casein delayed intestinal transit and increased inflammatory status measured by MPO activity, with both of these being negated by pre-treatment with naloxone, confirming that the effects were opioid-related [28]. In the same trial, DPP4 activity was also upregulated in the jejunum by the milk containing A1 beta-casein but this was identified to be by a non-opioid mechanism as it occurred independently of naloxone treatment.

The first human trial comparing the gastrointestinal effects of milks containing only A1 beta-casein in comparison with milks containing only A2 beta-casein, undertaken as a cross-over trial in Australia and published in 2014, found higher Bristol Stool readings with A1 beta-casein compared to A2 and that gut pain was strongly correlated with higher Bristol stool readings when participants were on the A1 diet [85]. Then, in 2015, a much more detailed crossover-design investigation in China, comparing milk containing a mix of A1 and A2 beta-casein (A1A2) with milk containing only A2 beta-casein (A2A2), found that the A1A2 milk resulted in significantly greater digestive discomfort, higher concentrations of inflammation-related biomarkers, longer gastrointestinal transit times by on average approximately 6 h, and lower levels of short-chain fatty acids [86]. The digestive discomfort symptoms on the A1A2 milk relative to baseline (after dairy washout) increased in both lactose-tolerant and lactose-intolerant subjects, with lactose status identified from urinary galactose, whereas when on the A2A2 milk, these symptoms did not increase relative to baseline for either lactose-tolerant or lactose-intolerant subjects. The authors concluded, inter alia, that given the relative benefits of the A2A2 milk for both lactose-tolerant and -intolerant subjects, some perceived symptoms of lactose intolerance may stem from inflammation relating to A1 beta-casein and its derivative bBCM7. Two further Chinese crossover studies, one of 600 adults [87] and another of 80 school children [81], have confirmed the previous digestive discomfort findings relating to A1 versus A2 beta-casein and also provided confirmatory evidence supporting interactions between A1 beta-casein and lactose intolerance that did not apply with the A2 beta-casein diet. A subsequent American study published in 2020 has confirmed the findings that discomfort symptoms among persons who consider themselves lactose intolerant are increased when the milk contains A1 beta-casein [87]. Additionally, in a subset of subjects who were identified as lactose maldigesters using a hydrogen breath test, the level of breath-hydrogen was higher when the diet contained A1 beta-casein, despite the milks containing no difference in lactose content. Accordingly, in explaining the consistent evidence for interactions between A1 beta-casein and lactose intolerance symptoms, there would seem to be at least two logical deductions from the evidence that are worthy of consideration. First, the delay in intestinal transit creates opportunities for enhanced fermentation of lactose that has not been digested by lactase. Second, inflammation associated with A1 beta-casein may reduce the residual ability to produce the lactase enzyme.

An area requiring further study includes differences in casein micelle structure and reduced chaperone ability in the gut of A1 versus A2 beta-casein identified in Australia by Raynes and colleagues [88]. The authors report that chaperone functionality is important for reducing aggregation of other proteins including whey proteins, with protein aggregation of potential relevance not only within the gut itself but linking through to a range of neurological decay conditions.

5.5. Other Conditions

A1 beta-casein has recently been implicated as a predisposing factor for asthma [89]. It has also been hypothesized that bBCM7 may influence fractures and obesity via mu-opioid pathways [90]. Milk has also been linked by epidemiology to multiple autoimmune conditions, including both Parkinson's [91] and multiple sclerosis [92,93]. However, specific causal agents such as bBCM7 are difficult to evaluate within either epidemiological or clinical settings.

The presence of opioid receptors had been identified by the late 1990s in the adrenal glands, kidney, lung, spleen, testis, ovary, and uterus [19]. Opioid receptors and opioid effects have also been evident since the 1990s in relation to the immune system [94], although aspects thereof remain to be elucidated [95]. The role of opioids and opioid receptors is also explicit in relation the endocrine system [96,97]. Mu-opioid receptors and opioid sensitivity are also associated with hepatic conditions [98,99]. Accordingly, with the opioid characteristics of bBCM7 well-established, together with comprehensive evidence of widespread presence of opioid receptors throughout the human body, there is a logical underpinning to a set of intriguing hypotheses for investigations across a broad range of inflammatory and autoimmune diseases.

Conversely, no published research has been found suggestive of any benefits of bBCM7 as a dietary component. However, there is a set of papers linked to Nanjing Agricultural University exploring the use of BCM7 as a drug to reduce the effects on various health parameters in rats with diabetes induced artificially by administration of streptozotocin [100–102].

6. Gliadin Peptides and Gliadorphin

The key gliadin peptide of opioid significance and where issues align with the casomorphins is gliadorphin-7, also often termed gliadomorphin and gluteomorphin. The amino-acid structure is tyrosine–proline–glutamine–proline–glutamine–proline–phenylalanine, and for simplicity this peptide is hereafter termed GD7. Key features in common between GD7 and bBCM7 are the Tyr-Pro at the N-terminus and two further proline amino acids in close succession thereafter (Figure 3). These features, as with bBCM7, will ensure opioid characteristics plus resilience to degradation of GD7 from the C-terminus. However, homology only extends to four of the seven amino acids in total, leading to the potential for considerable differences in specific opioid characteristics. As with bBCM7, shorter peptides deriving from GD7 are unlikely to be of importance within natural in vivo settings given the resilience to degradation from the C-terminus. However, given the diversity of gliadin proteins within the Triticeae, there is potential for other specific gliadorphin structures to be identified.

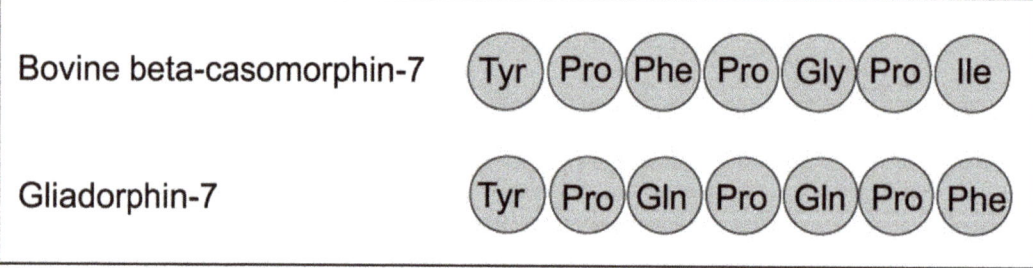

Figure 3. Comparing bovine beta-casomorphin-7 and gliadorphin-7.

In many respects, the investigatory situation with GD7 is considerably more complex and confusing than is the case with bBCM7. As a starting point, coeliac disease is associated with gluten in a much broader context than just GD7 [10]. Given the acute nature of coeliac disease, it has therefore inevitably overshadowed the study of more chronic and in some cases delayed conditions arising from GD7. Any trial removing gluten from the diet has inevitable confounding factors. These include issues such as fermentable short-chain carbohydrates (FODMAPs) [103] and glyphosate [104]. Additionally, the blinding of participants in GD7 investigations is scarcely possible given the need to remove all wheat, barley, and rye from the diet. In contrast, it has been possible to conduct blinded trials incorporating treatment and control of A1 versus A2 beta-casein without subjects automatically identifying the alternative diets and also without confounding from other variables.

Despite the dominance of coeliac research compared to non-coeliac gluten-intolerance research, there is evidence of serological differences between these two conditions, with IgG gliadin antibodies common but not always present in both groups, whereas IgG deamidated gliadin antibodies, IgA transglutaminase antibodies and endomysial antibodies are all typically found in coeliac subjects but not in non-coeliac intolerance subjects [105]. This highlights the fundamental difference between the two conditions.

An alternative investigational approach is therefore to draw on insights from casomorphin research, particularly in relation to bBCM7, and question whether there is comparable evidence for GD7 independent of a specific range of gluten-protein issues associated with coeliac disease.

A starting point is to recognize that in situations where bBCM7 is able to enter the circulatory system, relating particularly to intestinal permeability and in situations of decreased upregulation-potential for the brush-border DPP4, then the same conditions are likely to exist for GD7. Similarly, to the extent that GD7 is also a mu-opioid, or alternatively a delta-opioid, then it is likely to be attracted to the same organs as bBCM7, although not necessarily the same opioid receptors [106]. Different mechanisms by which these two peptides pass the blood/brain barrier have been identified, with Sun and Cade identifying that GD7 passage to the brain was restricted to diffusion through circumventricular organs while bBCM7 passes the BBB by carrier facilitation [71].

In relation to Type 1 diabetes, both milk and cereal diets have been implicated. For example, the non-obese diabetic (NOD) mouse strain was specifically bred as susceptible to cereal diets. The debate between A1 beta-casein and cereal diets as alternative triggers has at times been controversial [107,108]. However, once BCM7 and GD7 are considered as potential 'partners in crime' based on their peptide homology, combined with the accepted understanding that Type 1 diabetes is an autoimmune disease, then a different perspective is created.

In relation to psychological issues, there have long been theories that schizophrenia is related to cereals. Among other susceptibility factors, coeliac disease will create the underlying gut environment facilitating passage of high-proline peptides through the gut barrier. Accordingly, the neurological issues associated with coeliac disease and non-coeliac gluten intolerance such as 'brain fog' [109] are consistent with the specific peptides being either one or both of GD7 and bBCM7. It is also notable that a combined gluten-free and casein-free diet has been widely identified as relevant to autistic attributes. Similarly, when bBCM7 and GD7 were infused into rats, then both induced immunoreactivity in geniculate nuclei and the alveus hippocampus in a dose-related fashion, albeit with much higher doses required for GD7 than bBCM7, and with all effects prevented or reduced by naloxone treatment [76,106]. However, whereas bBCM7 elicited "bizarre behaviors", this did not occur with GD7 [106].

There is also an emerging literature linking gliadin antibodies to rheumatoid arthritis, with many and perhaps most of these cases not related to coeliac disease [110,111].

Evidence from Trivedi and colleagues [82] has demonstrated the commonality of effects of GD7 and bBCM7 decreasing cysteine uptake in cultured human neuronal and gastrointestinal epithelial cells via the activation of opioid receptors, albeit with bBCM7 effects being stronger. However, given that the major focus of their work was on casomorphins, there is considerable scope for further investigation of these issues with GD7. As with bBCM7, it is evident that the role of GD7 is worthy of consideration across the spectrum of autoimmune conditions.

There is no direct evidence that GD7 is a beneficial peptide for human health. However, it is part of the complex of gluten proteins that have important properties relating to the texture and form of cereal products. The importance of GD7 specifically to these attributes is not clear.

7. Links to Microbiota

There is a fast-developing literature in relation to microbiota and the gut–brain axis, with comprehensive recent reviews from Mayer et al. [112] and Martin et al. [113]. However, major questions remain to be answered as to the mechanisms by which crosstalk between the gut and brain might occur and also how that crosstalk is disrupted. Current evidence suggests that multiple mechanisms, including endocrine and neurocrine pathways, may be involved in gut microbiota-to-brain signaling and that the brain can in turn alter microbial composition and behavior via the autonomic nervous system [112]. Gut to brain connections are also linked to short-chain fatty acids [114].

In contrast to the generic gut–brain axis literature, the literature relating to both opioid drugs and food-derived opioids as modulators and disruptors of the gut–brain system is at a much earlier stage of development, but with a recent contribution from Spanish researchers representing a significant synthesis [115]. It is evident that food-derived opioids have the potential to be a generic and chronic source of system disruption in otherwise healthy populations. Within this framework, there is potential for dysbiosis and inflammation to be cross-influencing factors, but with food-derived opioids as the external source of system disruption.

Links between microbiota and food-derived opioids independent of the gut–brain axis are strongly evidential, albeit with the need for further investigations of both effects and specific mechanisms. To date, this existing evidence is not well-integrated into the gut–brain literature. Indeed, it is notable that the generic gut–brain axis literature has not placed a greater focus on external disruptors to the system. There may also be a need to take a broader system-based human biology perspective incorporating all internal organs and peripheral tissues that contain opioid receptors, given the fundamental messaging role of these receptors.

Differences in short-chain fatty-acid production between conventional milk containing an A1/A2 mix versus A2 milk with all beta-casein of the A2 variant were recorded in two blinded crossover Chinese trials [80,81], with considerably higher levels of short-chain fatty-acids, specifically butyrate, acetate, and propionic, when all beta-casein was A2, and with all differences to the A1-containing milk at very high levels of statistical significance ($p < 0.001$). The relevance of these results is that short-chain fatty-acids are produced by bacterial fermentation within the colon, and these fatty acids are therefore a proxy for specific microbial activity.

A recent Italian study [116] of diets containing milk from A2A2 cows versus milk containing a mix of A1 and A2 beta-casein provided to ageing mice identified consequential differences in microbiota, with A2 milk leading to higher levels of short-chain fatty acids including butyrate. This affected the gut immunological phenotype and favored $CD4^+$ T cell differentiation, resulting in improved gut villi morphology. The authors reported that this was the first known investigation of these issues within an ageing model. They concluded that A2A2 milk type may be suggested as a suitable strategy to achieve positive gut health outcomes in ageing populations.

A Danish study [117] found evidence for a low-gluten diet inducing changes in the intestinal microbiome of healthy Danish adults but the interpretation thereof is more complex given that these results can be confounded by FODMAP issues in wheat diets [103]. However, a recent study from Germany [118] that sought to distinguish between FODMAP and gluten issues in cereal diets concluded that both issues were relevant to non-coeliac gluten disorders, with gluten-free diets contributing independently of FODMAP issues. A recent Spanish study [119] found that a low-gliadin transgenic wheat produced a preferred microbe profile with higher butyrate-producing bacteria compared to a cereal-free gluten-free diet, with implications for reduced gut permeability.

A recent Italian review [120] concluded that for persons not exhibiting gluten sensitivity, a gluten-free diet can cause depletion of beneficial species, e.g., Bifidobacteria, in favor of opportunistic pathogens, e.g., Enterobacteriaceae and Escherichia coli, whereas in both coeliac and non-coeliac gluten sensitivity conditions, a gluten-free diet evokes a positive effect on gastrointestinal symptoms by helping to restore the microbiota population and by lowering pro-inflammatory species. A recent Mexican study [121] provides supporting evidence through the upregulation of *Pseudomonas* species in duodenal biopsies of patients with both coeliac and non-coeliac intolerances disorders, but particularly in non-coeliac gluten-intolerant patients, noting that *Pseudomonas* comprises strains with gluten-degrading capabilities. From an ecological perspective, contrasting microbiota evidence on a gluten-free diet between people who do and do not normally experience gluten sensitivity is not necessarily surprising, with specific gluten-degrading microbiota losing their competitive advantage in the absence of these opioid peptides within the diet.

There is increasing evidence that some microbiota have bacterial equivalents to human DPP4 [44,122], and this may include yogurt bacteria [123], with this creating the potential for attenuation of opioid peptides passing from the intestines to the circulatory system in individuals with a compromised intestinal barrier.

A recent Danish study [124] investigated whether gliadin would impact the metabolic effects of an obesogenic diet using a mouse model. Mice fed the gliadin-added high-fat diet displayed higher glycated hemoglobin and higher insulin resistance, more hepatic lipid accumulation, and smaller adipocytes than mice fed the gliadin-free high-fat diet. This was accompanied by alterations in the composition and activity of gut microbiota, gut barrier function, urine metabolome, and immune phenotypes within liver and adipose tissue. The authors concluded that gliadin disturbs the intestinal environment and affects metabolic homeostasis in obese mice, suggesting a detrimental effect of gliadin, and hence gluten intake, in normally gluten-tolerant subjects consuming a high-fat diet.

Beyond the specifics of the gut–brain axis, there is increasing evidence of the microbiome being relevant to a range of conditions. For example, the role of the microbiome in relation to Type 1 diabetes has recently become an increasing field of investigation [44,45,54,55], following earlier work implicating gut permeability as a key factor [42]. Similarly, there is detailed evidence that the microbiome is associated with cardiovascular conditions [125]. Given the almost ubiquitous presence of casomorphins and gliadorphins within diets, the question of whether the microbiome is a causal factor in these conditions independent of the food-derived opioids is unresolved. This can only be solved by bringing food-derived opioids, the microbiome, and these other conditions into an integrated research program.

More generally, the interpretive challenge with microbiota arises from the complexity of associations between the food-derived opioids, the short-chain fatty acids, the presence of inflammatory markers, the neurological effects of behavior and cognition, the complexity of crosstalk between the brain and the gut, and effects on many other organs that have opioid receptors. Within this overall complexity, the food-derived opioids are clearly an external flow into the system, with other factors such as microbiota having potential to be either directly or indirectly consequential and setting up cascading sequences of effects that then modulate and reinforce other specific outcomes. Whereas the knowledge of the role of the gut within food-derived opioid conditions can be considered as extensive albeit incomplete, the explicit role of specific microbiota, together with the molecular mechanisms and impacts of food-derived opioids within both the gut–brain axis and the broader human biological system, remain medical frontiers.

8. Conclusions

There is a broad range of evidential material linking food-derived opioids with delayed intestinal transit, intestinal inflammation, intestinal permeability, and an altered microbiome, with this being linked via opioid receptors and some other receptors to conditions affecting many organs. The diverse presence of opioid receptors within human tissue, combined with individual genetic differences, provides an explanation as to why the effects can be diverse. This then links to inflammatory and auto-immune outcomes in those organs. What remains to be elucidated is the precise nature of the interactions and influencing factors. Many auto-immune relationships remain speculative as to cause.

Whereas many of the short-term gut effects of bBCM7 can be investigated within clinical settings of double-blind random treatment-and-control investigations, this is more challenging with GD7 because of the need to isolate GD7 from other protein and non-protein components of cereals. In relation to the role of the microbiome, elucidation of the role is difficult given the complexity of the system containing direct and indirect effects, multiple interactions, and feedback loops. What is apparent is that the microbiome provides gut-condition indicators and gut-condition modulators, with this occurring in association with other factors and hence is occurring in a systemic framework. The biosynthesis of human DPP4 within the brush-border of the gut system, combined with bacterial DPP4 linked to the presence of particular bacteria within the microbiome, together with ability to upregulate DPP4 within the sera and other organs, are all likely to be of fundamental importance. When the microbiome is considered an ecological system, which itself is encompassed within a broader human system spanning the gut, brain, and internal organs with which it interacts, then a key question is what are the externally sourced causal modulators and disruptors of that system? It is in that context that more attention needs to be given to the food-derived opioids.

Specific strategies for reducing exposure to bBCM7 and GD7 are two-fold. Bovine BCM7 is relatively easy to remove from the food-system by producing cows that produce A2 rather than A1 beta-casein or alternatively placing more emphasis on milks from other species such as sheep and goats, plus an emphasis on human milk for babies. Removing GD7 from the diet is more difficult because currently it requires removing gluten and hence all cereals containing gluten from the diet. However, technical solutions such as genetic manipulation to alter one or two amino acids within the GD7 sequence may in the future become practical.

Funding: This research received no external funding.

Conflicts of Interest: The author consults internationally on agrifood systems projects, some of which relate to food-derived opioids. There has been no client support or client pre-publication awareness relating to the writing of this paper.

References

1. Clemente, J.C.; Ursell, L.K.; Parfrey, L.W.; Knight, R. The impact of the gut microbiota on human health: An integrative view. *Cell* **2012**, *148*, 1258–1270. [CrossRef] [PubMed]
2. Balakireva, A.V.; Zamyatnin, A.A. Properties of Gluten Intolerance: Gluten Structure, Evolution, Pathogenicity and Detoxification Capabilities. *Nutrients* **2016**, *8*, 644. [CrossRef]
3. Hardy, M.Y.; Russell, A.K.; Pizzey, C.; Jones, C.M.; Watson, K.A.; La Gruta, N.L.; Cameron, D.J.; Tye-Din, J.A. Characterisation of clinical and immune reactivity to barley and rye ingestion in children with coeliac disease. *Gut* **2020**, *69*, 830–840. [CrossRef] [PubMed]
4. Bromilow, S.; Gethings, L.A.; Buckley, M.; Bromley, M.; Shewry, P.; Langridge, J.I.; Mills, C.E.N. A curated gluten protein sequence database to support development of proteomics methods for determination of gluten in gluten-free foods. *J. Proteom.* **2017**, *163*, 67–75.
5. Kaneko, K.; Iwasaki, M.; Yoshikawa, M.; Ohinata, K. Orally administered soymorphins, soy-derived opioid peptides, suppress feeding and intestinal transit via gut mu(1)-receptor coupled to 5-HT(1A), D(2), and GABA(B) systems. *Am. J. Physiol. Gastrointest. Liver Physiol.* **2010**, *299*, G799–G805. [CrossRef]
6. Cassell, R.J.; Mores, K.L.; Zerfas, B.L.; Mahmoud, A.H.; Lill, M.A.; Trader, D.J.; van Rijn, R.M. Rubiscolins are naturally occurring G protein-biased delta opioid receptor peptides. *Eur. Neuropsychopharmacol.* **2019**, *29*, 450–456. [CrossRef] [PubMed]
7. Molberg, O.; Uhlen, A.K.; Jensen, T.; Flaete, S.L.; Fleckenstein, B.; Arentz-Hansen, M.; Raki, M.; Lundin, K.; Sollid, L. Mapping of gluten T-cell epitopes in the bread wheat ancestors: Implications for celiac disease. *Gastroenterology* **2005**, *12*, 393–401. [CrossRef] [PubMed]
8. Konic-Ristic, A.; Dodig, D.; Krstic, R.; Jelic, S.; Stankovic, I.; Ninkovic, A.; Radic, J.; Besu, I.; Bonaci-Nikolic, B.; Jojic, N.; et al. Different levels of humoral immunoreactivity to different wheat cultivars gliadin are present in patients with celiac disease and in patients with multiple myeloma. *BMC Immunol.* **2009**, *10*, 32. [CrossRef]
9. Henschen, A.; Lottspeich, F.; Brantl, V.; Teschemacher, H. Novel opioid peptides derived from casein (beta-casomorphins). II. Structure of active components from bovine casein peptone. *Hoppe-Seyler's Z. Physiol. Chem.* **1979**, *360*, 1217–1224.
10. Losowsky, M.S. A history of coeliac disease. *Dig. Dis.* **2008**, *26*, 112–120. [CrossRef]
11. Graf, L.; Horvath, K.; Walcz, E.; Berzetei, I.; Burnier, J. Effect of two synthetic alpha-gliadin peptides on lymphocytes in celiac disease: Identification of a novel class of opioid receptors. *Neuropeptides* **1987**, *9*, 113–122. [CrossRef]
12. Ul Haq, M.R.; Kapila, R.; Sharma, R.; Saliganti, V.; Kapila, S. Comparative evaluation of cow β-casein variants (A1/A2) consumption on Th2-mediated inflammatory response in mouse gut. *Eur. J. Nutr.* **2014**, *53*, 1039–1049. [CrossRef] [PubMed]
13. Eidson, L.N.; Murphy, A.Z. Blockade of Toll-like receptor 4 attenuates morphine tolerance and facilitates the pain-relieving properties of morphine. *J. Neurosci.* **2013**, *33*, 15952–15963. [CrossRef]
14. Sokolov, O.Y.; Pryanikova, N.A.; Kost, N.V.; Zolotarev, Y.A.; Ryukert', E.N.; Zozulya, A.A. Reactions between beta-casomorphins-7 and 5-HT2-serotonin receptors. *Bull. Exp. Biol. Med.* **2005**, *140*, 582–584. [CrossRef] [PubMed]

15. Yoshikawa, M.; Takahashi, M.; Yang, S. Delta opioid peptides derived from plant proteins. *Curr. Pharm. Des.* **2003**, *9*, 1325–1330. [CrossRef] [PubMed]
16. Tyagi, A.; Daliri, E.B.-M.; Kwami Ofosu, F.; Yeon, S.-J.; Oh, D.-H. Food-Derived Opioid Peptides in Human Health: A Review. *Int. J. Mol. Sci.* **2020**, *21*, 8825. [CrossRef] [PubMed]
17. Jordan, B.; Cvejic, S.; Devi, L. Opioids and Their Complicated Receptor Complexes. *Neuropsychopharmacology* **2000**, *23*, S5–S18. [CrossRef]
18. Hughes, J.; Beaumont, A.; Fuentes, J.A.; Malfroy, B.; Unsworth, C. Opioid peptides: Aspects of their origin, release and metabolism. *J. Exp. Biol.* **1980**, *89*, 239–255. [CrossRef]
19. Wittert, G.; Hope, P.; Pyle, D. Tissue distribution of opioid receptor gene expression in the rat. *Biochem. Biophys. Res. Commun.* **1996**, *218*, 877–881. [CrossRef]
20. Al-Hasani, R.; Bruchas, M.R. Molecular Mechanisms of Opioid Receptor-dependent Signaling and Behavior. *Anesthesiology* **2011**, *115*, 1363–1381. [CrossRef] [PubMed]
21. Pal, S.; Woodford, K.; Kukuljan, S.; Ho, S. Milk Intolerance, Beta-Casein and Lactose. *Nutrients* **2015**, *7*, 7285–7297. [CrossRef]
22. Brooke-Taylor, S.; Dwyer, K.; Woodford, K.; Kost, N. Systematic Review of the Gastrointestinal Effects of A1 Compared with A2 β-Casein. *Adv. Nutr.* **2017**, *8*, 739–748. [CrossRef] [PubMed]
23. Fiedorowicz, E.; Kaczmarski, M.; Cieślińska, A.; Sienkiewicz-Szłapka, E.; Jarmołowska, B.; Chwała, B.; Kostyra, E. β-casomorphin-7 alters μ-opioid receptor and dipeptidyl peptidase IV genes expression in children with atopic dermatitis. *Peptides* **2014**, *62*, 144–149. [CrossRef] [PubMed]
24. Brantl, V.; Teschemacher, H.; Blasig, J.´ Henschen, A.; Lottspeich, F. Opioid activities of beta-casomorphins. *Life Sci.* **1981**, *28*, 1903–1909. [CrossRef]
25. Jinsmaa, Y.; Yoshikawa, M. Enzymatic release of neocasomorphin and beta-casomorphin from bovine beta-casein. *Peptides* **1999**, *20*, 957–962. [CrossRef]
26. Saito, T.; Nakamura, T.; Kitazawa, H.; Kawai, Y.; Itoh, T. Isolation and structural analysis of antihypertensive peptides that exist naturally in gouda cheese. *J. Dairy Sci.* **2000**, *83*, 1434–1440. [CrossRef]
27. Deth, R.; Clarke, A.; Ni, J.; Trivedi, M. Clinical evaluation of glutathione concentrations after consumption of milk containing different subtypes of β-casein: Results from a randomized, cross-over clinical trial. *Nutr. J.* **2016**, *15*, 82. [CrossRef]
28. Barnett, M.P.; McNabb, W.C.; Roy, N.C.; Woodford, K.B.; Clarke, A.J. Dietary A1 beta-casein affects gastrointestinal transit time, dipeptidyl peptidase-4 activity, and inflammatory status relative to A2 beta-casein in Wistar rats. *Int. J. Food Sci. Nutr.* **2014**, *65*, 720–727. [CrossRef]
29. Ng-Kwai-Hang, K.F.; Grosclaude, F. Genetic Polymorphism of Milk Proteins. In *Advanced Dairy Chemistry—1 Proteins*; Springer: Boston, MA, USA, 2003.
30. Farrell, H.M., Jr.; Jimenez-Flores, R.; Bleck, G.T.; Brown, E.M.; Butler, J.E.; Creamer, L.K.; Hicks, C.L.; Hollar, C.M.; Ng-Kwai-Hang, K.F.; Swaisgood, H.E. Nomenclature of proteins of cow's milk-sixth revision. *J. Dairy Sci.* **2004**, *87*, 1641–1674.
31. Woodford, K.B. *Devil in the Milk*; Chelsea Green: White River Junction, VT, USA, 2009.
32. Koch, G.; Wiedemann, K.; Teschemacher, H. Opioid activities of human ß casomorphins. *Naunyn-Schmiedeberg's Arch. Pharmacol.* **1985**, *331*, 351–354. [CrossRef] [PubMed]
33. Jarmolowska, B.; Sidor, K.; Iwan, M.; Bielikowicz, K.; Kaczmarski, M.; Kostyra, E.; Kostyra, H. Changes of ß-casomorphin content in human milk during lactation. *Peptides* **2007**, *28*, 1982–1986. [CrossRef] [PubMed]
34. Laugesen, M.; Elliott, R. Ischaemic heart disease, Type 1 diabetes, and cow milk A1 ß-casein. *J. N. Zealand Med. Assoc.* **2003**, *116*, 1168.
35. Laugesen, M.; Elliott, R. The influence of consumption of A1 ß-casein on heart disease and Type 1 diabetes–the authors reply. *J. N. Zealand Med. Assoc.* **2003**, *116*, 1170.
36. Woodford, K.B. ; *Devil in the Milk*; Craig Potton Publishing: Nelson, New Zealand, 2007.
37. Gerstein, H.C. Cow's Milk Exposure and Type I Diabetes Mellitus: A critical overview of the clinical literature. *Diabetes Care* **1994**, *17*, 13–19. [CrossRef] [PubMed]
38. Gerstein, H.C.; VanderMeulen, J. The relationship between cow's milk exposure and type 1 diabetes. *Diabet. Med.* **1996**, *13*, 23–29. [CrossRef]
39. Akerblom, H.K.; Vaarala, O. Cow milk proteins, autoimmunity and type 1 diabetes. *Exp. Clin. Endocrinol. Diabetes* **1997**, *105*, 86–91. [CrossRef] [PubMed]
40. Pozzilli, P. Beta-casein in cow's milk: A major antigenic determinant for type 1 diabetes? *J. Endocrinol. Investig.* **1999**, *22*, 562–567. [CrossRef]
41. Padberg, S.; Schumm-Draeger, P.M.; Petzoldt, R.; Becker, F.; Federlin, K. The significance of A1 and A2 antibodies against beta-casein in type-1 diabetes mellitus. *Dtsch. Med. Wochenschr.* **1999**, *124*, 1518–1521. [CrossRef]
42. Vaarala, O.; Atkinson, M.A.; Neu, J. The "Perfect Storm" for Type 1 Diabetes. *Diabetes* **2008**, *57*, 2555–2562. [CrossRef]
43. Olivares, M.; Schüppel, V.; Hassan, A.M.; Beaumont, M.; Neyrinck, A.M.; Bindels, L.B.; Benítez-Páez, A.; Sanz, Y.; Haller, D.; Holzer, P.; et al. The Potential Role of the Dipeptidyl Peptidase-4-Like Activity from the Gut Microbiota on the Host Health. *Front. Microbiol.* **2018**, *9*, 1900. [CrossRef]
44. Sakurai, T.; Yamada, A.; Hashikura, N.; Odamaki, T.; Xiao, J.Z. Degradation of food-derived opioid peptides by bifidobacteria. *Benef. Microbes* **2018**, 675–682. [CrossRef] [PubMed]

45. Laparra, J.M.; Sanz, Y. Bifidobacteria inhibit the inflammatory response induced by gliadins in intestinal epithelial cells via modifications of toxic peptide generation during digestion. *J. Cell. Biochem.* 2010, *109*, 801–807. [CrossRef]
46. Sokolov, O.; Kost, N.; Andreeva, O.; Korneeva, E.; Meshavkin, V.; Tarakanova, Y.; Dadayan, A.; Zolotarev, Y.; Grachev, S.; Mikheeva, I.; et al. Autistic children display elevated urine levels of bovine casomorphin-7 immunoreactivity. *Peptides* 2014, *56*, 68–71. [CrossRef] [PubMed]
47. Wasilewska, J.; Sienkiewicz-Szłapka, E.; Kuźbida, E.; Jarmołowska, B.; Kaczmarski, M.; Kostyra, E. The exogenous opioid peptides and DPPIV serum activity in infants with apnoea expressed as apparent life-threatening events (ALTE). *Neuropeptides* 2011, *45*, 189–195. [CrossRef]
48. Chia, J.S.J.; McRae, J.L.; Kukuljan, S.; Woodford, K.; Elliott, R.B.; Swinburn, B.; Dwyer, K.M. A1 beta-casein milk protein and other environmental pre-disposing factors for type 1 diabetes. *Nutr. Diabetes* 2017, *7*, e274. [CrossRef]
49. Chia, J.; McRae, J.L.; Enjapoori, A.K.; Lefèvre, C.M.; Kukuljan, S.; Dwyer, K.M. Dietary Cows' Milk Protein A1 Beta-Casein Increases the Incidence of T1D in NOD Mice. *Nutrients* 2018, *10*, 1291. [CrossRef]
50. Beau, I.; Berger, A.; Servin, A.L. Rotavirus impairs the biosynthesis of brush-border-associated dipeptidyl peptidase IV in human enterocyte-like Caco-2/TC7 cells. *Cell. Microbiol.* 2007, *9*, 779–789. [CrossRef] [PubMed]
51. Claustre, J.; Toumi, F.; Trompette, A.; Jourdan, G.; Guignard, H.; Chayvialle, J.A.; Plaisancié, P. Effects of peptides derived from dietary proteins on mucus secretion in rat jejunum. *Am. J. Physiol. Gastrointest. Liver Physiol.* 2002, *283*, G521–G528. [CrossRef]
52. Trompette, A.; Claustre, J.; Caillon, F.; Jourdan, G.; Chayvialle, J.A.; Plaisancie, P. Milk bioactive peptides and beta-casomorphins induce mucus release in rat jejunum. *J. Nutr.* 2003, *133*, 3499–3503. [CrossRef]
53. Zoghbi, S.; Trompette, A.; Claustre, J.; El Homsi, M.; Garzon, J.; Jourdan, G.; Scoazec, J.Y.; Plaisancié, P. beta-Casomorphin-7 regulates the secretion and expression of gastrointestinal mucins through a mu-opioid pathway. *Am. J. Physiol. Gastrointest. Liver Physiol.* 2006, *290*, G1105–G1113. [CrossRef] [PubMed]
54. Gavin, P.G.; Hamilton-Williams, E.E. The gut microbiota in type 1 diabetes: Friend or foe? *Curr. Opin. Endocrinol. Diabetes Obes.* 2019, *26*, 207–212. [CrossRef]
55. Zhou, H.; Sun, L.; Zhang, S.; Zhao, X.; Gang, X.; Wang, G. Evaluating the Causal Role of Gut Microbiota in Type 1 Diabetes and Its Possible Pathogenic Mechanisms. *Front. Endocrinol.* 2020, *11*, 125. [CrossRef] [PubMed]
56. Ipp, E.; Dobbs, R.; Unger, R. Morphine and β-endorphin influence the secretion of the endocrine pancreas. *Nature* 1978, *276*, 190–191. [CrossRef]
57. Khawaja, X.Z.; Green, I.C.; Thorpe, J.R.; Titheradge, M.A. The occurrence and receptor specificity of endogenous opioid peptides within the pancreas and liver of the rat. Comparison with brain. *Biochem. J.* 1990, *267*, 233–240. [CrossRef] [PubMed]
58. Wen, T.; Peng, B.; Pintar, J. The MOR-1 Opioid Receptor Regulates Glucose Homeostasis by Modulating Insulin Secretion. *Mol. Endocrinol.* 2009, *23*, 671–678. [CrossRef] [PubMed]
59. Tudurí, E.; Beiroa, D.; Stegbauer, J.; Jerno, J.; López, M.; Diéguez, C.; Nogueiras, R. Acute stimulation of brain mu opioid receptors inhibits glucose-stimulated insulin secretion via sympathetic innervation. *Neuropharmacology* 2016, *110*, 322–332. [CrossRef]
60. Monetini, L.; Cavallo, M.G.; Manfrini, S.; Stefanini, L.; Picarelli, A.; Di Tola, M.; Petrone, A.; Bianchi, M.; La Presa, M.; Di Giulio, C.; et al. Antibodies to bovine beta-casein in diabetes and other autoimmune diseases. *Horm. Metab. Res.* 2002, *34*, 455–459. [CrossRef] [PubMed]
61. McLachlan, C.N. beta-casein A1, ischaemic heart disease mortality, and other illnesses. *Med. Hypotheses* 2001, *56*, 262–272. [CrossRef]
62. Tailford, K.A.; Berry, C.L.; Thomas, A.C.; Campbell, J.H. A casein variant in cow's milk is atherogenic. *Atherosclerosis* 2003, *170*, 13–19. [CrossRef]
63. Steinerova, A.; Korotvicka, M.; Racek, J.; Rajdl, D.; Trefil, L.; Stozicky, F.; Rokyta, A. Significant increase in antibodies against oxidized LDL particles (IgoxLDL) in three-month old infants who received milk formula. *Atherosclerosis* 2004, *173*, 147–148.
64. Steinerova, A.; Racek, J.; Korotvicka, M.; Stozicky, F. Beta casein A1 is a possible risk factor for atherosclerosis. *Atheroscler. Suppl.* 2009, *10*, e1464. [CrossRef]
65. Steinerova, A.; Stozicky, F.; Korotvicka, M.; Racek, J.; Tatzber, F. Does artificial suckling nutrition pose a risk of atherosclerosis at old age. *Cesko Slov. Pediatr.* 2006, *61*, 519–523.
66. Torreilles, J.; Guérin, M.C. Des peptides issus de la caséine peuvent provoquer l'oxydation des LDL humaines par un processus dépendant des peroxydases et indépendant des métaux [Casein-derived peptides can promote human LDL oxidation by a peroxidase-dependent and metal-independent process]. *Comptes Rendus Seances Soc. Biol. Fil.* 1995, *189*, 933–942.
67. Briggs, R.D.; Rubenberg, M.L.; O'Neal, R.M.; Thomas, W.A.; Hartroft, W.S. Myocardial infarction in patients treated with Sippy and other high-milk diets: An autopsy study of fifteen hospitals in the U.S.A. and Great Britain. *Circulation* 1960, *21*, 538–542. [CrossRef] [PubMed]
68. Sobanski, P.; Krajnik, M.; Shaqura, M.; Bloch-Boguslawska, E.; Schäfer, M.; Mousa, S.A. The presence of mu-, delta-, and kappa-opioid receptors in human heart tissue. *Heart Vessel.* 2014, *29*, 855–863. [CrossRef] [PubMed]
69. Barron, A. Opioid peptides and the heart. *Cardiovasc. Res.* 1999, *43*, 13–16. [CrossRef]
70. Muhamed, B.; Parks, T.; Sliwa, K. Genetics of rheumatic fever and rheumatic heart disease. *Nat. Rev. Cardiol.* 2020, *17*, 145–154. [CrossRef] [PubMed]
71. Sun, Z.; Zhang, Z.; Wang, X.; Cade, R.; Elmir, Z.; Fregly, M. Relation of beta-casomorphin to apnea in sudden infant death syndrome. *Peptides* 2003, *24*, 937–943. [CrossRef]

72. Hedner, J.; Hedner, T. beta-Casomorphins induce apnea and irregular breathing in adult rats and newborn rabbits. *Life Sci.* **1987**, *41*, 2303–2312. [CrossRef]
73. Pasi, A.; Mahler, H.; Lansel, N.; Bernasconi, C.; Messiha, F.S. beta-Casomorphin-immunoreactivity in the brain stem of the human infant. *Res. Commun. Chem. Pathol. Pharm.* **1993**, *80*, 305–322.
74. Kost, N.V.; Sokolov, O.Y.; Kurasova, O.B.; Dmitriev, A.D.; Tarakanova, J.N.; Gabaeva, M.V.; Zolotarev, Y.A.; Dadayan, A.K.; Grachev, S.A.; Korneeva, E.V.; et al. Beta-casomorphins-7 in infants on different type of feeding and different levels of psychomotor development. *Peptides* **2009**, *30*, 1854–1860. [CrossRef]
75. Cade, J.R.; Privette, M.R.; Fregly, M.; Rowland, N.; Sun, Z.; Zele, V. Autism and Schizophrenia: Intestinal Disorders. *Nutr. Neurosci.* **2000**, *3*, 57–72. [CrossRef] [PubMed]
76. Sun, Z.; Cade, J.R. A Peptide Found in Schizophrenia and Autism Causes Behavioral Changes in Rats. *Autism* **1999**, *3*, 85–95. [CrossRef]
77. Knivsberg, A.M.; Reichelt, K.L.; Hoien, T.; Nodland, M. A randomised, controlled study of dietary intervention in autistic syndromes. *Nutr. Neurosci.* **2002**, *5*, 251–261. [CrossRef] [PubMed]
78. Whiteley, P.; Haracopos, D.; Knivsberg, A.M.; Reichelt, K.L.; Parlar, S.; Jacobsen, J.; Seim, A.; Pedersen, L.; Schondel, M.; Shattock, P. The ScanBrit randomised, controlled, single-blind study of a gluten- and casein-free dietary intervention for children with autism spectrum disorders. *Nutr. Neurosci.* **2010**, *13*, 87–100. [CrossRef]
79. Jarmołowska, B.; Bukało, M.; Fiedorowicz, E.; Cieślińska, A.; Kordulewska, N.K.; Moszyńska, M.; Świątecki, A.; Kostyra, E. Role of Milk-Derived Opioid Peptides and Proline Dipeptidyl Peptidase-4 in Autism Spectrum Disorders. *Nutrients* **2019**, *11*, 87. [CrossRef]
80. Jianqin, S.; Leiming, X.; Lu, X.; Yelland, G.W.; Ni, J.; Clarke, A.J. Effects of milk containing only A2 beta casein versus milk containing both A1 and A2 beta casein proteins on gastrointestinal physiology, symptoms of discomfort, and cognitive behavior of people with self-reported intolerance to traditional cows' milk. *Nutr. J.* **2015**, *15*, 35. [CrossRef]
81. Sheng, X.; Li, Z.; Ni, J.; Yelland, G. Effects of Conventional Milk Versus Milk Containing Only A2 β-Casein on Digestion in Chinese Children: A Randomized Study. *J. Pediatr. Gastroenterol. Nutr.* **2019**, *69*, 375–382. [CrossRef]
82. Trivedi, M.S.; Shah, J.S.; Al-Mughairy, S.; Hodgson, N.W.; Simms, B.; Trooskens, G.A.; Van Criekinge, W.; Deth, R.C. Food-derived opioid peptides inhibit cysteine uptake with redox and epigenetic consequences. *J. Nutr. Biochem.* **2014**, *25*, 1011–1018. [CrossRef] [PubMed]
83. Trivedi, M.; Shah, J.; Hodgson, N.; Byun, H.M.; Deth, R. Morphine induces redox-based changes in global DNA methylation and retrotransposon transcription by inhibition of excitatory amino acid transporter type 3-mediated cysteine uptake. *Mol. Pharm.* **2014**, *85*, 747–757. [CrossRef]
84. Trivedi, M.; Zhang, Y.; Lopez-Toledano, M.; Clarke, A.; Deth, R. Differential neurogenic effects of casein-derived opioid peptides on neuronal stem cells: Implications for redox-based epigenetic changes. *J. Nutr. Biochem.* **2016**, *37*, 39–46. [CrossRef]
85. Ho, S.; Woodford, K.; Kukuljan, S.; Pal, S. Comparative effects of A1 *versus* A2 beta-casein on gastrointestinal measures: A blinded randomised cross-over pilot study. *Eur. J. Clin. Nutr.* **2014**, *68*, 994–1000. [CrossRef] [PubMed]
86. He, M.; Sun, J.; Jiang, Z.Q.; Yang, Y.X. Effects of cow's milk beta-casein variants on symptoms of milk intolerance in Chinese adults: A multicentre, randomised controlled study. *Nutr. J.* **2017**, *16*, 72. [CrossRef]
87. Ramakrishnan, M.; Eaton, T.K.; Sermet, O.M.; Savaiano, D.A. Milk Containing A2 β-Casein ONLY, as a Single Meal, Causes Fewer Symptoms of Lactose Intolerance than Milk Containing A1 and A2 β-Caseins in Subjects with Lactose Maldigestion and Intolerance: A Randomized, Double-Blind, Crossover Trial. *Nutrients* **2020**, *12*, 3855. [CrossRef]
88. Raynes, J.K.; Day, L.; Augustin, M.A.; Carver, J.A. Structural differences between bovine A(1) and A(2) β-casein alter micelle self-assembly and influence molecular chaperone activity. *J. Dairy Sci.* **2015**, *98*, 2172–2182. [CrossRef] [PubMed]
89. Yadav, S.; Yadav, N.D.S.; Gheware, A.; Kulshreshtha, A.; Sharma, P.; Singh, V.P. Oral Feeding of Cow Milk Containing A1 Variant of β Casein Induces Pulmonary Inflammation in Male Balb/c Mice. *Sci. Rep.* **2020**, *10*, 8053. [CrossRef]
90. Aslam, H.; Ruusunen, A.; Berk, M.; Loughman, A.; Rivera, L.; Pasco, J.A.; Jacka, F.N. Unravelled facets of milk derived opioid peptides: A focus on gut physiology, fractures and obesity. *Int. J. Food Sci. Nutr.* **2020**, *71*, 36–49. [CrossRef]
91. Jiang, W.; Ju, C.; Jiang, H.; Zhang, D. Dairy foods intake and risk of Parkinson's disease: A dose-response meta-analysis of prospective cohort studies. *Eur. J. Epidemiol.* **2014**, *29*, 613–619. [CrossRef] [PubMed]
92. Malosse, D.; Perron, H.; Sasco, A.; Seigneurin, J.M. Correlation between milk and dairy product consumption and multiple sclerosis prevalence: A worldwide study. *Neuroepidemiology* **1992**, *11*, 304–312. [CrossRef] [PubMed]
93. Malosse, D.; Perron, H. Correlation analysis between bovine populations, other farm animals, house pets, and multiple sclerosis prevalence. *Neuroepidemiology* **1993**, *12*, 15–27. [CrossRef]
94. Bidlack, J.M. Detection and function of opioid receptors on cells from the immune system. *Clin. Diagn. Lab. Immunol.* **2000**, *7*, 719–723. [CrossRef]
95. Eisenstein, T.K. The Role of Opioid Receptors in Immune System Function. *Front. Immunol.* **2019**, *10*, 2904. [CrossRef]
96. Kapas, S.; Purbrick, A.; Hinson, J.P. Action of opioid peptides on the rat adrenal cortex: Stimulation of steroid secretion through a specific μ opioid receptor. *J. Endocrinol.* **1995**, *144*, 503–510. [CrossRef] [PubMed]
97. Rhodin, A.; Stridsberg, M.; Gordh, T. Opioid endocrinopathy: A clinical problem in patients with chronic pain and long-term oral opioid treatment. *Clin. J. Pain* **2010**, *26*, 374–380. [CrossRef] [PubMed]

98. Bergasa, N.V.; Rothman, R.B.; Mukerjee, E.; Vergalla, J.; Jones, E.A. Up-regulation of central mu-opioid receptors in a model of hepatic encephalopathy: A potential mechanism for increased sensitivity to morphine in liver failure. *Life Sci.* **2002**, *70*, 1701–1708. [CrossRef]
99. Ebrahimkhani, M.R.; Kiani, S.; Oakley, F.; Kendall, T.; Shariftabrizi, A.; Tavangar, S.M.; Moezi, L.; Payabvash, S.; Karoon, A.; Hoseininik, H.; et al. Naltrexone, an opioid receptor antagonist, attenuates liver fibrosis in bile duct ligated rats. *Gut* **2006**, *551*, 606–1616. [CrossRef] [PubMed]
100. Yin, H.; Miao, J.; Zhang, Y. Protective effect of β-casomorphin-7 on type 1 diabetes rats induced with streptozotocin. *Peptides* **2010**, *31*, 1725–1729. [CrossRef]
101. Yin, H.; Miao, J.; Ma, C.; Sun, G.; Zhang, Y. β-Casomorphin-7 cause decreasing in oxidative stress and inhibiting NF-κB-iNOS-NO signal pathway in pancreas of diabetes rats. *J. Food Sci.* **2012**, *77*, 278–282. [CrossRef]
102. Zhang, W.; Miao, J.; Ma, C.; Han, D.; Zhang, Y. β-Casomorphin-7 attenuates the development of nephropathy in type 1 diabetes via inhibition of epithelial-mesenchymal transition of renal tubular epithelial cells. *Peptides* **2012**, *36*, 186–191. [CrossRef]
103. Fasano, A.; Sapone, A.; Zevallos, V.; Schuppan, D. Nonceliac Gluten Sensitivity. *Gastroenterology* **2015**, *148*, 1195–1204. [CrossRef]
104. Barnett, J.A.; Gibson, D.L. Separating the Empirical Wheat from the Pseudoscientific Chaff: A Critical Review of the Literature Surrounding Glyphosate, Dysbiosis and Wheat-Sensitivity. *Front. Microbiol.* **2020**, *11*, 556729. [CrossRef]
105. Volta, U.; Tovoli, F.; Cicola, R.; Parisi, C.; Fabbri, A.; Piscaglia, M.; Fiorini, E.; Caio, G. Serological Tests in Gluten Sensitivity (Nonceliac Gluten Intolerance). *J. Clin. Gastroenterol.* **2012**, *46*, 680–685. [CrossRef]
106. Sun, Z.; Cade, R. Findings in normal rats following administration of gliadorphin-7 (GD-7). *Peptides* **2003**, *24*, 321–323. [CrossRef]
107. Norris, J.M.; Barriga, K.; Klingensmith, G.; Hoffman, M.; Eisenbarth, G.S.; Erlich, H.A.; Rewers, M. Timing of initial cereal exposure in infancy and risk of islet autoimmunity. *JAMA* **2003**, *290*, 1713–1720. [CrossRef]
108. Scott, F.W. Food induced type 1 diabetes in the BB rat. *Diabetes Metab. Rev.* **1996**, *12*, 341–359. [CrossRef]
109. Makhlouf, S.; Messelmani, M.; Zaouali, J.; Mrissa, R. Cognitive impairment in celiac disease and non-celiac gluten sensitivity: Review of literature on the main cognitive impairments, the imaging and the effect of gluten free diet. *Acta Neurol. Belg.* **2018**, *118*, 21–27. [CrossRef] [PubMed]
110. Koszarny, A.; Majdan, M.; Suszek, D.; Dryglewska, M.; Tabarkiewicz, J. Autoantibodies against gliadin in rheumatoid arthritis and primary Sjögren's syndrome patients. *Wiad. Lek.* **2015**, *68*, 242–247. [PubMed]
111. Yang, Y.; Deshpande, P.; Krishna, K.; Ranganathan, V.; Jayaraman, V.; Wang, T.; Bei, K.; Rajasekaran, J.; Krishnamurthy, H. Overlap of Characteristic Serological Antibodies in Rheumatoid Arthritis and Wheat-Related Disorders. *Dis. Markers* **2019**, *4089178*. [CrossRef]
112. Mayer, E.; Tillisch, K.; Gupta, A. Gut/brain axis and the microbiota. *J. Clin. Investig.* **2015**, *125*, 926–938. [CrossRef]
113. Martin, C.R.; Osadchiy, V.; Kalani, A.; Mayer, E.A. The Brain-Gut-Microbiome Axis. *Cell. Mol. Gastroenterol. Hepatol.* **2018**, *6*, 133–148. [CrossRef] [PubMed]
114. Silva, Y.P.; Bernardi, A.; Frozza, R.L. The Role of Short-Chain Fatty Acids from Gut Microbiota in Gut-Brain Communication. *Front. Endocrinol. (Lausanne)* **2020**, *11*, 25. [CrossRef]
115. Rueda-Ruzafa, L.; Cruz, F.; Cardona, D.; Hone, A.J.; Molina-Torres, G.; Sánchez-Labraca, N.; Roman, P. Opioid system influences gut-brain axis: Dysbiosis and related alterations. *Pharmacol. Res.* **2020**, *159*, 104928. [CrossRef] [PubMed]
116. Guantario, B.; Giribaldi, M.; Devirgiliis, C.; Finamore, A.; Colombino, E.; Capucchio, M.T.; Evangelista, R.; Motta, V.; Zinno, P.; Cirrincione, S.; et al. A Comprehensive Evaluation of the Impact of Bovine Milk Containing Different Beta-Casein Profiles on Gut Health of Ageing Mice. *Nutrients* **2020**, *12*, 2147. [CrossRef] [PubMed]
117. Hansen, L.B.S.; Roager, H.M.; Søndertoft, N.B.; Gøbel, R.J.; Kristensen, M.; Vallès-Colomer, M.; Vieira-Silva, S.; Ibrügger, S.; Lind, M.V.; Mærkedahl, R.B.; et al. A low-gluten diet induces changes in the intestinal microbiome of healthy Danish adults. *Nat. Commun.* **2018**, *9*, 4630. [CrossRef] [PubMed]
118. Dieterich, W.; Schuppan, D.; Schink, M.; Schwappacher, R.; Wirtz, R.; Abbas Agaimy, A.; Neurath, M.F.; Zopf, Y. Influence of low FODMAP and gluten-free diets on disease activity and intestinal microbiota in patients with non-celiac gluten sensitivity. *Clin. Nutr.* **2019**, *38*, 697–707. [CrossRef] [PubMed]
119. Haro, C.; Villatoro, M.; Vaquero, L.; Pastor, J.; Giménez, M.J.; Ozuna, C.V.; Sánchez-León, S.; García-Molina, M.D.; Segura, V.; Comino, I.; et al. The Dietary Intervention of Transgenic Low-Gliadin Wheat Bread in Patients with Non-Celiac Gluten Sensitivity (NCGS) Showed No Differences with Gluten Free Diet (GFD) but Provides Better Gut Microbiota Profile. *Nutrients* **2018**, *10*, 1964. [CrossRef]
120. Caio, G.; Lungaro, L.; Segata, N.; Guarino, M.; Zoli, G.; Volta, U.; De Giorgio, R. Effect of Gluten-Free Diet on Gut Microbiota Composition in Patients with Celiac Disease and Non-Celiac Gluten/Wheat Sensitivity. *Nutrients* **2020**, *12*, 1832. [CrossRef]
121. Garcia-Mazcorro, J.F.; Rivera-Gutierrez, X.; Cobos-Quevedo, O.D.J.; Grube-Pagola, P.; Meixueiro-Daza, A.; Hernandez-Flores, K.; Cabrera-Jorge, F.J.; Vivanco-Cid, H.; Dowd, S.E.; Remes-Troche, J.M. First Insights into the Gut Microbiota of Mexican Patients with Celiac Disease and Non-Celiac Gluten Sensitivity. *Nutrients* **2018**, *10*, 1641. [CrossRef]
122. Janer, C.; Arigoni, F.; Lee, B.H.; Peláez, C.; Requena, T. Enzymatic ability of *Bifidobacterium animalis* subsp. *lactis* to hydrolyze milk proteins: Identification and characterization of endopeptidase O. *Appl. Environ. Microbiol.* **2005**, *71*, 8460–8465. [CrossRef]
123. Jin, Y.; Yu, Y.; Qi, Y.; Wang, F.; Yan, J.; Zou, H. Peptide profiling and the bioactivity character of yogurt in the simulated gastrointestinal digestion. *J. Proteom.* **2016**, *141*, 24–46. [CrossRef]

124. Zhang, L.; Andersen, D.; Roager, H.; Bahl, M.L.; Hansen, C.H.F.; Danneskiold-Samsøe, N.B.; Kristiansen, K.; Radulescu, I.D.; Sina, C.; Frandsen, H.L.; et al. Effects of Gliadin consumption on the Intestinal Microbiota and Metabolic Homeostasis in Mice Fed a High-fat Diet. *Sci. Rep.* **2017**, *7*, 44613. [PubMed]
125. Peng, J.; Xiao, X.; Hu, M.; Zhang, X. Interaction between gut microbiome and cardiovascular disease. *Life Sci.* **2018**, *214*, 153–157. [CrossRef] [PubMed]

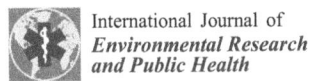

Project Report

Evaluation of Changes in Gut Microbiota in Patients with Crohn's Disease after Anti-Tnfα Treatment: Prospective Multicenter Observational Study

Laura Sanchis-Artero [1], Juan Francisco Martínez-Blanch [2,*], Sergio Manresa-Vera [2], Ernesto Cortés-Castell [3], Josefa Rodriguez-Morales [1] and Xavier Cortés-Rizo [1]

1. Inflammatory Bowel Disease Unit, Department of Digestive Diseases, Hospital of Sagunto, Av. Ramón y Cajal s/n, 46520 Sagunto, Valencia, Spain; laurasanchisartero@gmail.com (L.S.-A.); prmorales06@yahoo.es (J.R.-M.); xacori@gmail.com (X.C.-R.)
2. Genomics Laboratory, ADM-Lifesequencing, Parque Científico Universidad de Valencia, Catedrático Agustín Escardino Benlloch, 9, Edifício 2, 46980 Paterna, Valencia, Spain; sergiomanre@gmail.com
3. Department of Pharmacology, Pediatrics and Organic Chemistry Miguel Hernández University, Carretera de Valencia—Alicante S/N, 03550 San Juan de Alicante, Alicante, Spain; ernesto.cortes@umh.es
* Correspondence: juan.martinezblanch@adm.com

Received: 4 June 2020; Accepted: 10 July 2020; Published: 15 July 2020

Abstract: *Background:* Crohn's disease is believed to result from the interaction between genetic susceptibility, environmental factors and gut microbiota, leading to an aberrant immune response. The objectives of this study are to evaluate the qualitative and quantitative changes in the microbiota of patients with Crohn's disease after six months of anti-tumor-necrosis factor (anti-TNFα) (infliximab or adalimumab) treatment and to determine whether these changes lead to the recovery of normal microbiota when compared to a control group of healthy subjects. In addition, we will evaluate the potential role of the *Faecalibacterium prausnitzii/Escherichia coli* and *Faecalibacterium prausnitzii/Clostridium coccoides* ratios as indicators of therapeutic response to anti-TNFα drugs. *Methods/Design:* This prospective multicenter observational study will comprise a total of 88 subjects: 44 patients with Crohn's disease scheduled to start anti-TNFα treatment as described in the drug specifications to control the disease and 44 healthy individuals who share the same lifestyle and eating habits. The presence of inflammatory activity will be determined by the Harvey-Bradshaw index, analytical parameters in blood, including C-reactive protein, and fecal calprotectin levels at commencement of the study, at three months and at six months, allowing the classification of patients into responders and non-responders. Microbiota composition and the quantitative relationship between *Faecalibacterium prausnitzii* and *Escherichia coli* and between *Faecalibacterium prausnitzii* and *Clostridium coccoides group* as indicators of dysbiosis will be studied at inclusion and six months after initiation of treatment using ultra sequencing with Illumina technology and comparative bioinformatics analysis for the former relationship, and digital droplet PCR using stool samples for the latter. Upon inclusion, patients will complete a survey of dietary intake for the three days prior to stool collection, which will be repeated six months later in a second collection to minimize dietary bias. *Discussion:* In this study, massive sequencing, a reliable new tool, will be applied to identify early biomarkers of response to anti-TNF treatment in patients with Crohn's disease to improve clinical management of these patients, reduce morbidity rates and improve efficiency.

Keywords: gut microbiota; anti-TNFα; Crohn's disease; *Faecalibacterium prausnitzii*; *Escherichia coli* and *Clostridium coccoides* group

1. Background

Gut microbiota is defined as the total number of living microorganisms (bacteria, fungi, archaea, viruses and others) present in the intestine. The gut microbiome is a taxonomic characterization of microbial diversity including the set of genomes and, via genes, their physicochemical capabilities [1,2]. In healthy individuals, the gut bacterial microbiota is composed of more than 10^{18} different microorganisms. The vast majority of these are bacteria, with some 1100 more prevalent species; of these an estimated 160 species of bacteria are specific to each individual [3].

The microbiome, therefore, is a highly complex structure, involving thousands of microorganisms belonging to very different taxonomic classifications and, consequently, millions of associations between them, making its study a great challenge [4]. Through advances in bioinformatics, in 2003 the human genome was decoded, a milestone in science. Since then, much attention has been focused on deciphering this extensive network of microbes, the microbiota, also known as the second human genome, or as another organ. These microbes coexist with us and have a larger total number of genes than the human genome. In short, there is no simple description of these structures. However, due to their importance, considerable interest has been generated in the identification of patterns associated with human health and disease states which may even lead to the development of microbiota-based diagnostics and therapies as well as having implications for nutritional or pharmaceutical interventions [2]. To this end, reproducible patterns of gut microbiome variation have been observed in healthy adults, determining the existence of three major microbiota communities, based on the predominance or absence of species of the key genera [5]. Any other combination of key genera or genera not described by Arumugam et al. [5], together with a reduction in biodiversity, is considered dysbiosis [6,7]. Numerous technologies have been applied with the aim of examining the gut microbiota, which has resulted in the capacity and cost of microbiota research being significantly reduced in recent years, mainly due to advances in massive sequencing technologies such as next-generation sequencing. These techniques allow information of interest to be obtained quickly and efficiently by sequencing regions of the prokaryotic 16S ribosomal RNA gene [8].

In inflammatory bowel disease (IBD), the role of the microbiota in disease development and onset is very clear. While it is true that to date no specific pathogen has been conclusively identified as a trigger, we do know that, for the disease to develop, dysbiosis or a definitive change in the intestinal microbiota must occur and is likely to be the defining event in the development of Crohn's disease (CD). In IBD, it has been documented that the gut microbiota bacterial composition transitions from saprophytic to predominantly pathogenic [9]. Indeed, there is evidence of a significant increase in *Escherichia coli* concentrations, including pathogenic variants, in CD patients with ileal involvement [10]. It unknown at present whether dysbiosis is a cause or a consequence of the development of CD. It appears that the combination of a genetic predisposition and an alteration in gut microbiota are the final triggers of a chronic IBD-type inflammatory process. Specifically, we know that the disease develops in genetically susceptible individuals through dysregulation of homeostasis between commensal microbiota and/or other environmental elements and an altered immune response in the patient. An error in the interpretation of the stimulus or in the regulation of the immune response leads to an imbalance between pro- and anti-inflammatory factors, perpetuating the inflammatory process [11].

The gut microbiota play a crucial role in the development of the immune system and maintenance of the intestinal epithelial barrier. Inflamed ileal mucosa in CD patients shows increased production of tumor necrosis factor-α (TNFα), compared to normal ileum, induced by a dysbiosis in the gut microbiota, with a significant increase in bacteria that stimulate TNF production. Numerous bacteria in the commensal microbiota inhibit the release of TNF and other pro-inflammatory cytokines, e.g., bacteria that produce short-chain fatty acids (SCFA), inducing a potent anti-inflammatory effect in the intestinal mucosa. In contrast, other types of bacteria, such as *Escherichia coli ECOR-26*, which have been linked to CD, induce increased TNF release and stimulation of IL-10 release [12]. Current hypotheses in favor of a higher release of TNFα induced by intestinal dysbiosis support the idea that restoration of a less pathogenic microbe in the intestinal mucosa (inducing a reduced release of TNF and other pro-inflammatory cytokines) could lead to better disease control [13].

Today, anti-TNF therapy is one of the therapeutic pillars in the management of CD, but these drugs only treat the consequences of the disease and not the possible cause. Approximately one quarter of CD patients will be primary non-responders to anti-TNF agents, and one third of responders will experience a loss of response over time [14]. To improve treatment effectiveness, it is essential to study why these patients do not have an optimal response.

Traditionally, the prognosis and monitoring of treatments in patients with CD have been limited to the control of clinical symptoms (e.g., through the Harvey-Bradshaw Index [HBI]: see Table 1) accompanied by imaging techniques (primarily endoscopy and magnetic resonance imaging). However, these tools for assessing disease activity have many drawbacks and limitations. Among them, clinical scoring systems are highly subjective and can be misleading in this disease, characterized by alternating periods of exacerbation and remission [15,16]. Ileo-colonoscopy with biopsies is the current gold standard for the diagnosis and evaluation of inflammatory activity, with the great disadvantage that it is an invasive procedure [17] and that it is not always possible to reach the diseased area. In an attempt to identify non-invasive markers, fecal calprotectin (FC), a protein originating from the migration of neutrophils to the intestinal mucosa, was introduced as an indirect trait of intestinal inflammation, allowing more objective monitoring than clinical indices, although with low specificity and low positive predictive value depending on the chosen cut-off point [18,19].

Table 1. Harvey-Bradshaw Index (HBI).

General Well-Being (Previous Day)	0 (Very Well)	1 (Slightly Below Par)	2 (Poor)	3 (Very Poor)	4 (Terrible)
Abdominal pain	0 (none)	1 (mild)	2 (moderate)	3 (severe)	
Number of liquid or soft stools per day (previous day)					
Complications (score 1 per item)	Arthritis/ arthralgia	Iritis/ uveitis	Erythema nodosum/ aphthous ulcers/Pyoderma gangrenosum	Anal fissure new fistula/ abscess	
Abdominal mass	0 (none)	1 (dubious)	2 (definite)	3 (definite + tender)	

Remission ≤ 4 points; mild disease 5–6 points; moderate disease 6–12 points; severe disease > 12 points.

Currently, the role of bacterial gut microbiota is described as a key factor in the development of CD. Various authors defend the reduction in biodiversity and abundance of the phyla *Bacteroidetes* and *Firmicutes* such as *Faecalibacterium prausnitzii* (SCFA-producing bacteria), as well as an increase in the phylum *Proteobacteria* such as *Escherichia coli*, characteristic of patients with this disease compared to healthy individuals [6,7,20]; a decrease in abundance of this species has even been observed after anti-TNF treatment [20]. In this line, one study has identified certain specific microbial profiles that correlate with the recurrence of disease after achieving remission with infliximab treatment [14]. Several studies have also shown that the greater abundance of SCFA-producing bacteria predicted the effectiveness of infliximab [21,22] and another study associated the greater abundance of SCFA with a sustained response to this treatment [23].

A greater understanding of the composition of the bacterial gut microbiota in CD patients, such as the persistence of a significant proportion of certain pathogenic bacteria or low bacterial biodiversity, would make it possible to determine the role of gut microbiota in therapeutic responses and to establish biomarkers of response and relapse, as well as to determine whether it is necessary to restore intestinal normo-biosis in these patients. In addition, different gut microbiota profiles can be found, which enable us to predict the response to different therapeutic lines, thus being more efficient from the outset.

Accordingly, this study has been designed to analyze biomarkers of response to anti-TNF treatment in CD through gut microbiota as an alternative non-invasive tool for predicting treatment response.

2. Methods

2.1. Ethics, Consent and Permission

The final protocol was approved by the Sagunto Hospital Clinical Research Ethics Committee, in accordance with applicable national and local laws and requirements. The study was classified by the Spanish Agency for Medicine and Health Products as a prospective follow-up post-authorization study.

The study adheres to the European guidelines for the protection of human research subjects, the Declaration of Helsinki and the recommendations of the European Network of Centres for Pharmacoepidemiology and Pharmacovigilance. Approval was obtained from all local ethics committees at all participating centers. Prior to inclusion, each patient will receive a detailed report on the nature, scope and possible consequences of the study from a physician and then will provide written informed consent. No action specifically required for the study will be taken without the valid consent of the patient.

2.2. Investigators

This multicenter study in the Valencian Community (Spain) includes eight academic medical centers. The patients will be recruited by the respective participating centers of the Public Health System of the Valencian Community, in which there are approximately 15,000 patients with IBD [24]. All the researchers will be gastroenterologists with experience in the follow-up and treatment of patients with CD. The centers participating in the study will have a total load of 3600 patients with CD, 10–15% of whom will be candidates for biological treatment according to estimated data from each center.

2.3. Study Objectives

The main objective of this study is to evaluate the modification of the gut microbiota in CD patients prior to and six months after anti-TNF therapy (infliximab or adalimumab). The secondary objectives are to evaluate the association between the changes in microbiota and the clinical, biological and endoscopic response of the patients; to correlate the normalization of the gut microbiota with the response to anti-TNF treatment; to determine the level of biodiversity of the fecal microbiota at the inclusion and completion of the study in each participant; to evaluate the potential role of the *Faecalibacterium prausnitzii/Escherichia coli* and *Faecalibacterium prausnitzii/Clostridium coccoides* ratios as an indicator of therapeutic response; and finally, to describe the clinical, biological and epidemiological characteristics of the patients included in the study prior to and six months after anti-TNF treatment.

2.4. Primary Study Variable

Normalization of gut microbiota after treatment: percentage of patients with dysbiosis of the gut microbiota before the introduction of anti-TNF therapy whose microbiota is normalized after six months of treatment. Dysbiosis is defined as a gut microbiota pattern different from the established patterns of normality according to Arumugam et al. [5]: enterotype 1 (ET B) predominantly contains *Bacteroides*, enterotype 2 (ET P) is characterized by the high abundance of *Prevotella* inversely correlated with *Bacteroides*, and enterotype 3 (ET F) can be distinguished by the presence of *Firmicutes*, highlighting the genus *Ruminococcus*.

2.5. Secondary Study Variables

Percentage of patients with dysbiosis at inclusion (after initiation of anti-TNF treatment) and at study completion, measured as dichotomous qualitative variables.

Levels of biodiversity of the fecal microbiota for the microbiome analyzed are defined as follows: low biodiversity is a total of five or fewer species, medium biodiversity is a total of between 6 and 10 species, and high biodiversity is a total of 11 or more species present.

Determine the increase in biodiversity pre- and post-anti-TNF treatment, defining an improvement as an increase in the number of species greater than or equal to five with respect to baseline.

Determine the relationship between *Faecalibacterium prausnitzii/Escherichia coli* and *Faecalibacterium prausnitzii/Clostridium coccoides* pre- and post-anti-TNF treatment.

Associate the presence and type of modifications in the gut microbiota after anti-TNF treatment with the clinical and biological response of the patient during the study.

Definitions:

- Clinical remission: HBI ≤4 (Table 1)
- Clinically active disease: HBI >4
- Clinical response: when the HBI falls by three or more points.
- Relapse: increased activity assessed by clinical, laboratory, radiology or endoscopic findings leading to a change in treatment to control the disease or an HBI > 4.
- Biological remission: C-reactive protein (CRP) < 5 mg/L and (FC) < 250 µg/g.
- Active biological disease: CRP ≥ 5 mg/L and FC ≥ 250 µg/g.
- Overall response: the evaluation of clinical response will be established subjectively by the responsible physician according to clinical and analytical parameters, classifying patients as non-responders, responders without remission and responders in remission.

Clinical, demographic and complementary test variables included in the study protocol (Table 2):

- Epidemiological characteristics: age, sex, smoking habits and body mass index.
- Clinical characteristics: date of diagnosis and disease pattern, Montreal classification, activity index, presence of extra-intestinal manifestations, pharmacological history, concomitant medication, adverse effects, presence/absence of initial and final overall response, and clinical decisions derived from this response.
- Anti-TNF treatment data: indication, type, start date, induction pattern, maintenance pattern, specify whether anti-TNF drugs were used prior to 24 weeks before inclusion and reason for discontinuation.
- Complementary examinations for each patient:
    - Laboratory tests: complete blood count, erythrocyte sedimentation rate, CRP, fibrinogen, ferritin, transferrin saturation index, total proteins, albumin, urea, creatinine, GOT/AST (Aspartate Aminotransferase), GPT/ALT (Alanine Aminotransferase), GGT (Gamma-glutamyl transpeptidase), ALP (Alkaline Phosphatase), cholesterol and triglycerides
    - FC
    - Stool culture, parasites and *Clostridium difficile* toxin in feces
    - Stool collection for microbiota analysis
    - Radiological (ultrasound/computerized tomography/magnetic resonance imaging) and/or endoscopic testing if available prior to treatment (at least 12 weeks prior to inclusion) or 6 months after treatment.
    - 72-h dietary record prior to stool sample collection for microbiota analysis. Patients will be provided with a daily survey in which they must record food and beverage intake, specifying characteristics, quantity and brands of packaged products.
    - Record of adherence to the Mediterranean diet. Together with the dietary record, the patients will also complete a validated survey of adherence to the Mediterranean diet [25] classifying this adherence as low (0–6 points), moderate (7–10 points) or high (11–14 points).

Table 2. Summary of variables to be collected during the study.

Study Variables
Primary: Normalization of gut microbiota (after anti-TNF treatment) (yes/no)
Secondary variables: **A. Gut microbiota** - Initial dysbiosis (yes/no) - Final dysbiosis (yes/no) - Initial biodiversity level (low/medium/high) - Final biodiversity level (low/medium/high) - Increase in biodiversity (yes/no) - Initial *Faecalibacterium prausnitzii/Escherichia coli* - Final *Faecalibacterium prausnitzii/Escherichia coli* - Initial *Faecalibacterium prausnitzii/Clostridium coccoides* group - Final *Faecalibacterium prausnitzii/Clostridium coccoides* group **B. Clinical-biological parameters:** - Initial Harvey-Bradshaw Index - Final Harvey-Bradshaw Index - Initial C-reactive protein (mg/l) - Final C-reactive protein (mg/l) - Initial fecal calprotectin (µg/g) - Final fecal calprotectin (µg/g) **C. Epidemiological data** - Age (years) - Sex (male/female) - Time from diagnosis to anti-TNF treatment (months) - Body Mass Index (kg/m^2) - Smoking habit (yes/no) - 72-h dietary record - Adherence to Mediterranean diet

2.6. Study Design

This prospective, observational, multicenter study will include patients with CD who require anti-TNF therapy to control IBD. Anti-TNF (infliximab or adalimumab) treatment will be initiated under medical prescription according to the drug data sheet and the MAISE (drugs with a high health or economic impact) of the Valencian Health Agency. Administration of treatment will be performed in routine clinical practice and will not be promoted by this study. Fecal samples will be collected for gut microbiota analysis prior to exposure to the anti-TNF drug and six months after commencement of treatment. The patients will be monitored prospectively by their responsible physician during routine clinical practice during the first six months of anti-TNF treatment, recording the presence of inflammatory activity and whether there was no response, partial response or clinical remission at three months and at the end of the study follow-up.

Data to be recorded will include the presence of inflammatory activity (through calculation of the HBI), laboratory analytical data (complete blood count, general biochemistry, CRP) and the FC value prior to and three and six months after anti-TNF drug exposure, as well as treatments at the time of inclusion and any treatment changes throughout the duration of the study. The patient will be instructed to avoid taking probiotics and antibiotics during the study period. However, if antibiotics have to be taken, the patient must contact the study coordinator. In all cases, the second stool sample for mass sequencing will be performed after four weeks without treatment with probiotics/antibiotics, maintaining the same dietary conditions to avoid variability.

Whenever available, radiological and endoscopic activity data used in clinical practice to assess disease activity will be collected when performed, up to 12 weeks prior to patient inclusion and during the study.

Patients who undergo surgical resection within the study period will remain included but will be classified as non-responders to anti-TNF. Prior to surgery, clinical evaluation will be performed and blood and stool samples collected for fecal microbiota analysis, identical to the last determination at week 24 performed per protocol.

The patients will be provided with a 72-h dietary survey designed to record their dietary intake three days prior to stool collection at inclusion, repeated at six months to minimize bias concerning diet. Similarly, patients must complete a validated survey of adherence to the Mediterranean diet at inclusion and at six months to assess significant changes in their eating habits. An outline of the different data collection phases is shown in Figure 1.

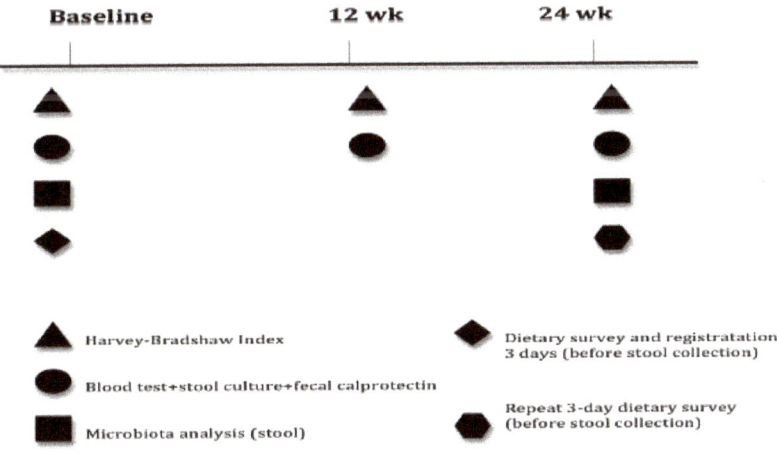

Figure 1. Overall study design.

2.7. Inclusion Criteria

All the patients must be adults (aged ≥ 18 years) diagnosed with CD with a clinical course of moderate-severe disease requiring anti-TNF treatment, in whom the indication for such treatment was inflammatory bowel activity.

2.8. Exclusion Criteria

Excluded from the study will be all patients who had taken antibiotics, probiotics, or proton pump inhibitors four weeks prior to the start of the study and stool collection; patients with chronic hepatitis C virus and chronic HIV infection; indication for anti-TNF treatment for reasons other than control of their luminal disease (e.g., enteropathic arthropathy, perianal disease, or prevention of recurrence); patients with previous ileum or colon surgery; and patients who will have received previous anti-TNF treatment in the 24 weeks prior to the start of the study.

2.9. Sample Size Considerations

Few studies have evaluated the variability in gut microbiota after anti-TNF therapy in adult patients with IBD [14,21–23,26–30]. However, from the results obtained it is not possible to determine the exact percentage of expected variability. Accepting an alpha risk of 0.05 and a beta risk of 0.2 in a bilateral contrast, 44 subjects will be required assuming that the initial proportion of events is 0.95 (degree of dysbiosis in the population at the start of the study) and 0.70 at the end. A loss to follow-up rate of 10% has been estimated.

2.10. Planning of the Sample Collection

The participating centers will be responsible for taking samples and determining conventional analytical and fecal data (complete blood count, stool samples, parasitology, FC, etc.) within routine clinical practice. The specific samples for the analysis of microbiota to be conducted externally will be collected by the patients themselves. The samples must be frozen after collection (by the patient in his or her freezer) until they are delivered to the laboratory of the hospital of origin, where they will be stored at −20 °C. The samples will subsequently be centralized.

2.11. Sequencing and Bioinformatics

The samples will be coded and the bacterial microbiota present will be analyzed using capture of the v3-v4 region of the 16S rRNA subunit [8], ultra-sequencing with Library Illumina 15044223 B protocol (ILLUMINA) comparative bioinformatics analysis. From 200 mg of stool, DNA will be obtained through a combination of mechanical and enzymatic lysis, and purified using the PowerFecal Pro DNA isolation (Qiagen) protocol with modifications. The DNA will be processed and prepared for sequencing. The sequences obtained will be filtered by parameters of quality (threshold value Q20) and length (sequences greater than 250 nucleotides). This strategy avoids erroneous ascriptions that generate an incorrect distribution of taxa. The minimum number of readings per sample will be 5000 and the mean length greater than 400 nt. A rarefaction analysis will be performed on the sample sequences to assess saturation for microbial biodiversity. Subsequently, the analysis of taxonomic identification at different taxonomic levels will be performed using the Microbiome bioinformatics with QIIME 2 2019.4 protocol [31] (Figure 2).

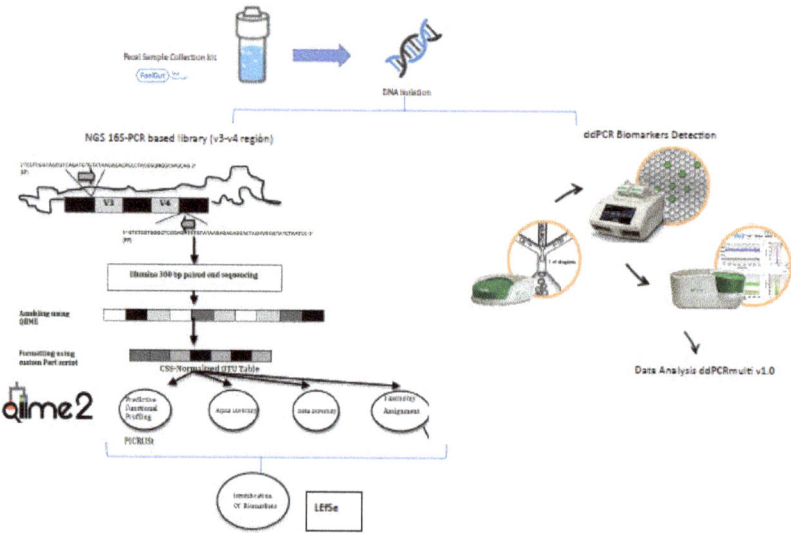

Figure 2. Sequencing and bioinformatics scheme.

2.12. Identification and Evaluation of Potential Biomarkers

To identify potential non-invasive biomarkers from the characterization of the intestinal microbiome in various stages of CD, we will use LEfSe (Linear Discriminant Analysis Effect Size), an algorithm designed for the discovery of metagenomic biomarkers through class comparison, biological consistency testing and effect size estimation [32].

Due to the need to develop a rapid method of analysis such as the ratios of *Faecalibacterium prausnitzii/Escherichia coli* and *Faecalibacterium prausnitzii/Clostridium coccoides* group, a triplex digital droplet PCR will be implemented to allow the absolute quantification of the *Faecalibacterium prausnitzii*, *Escherichia coli* and *Clostridium coccoides* species, as well as the total number of bacteria present in a given sample through the 16S rRNA gene, all with a minimum volume and in a single reaction. Therefore, the appropriate primers and probes have been selected to perform this digital droplet PCR (Table 3), as well as to optimize the different concentrations and hybridization temperatures, based on numerous relevant studies [20,33–36].

Table 3. Primers and probes used in digital droplet PCR [20,35,36].

Target	Primers and Probe	Sequences 5'-3'	Reference
F. prausnitzii	Fpra_428_F Fpra_583_R Fpra_493_PR	TGTAAACTCCTGTTGTTGAGGAAGATAA GCGCTCCCTTTACACCCA FAM/CAAGGAAGTGACGGCTAACTACGTGCCAG/IABkFQ	[20]
E. coli	Ecoli_395_F Ecoli_490_R Ecoli_437_PR	CATGCCGCGTGTATGAAGAA CGGGTAACGTCAATGAGCAAA FAM/TATTAACTTTACTCCCTTCCTCCCCGCTGAA/IABkFQ	[35]
C. coccoides	F_Ccoc_07 R_Ccoc_14 P_Erec_482	GACGCCGCGTGAAGGA AGCCCCAGCCTTTCACAT VIC/CGGTACCTGACTAAGAAG/IABkFQ	[36]
Bacteria	F_Bact_1369 R_Prok_1492 P_TM_1389F	CGGTGAATACGTTCCCGG TACGGCTACCTTGTTACGACTT FAM/CTTGTACACACCGCCCGTC/IABkFQ	[36]

2.13. Anti-TNF Dosage and Safety Evaluation

Anti-TNFs are monoclonal antibodies that neutralize pro-inflammatory cytokine tumor necrosis factor (TNF) involved in the inflammatory cascade of CD and other immune-mediated diseases. The anti-TNFs used are infliximab and adalimumab by indication for induction of remission in patients with moderate-severe CD. The administered doses of anti-TNFs are those listed in the data sheet, both at induction and maintenance doses. Infliximab dose regimen for adult patients with CD 5 mg/kg is given as an IV induction regimen at 0, 2, and 6 weeks followed by a maintenance regimen of 5 mg/kg IV every 8 weeks thereafter; treatment with 10 mg/kg IV may be considered for patients who respond and then lose their response. Adalimumab dose regimen for adult patients with CD is 160 mg initially on Day 1 (given in one day or split over two consecutive days), followed by 80 mg two weeks later (Day 15). Two weeks later (Day 29) they begin a maintenance dose of 40 mg every other week. During the prospective follow-up, according to usual clinical practice, the gastroenterologist responsible will modify or maintain a maintenance pattern according to the response to the drug by means of clinical (HBI) and analytical (fecal C-reactive protein and calprotectin) variables, which will be recorded in each patient's data collection notebook.

To identify any adverse effects associated with the administration of the anti-TNFα drug, a combination of physical examination, recording of vital signs (BP, pulse, temperature), and questionnaires are evaluated after administration (30 min later) and at follow-up visits at weeks 12 and 24. These questionnaires inquire about possible adverse effects related to adverse reactions to infliximab and adalimumab drugs (nausea, headache, dizziness, fever, hives, reactions at the infusion site, nervous system disorders, cardiac arrhythmia or myocardial ischemia, hypertensive or hypotensive events, skin reactions, gastrointestinal disorders, infections, hypersensitivity or anaphylaxis). In addition, patients are asked open-ended questions about their general well-being to request notification of any other adverse effects not listed in the data sheet. In order to assess the causality of adverse effects related to infliximab and adalimumab, the ADR (Adverse Drug Reaction) Naranjo probability scale is applied [37].

Laboratory parameters, including white blood cell count, liver transaminase levels, phosphate levels, and kidney function are studied prior to anti-TNF treatment and at the 12-week and 24-week follow-up (post-anti-TNF).

2.14. Statistical Analysis

As this is an observational non-interventional study, there may be confounding factors between treatment allocation and outcomes in analyses of comparative response rates and samples may be included of patients that do not represent real-world clinical practices. Accordingly, all analyses in this study will be considered to be of an exploratory nature. Statistical analysis will be performed with SPSS v.22 software version 9.2 or later.

Population characteristics (including demographic characteristics, medical conditions, disease duration, types of treatment used at the start of the study and other variables collected in the data collection logbook) and all primary and secondary endpoints will be summarized by indicating the mean, standard deviation, minimum value, maximum value, median, 25th and 75th percentile and 95% confidence interval (CI) of the mean for continuous variables, and the absolute and relative frequencies, with a 95% CI of the proportion for categorical data. In the bivariate analysis, the chi-square test will be used to determine differences in proportions and Student's *t*-test for paired data before and after the administration of anti-TNF treatment.

The statistical analyses conducted throughout this study on bioinformatics data management to determine significant differences between established groups, their corresponding graphs and the study of ROC curves (AUC values) will be performed using GraphPad Prism software version 8.2.0. STAMP (Statistical Analysis of Metagenomic Profiles), another bioinformatics tool based on Python, will also be used. STAMP was specifically designed for statistical processing and creation of plots from large amounts of biological data [38].

3. Discussion

The gut microbiome has a highly complex structure, involving thousands of microorganisms belonging to very different taxonomic classifications with millions of relationships between them, making its study a great challenge. In IBD, no specific pathogen has been definitively identified, but the gut microbiota as a whole has been shown to be pathogenic, contributing to the development of a deregulated inflammatory response in susceptible hosts. Several authors defend the suggestion that there is a reduction in biodiversity and abundance of *Bacteroidetes* and *Firmicutes*, as well as an increase in *Proteobacteria*, characteristic of patients compared to healthy individuals [6,7].

Treatment for CD is selected according to the severity of the disease and the response to previous therapies. Among the drugs used are biological treatments based on TNFα monoclonal antibodies such as infliximab and adalimumab, developed for the induction and maintenance of remission, allowing the control of symptoms and an improvement in the quality of life of responders, as well as changes in the natural course of the disease [38–40]. Nonetheless, although approximately one third of patients do not respond to these inhibitory therapies, we currently do not have a non-invasive biomarker that serves as a tool to predict this response, and invasive methods such as colonoscopy continue to be the gold standard for assessing therapeutic response.

In this prospective observational study, a new tool, massive sequencing of bacterial DNA, will be applied to the study of a clinical problem that affects an important number of patients. This will enable both the identification of early biomarkers of response in patients with CD after anti-TNF treatment as well as the prediction of therapeutic response from the start to thus improve the clinical management of these patients, reduce morbidity rates and increase efficiency. Since this is a longitudinal study, the patients will be analyzed before and after exposure to anti-TNF treatment, and the data will be paired, thereby diminishing the effect of the high variability of gut microbiota.

We know that the composition of the microbiota varies due to multiple external factors, particularly diet, and that a dietary intervention of just three days can cause a change in enterotype [41,42]. Nevertheless, after ten days, the enterotypes stabilized in one study suggesting a tendency to return to the original state [41]. Even so, we added to the protocol a 3-day dietary record prior to stool collection for microbiota analysis and will repeat this dietary record prior to the second assessment after six months of anti-TNF treatment to minimize significant diet-induced changes. An additional measure to objectively determine whether significant changes in the eating behavior of patients occur during the six months of the study will be undertaken through completion of a validated survey on adherence to the Mediterranean diet, both at inclusion and completion of the study. Given that long-term disturbances have a more profound effect, with a one-year diet modification having a strong impact on the *Bacteroidetes/Firmicutes ratio* [41,43], this may lead to changes in enterotype.

The proposed design takes diet into consideration and is therefore novel with respect to similar studies published to date, which did not evaluate this factor known to modify the composition of the microbiota. This study may provide additional evidence regarding potential non-invasive tools such as biomarkers of the response before and after anti-TNF therapy in CD as a starting point for future clinical trials. These trials could determine the most effective treatment among not only these therapies but all therapies used in the management of CD based on patient microbiota and provide more appropriate, inexpensive and non-invasive tools for predicting clinical response to treatment.

4. Conclusions

Currently, the role of bacterial gut microbiota is described as a key factor in the development of Crohn's disease, we do know that, for the disease to develop, dysbiosis or a definitive change in the intestinal microbiota must occur. This study may provide additional evidence regarding potential non-invasive tools such as microbiota-based biomarkers of the response before and after anti-TNF therapy in Crohn's disease as a starting point for future clinical trials. These trials could determine the most effective treatment among not only these therapies but all therapies used in the management of Crohn's disease based on patient microbiota and provide more appropriate, inexpensive and non-invasive tools for predicting clinical response to treatment, reduce morbidity rates and improve efficiency.

Author Contributions: L.S.-A. participated in the design of the study and drafted the manuscript, revising for important intellectual content, and fully approved the final version for submission. J.F.M.-B. participated in the design of the study, contributed to the statistical analysis plan and was also involved in the drafting of the manuscript. S.M.-V. participated in design of the study related to gut microbiota analysis and contributed to the statistical analysis plan. E.C.-C. participated in the design of the study, contributed to the statistical analysis plan and was also involved in the drafting of the manuscript, revising for important intellectual content, and fully approved the final version for submission. J.R.-M. participated in the design of the study and its coordination. X.C.-R. conceived of the study and was involved in the overall design and helped to draft the manuscript revising for important intellectual content, and fully approved the final version for submission. All authors have read and agreed to the published version of the manuscript.

Funding: This research received no external funding.

Acknowledgments: The authors thank Maria Repice and Ian Johnstone for their help with the English version of the text.

Conflicts of Interest: The authors declare that there are no conflicts of interest to disclose.

Abbreviations

CD	Crohn's disease
CI	confidence interval
CRP	C-reactive protein
ET	enterotype
FC	fecal calprotectin
HBI	Harvey-Bradshaw Index
IBD	inflammatory bowel disease
RNA	ribonucleic acid
SCFA	short chain fatty acids
STAMP	Statistical Analysis of Metagenomic Profiles
TNF	Tumor necrosis factor

References

1. Amon, P.; Sanderson, I. What is the microbiome? *Arch. Dis. Child. Educ. Pract. Ed.* **2017**, *102*, 258–261. [CrossRef] [PubMed]
2. Young, V.B. The role of the microbiome in human health and disease: An introduction for clinicians. *BMJ* **2017**, *356*, j831. [CrossRef] [PubMed]
3. Qin, J.; Li, R.; Raes, J.; Arumugam, M.; Burgdorf, K.S.; Manichanh, C.; Nielsen, T.; Pons, N.; Levenez, F.; Yamada, T.; et al. A human gut microbial gene catalogue established by metagenomic sequencing. *Nature* **2010**, *464*, 59–65. [CrossRef] [PubMed]
4. Methé, B.A.; Nelson, K.E.; Pop, M.; Creasy, H.H.; Giglio, M.G.; Huttenhower, C.; Gevers, D.; Petrosino, J.F.; Abubucker, S.; Badger, J.H.; et al. A framework for human microbiome research. *Nature* **2012**, *486*, 215–221. [CrossRef]
5. Arumugam, M.; Raes, J.; Pelletier, E.; Le Paslier, D.; Yamada, T.; Mende, D.R.; Fernandes, G.R.; Tap, J.; Bruls, T.; Batto, J.M.; et al. Enterotypes of the human gut microbiome. *Nature* **2011**, *473*, 174–180. [CrossRef]
6. Zuo, T.; Ng, S.C. The Gut Microbiota in the Pathogenesis and Therapeutics of Inflammatory Bowel Disease. *Front. Microbiol.* **2018**, *9*, 2247. [CrossRef]
7. Collins, S.M. A role for the gut microbiota in IBS. *Nat. Rev. Gastroenterol. Hepatol.* **2014**, *11*, 497–505. [CrossRef]
8. Klindworth, A.; Pruesse, E.; Schweer, T.; Peplies, J.; Quast, C.; Horn, M.; Glöckner, F.O. Evaluation of general 16S ribosomal RNA gene PCR primers for classical and next-generation sequencing-based diversity studies. *Nucleic Acids Res.* **2013**, *41*, 1–11. [CrossRef]
9. Kaur, N.; Chen, C.C.; Luther, J.; Kao, J.Y. Intestinal dysbiosis in inflammatory bowel disease. *Gut Microbes* **2011**, *2*, 211–216. [CrossRef]
10. Erickson, A.R.; Cantarel, B.L.; Lamendella, R.; Darzi, Y. Integrated metagenomics/metaproteomics reveals human host-microbiota signatures of Crohn's disease. *PLoS ONE* **2012**, *7*, e49138. [CrossRef]
11. Manichanch, C.; Borruel, N.; Casellas, F.; Guarner, F. The gut microbiota in IBD. *Nat. Rev. Gastroenterol. Hepatol.* **2012**, *9*, 599–608. [CrossRef] [PubMed]
12. Da Silva, A.C.; Gomes, F.; Sassaki, Y.; Rodrigues, J. Escherichia coli from Crohn's disease patient displays virulence features of enteroinvasive (EIEC), enterohemorragic (EHEC), and enteroaggregative (EAEC) pathotypes. *Gut Pathog.* **2015**, *7*, 2. [CrossRef] [PubMed]
13. Borruel, N.; Carol, M.; Casellas, F.; Antolín, M.; De Lara, F.; Espín, E.; Naval, J.; Guarner, F.; Malagelada, J.R. Increased mucosal tumour necrosis factor alpha production in Crohn's disease can be downregulated ex vivo by probiotic bacteria. *Gut* **2002**, *51*, 659–664. [CrossRef] [PubMed]
14. Rajca, S.; Grondin, V.; Louis, E.; Vernier-Massouille, G.; Grimaud, J.-C.; Bouhnik, Y.; Laharie, D.; Dupas, J.-L.; Pillant, H.; Picon, L.; et al. Alterations in the intestinal microbiome (dysbiosis) as a predictor of relapse after infliximab withdrawal in Crohn's disease. *Inflamm. Bowel Dis.* **2014**, *20*, 978–986. [CrossRef] [PubMed]
15. Peyrin-Biroulet, L.; Reinisch, W.; Colombel, J.F.; Mantzaris, G.J.; Kornbluth, A.; Diamond, R.; Rutgeerts, P.; Tang, L.K.; Cornillie, F.J.; Sandborn, W.J. Clinical disease activity, C-reactive protein normalisation and mucosal healing in Crohn's disease in the SONIC trial. *Gut* **2014**, *63*, 88–95. [CrossRef] [PubMed]
16. Harvey, R.; Bradshaw, J. A simple index of Crohn's disease activity. *Lancet* **1980**, *1*, 514. [CrossRef]
17. Rogler, G.; Vavricka, S.; Schoepfer, A.; Lakatos, P.L. Mucosal healing and deep remission: What does it mean? *World J. Gastroenterol.* **2013**, *19*, 7552–7560. [CrossRef]
18. Roseth, A.G.; Aadland, E.; Grzyb, K. Normalization of faecal calprotectin: A predictor of mucosal healing in patients with inflammatory bowel disease. *Scand. J. Gastroenterol.* **2004**, *39*, 1017–1020. [CrossRef]
19. Sipponen, T.; Savilahti, E.; Kolho, K.L.; Nuutinen, H.; Turunen, U.; Färkkilä, M. Crohn's disease activity assessed by fecal calprotectin and lactoferrin: Correlation with Crohn's disease activity index and endoscopic findings. *Inflamm. Bowel Dis.* **2008**, *14*, 40–46. [CrossRef]
20. Lopez-Siles, M.; Martinez-Medina, M.; Busquets, D.; Sabat-Mir, M.; Duncan, S.H.; Flint, H.J.; Aldeguer, X.; Garcia-Gil, L.J. Mucosa-associated Faecalibacterium prausnitzii and Escherichia coli co-abundance can distinguish Irritable Bowel Syndrome and Inflammatory Bowel Disease phenotypes. *Appl. Environ. Microbiol.* **2015**, *81*, 7582–7592. [CrossRef]

21. Zhou, Y.; Xu, Z.Z.; He, Y.; Yang, Y.; Liu, L.; Lin, Q.; Nie, Y.; Li, M.; Zhi, F.; Liu, S.; et al. Gut Microbiota Offers Universal Biomarkers across Ethnicity in Inflammatory Bowel Disease Diagnosis and Infliximab Response Prediction. *mSystems* **2018**, *3*, 1–14. [CrossRef]
22. Magnusson, M.K.; Strid, H.; Sapnara, M.; Lasson, A.; Bajor, A.; Ung, K.-A.; Öhman, L. Anti-TNF therapy response in patients with ulcerative colitis is associated with colonic antimicrobial peptide expression and microbiota composition. *J. Crohns Colitis* **2016**, *10*, 943–952. [CrossRef]
23. Wang, Y.; Gao, X.; Ghozlane, A.; Hu, H.; Li, X.; Xiao, Y.; Li, D.; Yu, G.; Zhang, T. Characteristics of faecal microbiota in paediatric Crohn's disease and their dynamic changes during infliximab therapy. *J. Crohns Colitis* **2017**, *1*, 1–10. [CrossRef] [PubMed]
24. Puig, L.; Ruiz de Morales, J.G.; Dauden, E.; Andreu, J.L.; Cervera, R.; Adán, A.; Marsal, S.; Escobar, C.; Hinojosa, J.; Palau, J.; et al. La prevalencia de diez enfermedades inflamatorias inmunomediadas (IMID) en España. *Rev. Esp. Salud Pública* **2019**, *93*, 25.
25. Martínez-González, M.A.; Salas-Salvadó, J.; Estruch, R.; Corella, D.; Fitó, M.; Ros, E. Predimed Investigators. Benefits of the Mediterranean Diet: Insights from the PREDIMED Study. *Prog. Cardiovasc. Dis.* **2015**, *58*, 50–60. [CrossRef]
26. Lewis, J.D.; Chen, E.Z.; Baldassano, R.N.; Otley, A.R.; Griffiths, A.M.; Lee, D.; Bittinger, K.; Bailey, A.; Friedman, E.S.; Hoffmann, C.; et al. Inflammation, Antibiotics, and Diet as Environmental Stressors of the Gut Microbiome in Pediatric Crohn's Disease. *Cell Host Microbe* **2015**, *18*, 489–500. [CrossRef] [PubMed]
27. Scaldaferri, F.; Gerardi, V.; Pecere, S.; Petito, V.; Lopetuso, L.R.; Zambrano, D.; Schiavoni, E.; D'Ambrosio, D.; di Agostini, A.; Laterza, L.; et al. Anti-TNF-α induction regimen modulates gut microbiota molecular composition while inducing clinical response in Crohn's Disease patients: Toward a personalized Medicine. *Gastroenterology* **2015**, *148*, S-852. [CrossRef]
28. Kolho, K.L.; Korpela, K.; Jaakkola, T.; Pichai, M.V.; Zoetendal, E.G.; Salonen, A.; De Vos, W.M. Fecal microbiota in pediatric inflammatory bowel disease and its relation to inflammation. *Am. J. Gastroenterol.* **2015**, *110*, 921–930. [CrossRef]
29. Busquets, D.; Mas-de-Xaxars, T.; Lpez-Siles, M.; Martínez-Medina, M.; Bahí, A.; Sàbat, M.; Louvriex, R.; Miquel-Cusachs, J.O.; Garcia-Gil, J.L.; Aldeguer, X. Anti-tumour necrosis factor treatment with adalimumab induces changes in the microbiota of Crohn's Disease. *J. Crohns Colitis* **2015**, *9*, 899–906. [CrossRef]
30. Ribaldone, D.G.; Caviglia, G.P.; Abdulle, A.; Pellicano, R.; Ditto, M.C.; Morino, M.; Fusaro, E.; Saracco, G.M.; Bugianesi, E.; Astegiano, M. Adalimumab Therapy Improves Intestinal Dysbiosis in Crohn's Disease. *J. Clin. Med.* **2019**, *8*, 1646. [CrossRef]
31. Bolyen, E.; Rideout, J.R.; Dillon, M.R.; Bokulich, N.A.; Abnet, C.C.; Al-Ghalith, G.A.; Alexander, H.; Alm, E.J.; Arumugam, M.; Asnicar, F.; et al. Reproducible, interactive, scalable and extensible microbiome data science using QIIME 2. *Nat. Biotechnol.* **2019**, *37*, 852–857. [CrossRef] [PubMed]
32. Segata, N.; Izard, J.; Waldron, L.; Gevers, D.; Miropolsky, L.; Garrett, W.S.; Huttenhower, C. Metagenomic biomarker discovery and explanation. *Genome Biol.* **2011**, *12*, R60. [CrossRef] [PubMed]
33. Dobnik, D.; Štebih, D.; Blejec, A.; Morisset, D.; Žel, J. Multiplex quantification of four DNA targets in one reaction with Bio-Rad droplet digital PCR system for GMO detection. *Sci. Rep.* **2016**, *6*, 1–9. [CrossRef] [PubMed]
34. Postel, M.; Roosen, A.; Laurent-Puig, P.; Taly, V.; Wang-Renault, S.F. Droplet-based digital PCR and next generation sequencing for monitoring circulating tumor DNA: A cancer diagnostic perspective. *Expert Rev. Mol. Diagn.* **2018**, *18*, 7–17. [CrossRef] [PubMed]
35. Huijsdens, X.W.; Linskens, R.K.; Mak, M.; Meuwissen, S.G.; Vandenbroucke-Grauls, C.M.; Savelkoul, P.H. Quantification of Bacteria Adherent to Gastrointestinal Mucosa by Real-Time PCR. *J. Clin. Microbiol.* **2002**, *40*, 4423–4427. [CrossRef]
36. Furet, J.P.; Firmesse, O.; Gourmelon, M.; Bridonneau, C.; Tap, J.; Mondot, S.; Dore, J.; Corthier, G. Comparative assessment of human and farm animal faecal microbiota using real-time quantitative PCR. *FEMS Microbiol. Ecol.* **2009**, *68*, 351–362. [CrossRef] [PubMed]
37. Naranjo, C.A.; Busto, U.; Sellers, E.M.; Sandor, P.; Ruiz, I.; Roberts, E.A.; Janecek, E.; Domecq, C.; Greenblatt, D.J. A method for estimating the probability of adverse drug reactions. *Clin. Pharmacol. Ther.* **1981**, *30*, 239–245. [CrossRef]
38. Parks, D.H.; Tyson, G.W.; Hugenholtz, P.; Beiko, R.G. STAMP: Statistical analysis of taxonomic and functional profiles. *Bioinformatics* **2014**, *30*, 3123–3124. [CrossRef] [PubMed]

39. Monif, G.R. Understanding Therapeutic Concepts in Crohn's Disease. *Clin. Med. Insights Gastroenterol.* **2018**, *11*, 1–3. [CrossRef]
40. Na, S.Y.; Moon, W. Perspectives on Current and Novel Treatments for Inflammatory Bowel Disease. *Gut Liver* **2019**, *13*, 604–616. [CrossRef] [PubMed]
41. Wu, G.D.; Chen, J.; Hoffmann, C.; Bittinger, K.; Chen, Y.-Y.; Keilbaugh, S.A.; Bewtra, M.; Knights, D.; Walters, W.A.; Knight, R.; et al. Linking long-term dietary patterns with gut microbial enterotypes. *Science* **2011**, *334*, 105–108. [CrossRef] [PubMed]
42. Kovatcheva-Datchary, P.; Nilsson, A.; Akrami, R.; Lee, Y.S.; de Vadder, F.; Arora, T.; Hallen, A.; Martens, E.; Björck, I.; Bäckhed, F. Dietary Fiber-Induced Improvement in Glucose Metabolism Is Associated with Increased Abundance of Prevotella. *Cell Metab.* **2015**, *22*, 971–982. [CrossRef] [PubMed]
43. Ley, R.E.; Turnbaugh, P.J.; Klein, S.; Gordon, J.I. Human gut microbes associated with obesity. *Nature* **2006**, *444*, 1022–1023. [CrossRef] [PubMed]

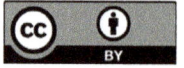

© 2020 by the authors. Licensee MDPI, Basel, Switzerland. This article is an open access article distributed under the terms and conditions of the Creative Commons Attribution (CC BY) license (http://creativecommons.org/licenses/by/4.0/).

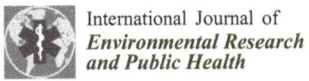

Article

Feasibility of an At-Home Adult Stool Specimen Collection Method in Rural Cambodia

Jordie A. J. Fischer [1,2] and Crystal D. Karakochuk [1,2,*]

[1] Food, Nutrition, and Health, The University of British Columbia, Vancouver, BC V6T 1Z4, Canada; jordie.fischer@ubc.ca
[2] Healthy Starts, BC Children's Hospital Research Institute, Vancouver, BC V5Z 4H4, Canada
* Correspondence: crystal.karakochuk@ubc.ca

Abstract: The human microbiome has received significant attention over the past decade regarding its potential impact on health. Epidemiological and intervention studies often rely on at-home stool collection methods designed for high-resource settings, such as access to an improved toilet with a modern toilet seat. However, this is not always appropriate or applicable to low-resource settings. Therefore, the design of a user-friendly stool collection kit for low-resource rural settings is needed. We describe the development, assembly, and user experience of a simple and low-cost at-home stool collection kit for women living in rural Cambodia as part of a randomized controlled trial in 2020. Participants were provided with the stool collection kit and detailed verbal instruction. Enrolled women (n = 480) provided two stool specimens (at the start of the trial and after 12 weeks) at their home and brought them to the health centre that morning in a sterile collection container. User specimen collection compliance was high, with 90% (n = 434) of women providing a stool specimen at the end of the trial (after 12 weeks). This feasible and straightforward method has strong potential for similar or adapted use among adults residing in other rural or low-resource contexts.

Keywords: stool; stool collection; Cambodia; sample collection; rural health; gut microbiome; collection kit

1. Introduction

There has been a growing interest in understanding the composition of the human gut microbiome and its linkages with all areas of health [1]. This has led to increased microbial community analysis, using techniques including 16 s rRNA gene sequencing, quantitative PCR, and culture-based methods [2,3]. Increasingly, large-scale observational and intervention studies have aimed to collect stool specimens to provide data in this rapidly evolving field of microbiology.

In both clinical practice and research studies, it has become increasingly common for stool specimen collection to be completed at an individual's home and then shipped to the laboratory [4,5]. At-home stool collection kits are often designed for a modern toilet seat and depend on a reliable national priority mail delivery system, [5,6] such as the widely used OMNIgene•GUT (DNA Genotek, Ottawa, ON, Canada) along with the OM-AC1 toilet accessory, a flushable collection paper secured to the toilet seat with adhesive strips [7].

Nevertheless, there is limited data concerning practical methods for collecting stool specimens for microbiome analyses in settings outside of the high-resource contexts, specifically for those without modern toilet seats or reliable shipment options. Thus, in an effort to characterize the human microbiome across the full range of the human experience, populations in low-resource settings continue to be underrepresented [8]. In the context of large studies in low-resource settings, specimen transportation and refrigeration, contamination, and acceptable collection may pose challenges. Designing a simple, user-friendly stool specimen collection kit for use in these challenging environments is imperative.

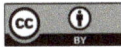

Here, we report on study tools developed and used to collect neat stool specimens from women in rural Cambodia, used as a part of a randomized controlled trial that aimed to evaluate the potential harms of iron supplementation [9]. We discuss the feasibility and acceptability of our convenient at-home stool collection methods that have the potential to be implemented in similar low-resource locations.

2. Materials and Methods

2.1. Study Participants and Setting

This stool specimen collection methodology was designed as a part of a randomized controlled trial in rural Kampong Thom province, Cambodia, with ethics granted from the Clinical Research Ethics Board at the University of British Columbia in Vancouver, Canada (H18-02610), and the National Ethics Committee for Health Research in Phnom Penh, Cambodia (273-NECHR). All participants provided written informed consent before participating in the study, including the collection of baseline and 12-week venous blood, neat stool, and fecal swab specimen. Full details of the original study can be found elsewhere [9], and the trial was registered at clinicaltrials.gov (NCT04017598). Between December 2019 and January 2020, women were recruited, and n = 480 non-pregnant women of reproductive age (18–45 years) were randomized to 12 weeks of daily oral iron supplementation in the form of either 60 mg ferrous sulfate (n = 161), 18 mg ferrous bisglycinate (n = 158), or placebo (n = 161). Venous blood specimens and neat stool specimens were collected at baseline and after 12 weeks.

Enrolled women did not have access to modern toilets with toilet seats nor household refrigeration. The most common type of sanitation facility available at most households was pour-flush to a septic tank or pit latrines (91% [437/480]).

2.2. Stool Collection Protocol

Development of the stool collection methodology took place in discussion with local public health staff highly experienced in rural specimen collection and knowledgeable about resource limitations of the study location (i.e., toilet facilities). Research staff were trained on the use of the stool collection kits and the procedures to disperse and collect the specimens from research participants. At the initial study visit, following administration of the baseline questionnaire, study staff provided the participants with the stool collection kit, verbally explained how to properly collect the specimen in Khmer (local Cambodian language), and dispose of collection materials. Women were also provided with a written copy of the same instructions regarding stool collection to take home via a simple Khmer-translated infographic. They were instructed to bring their stool specimen back to the local health centre the following day.

The stool collection kit was labelled with the participant ID number. It contained the following items: 30 mL clear polystyrene stool collection container with a screw-on blue lid and attached spoon, gloves, Khmer translated infographics and a metal pot (Figure 1). The metal pots were stored in heavy-duty plastic bags to prevent contamination before distribution to participants.

The verbal instructions as provided in staff training and written infographic (Figure 2) were communicated to study participants as follows:

1. Collect first stool the morning of your health centre visit.
2. Put on gloves provided in the stool collection bag.
3. Squat or sit over the provided metal pot.
4. Ensure that the pot is not touching toilet water—make sure no water, other liquids or materials get into the pot.
5. Defecate into the pot. A small amount of stool is ok.
6. Open the stool container tube by unscrewing the blue lid.
7. Use scoop attached to blue lib to collect a small portion of stool from the pot (size of cashew nut).

8. Place stool specimen and scoop into the stool collection tube and screw tight to secure lid.
9. Place the tube into the stool collection bag with your personal ID number.
10. Dispose of or clean the metal pot thoroughly with soap and hot water.
11. Thoroughly wash hands with soap and hot water.
12. Bring stool specimen to study nurse at the health centre on the same morning.

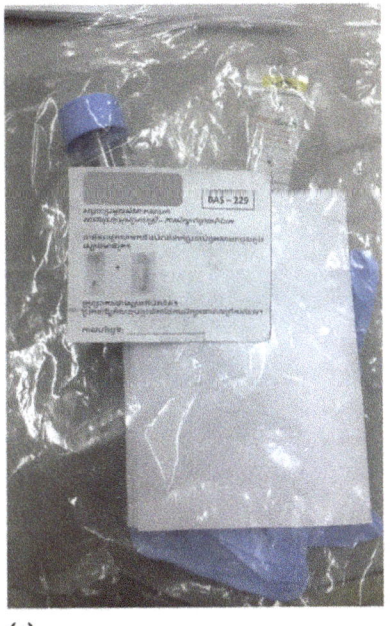 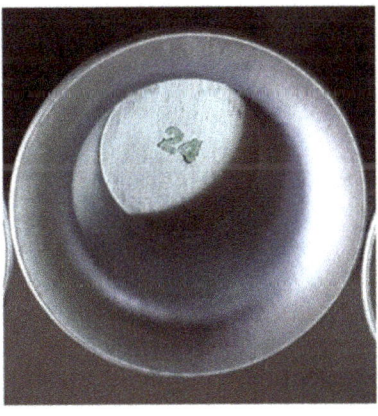

(a) (b)

Figure 1. Stool Collection Kit: (**a**) Resealable participant labelled bag, infographic, gloves, 30 mL clear polystyrene stool collection container; (**b**) Metal collection pot.

Women collected their stool specimens at their home and brought the completed kit back to the health center within ~2 h of defecation in the provided clear resealable plastic bag. Many participants opted to place the transparent bag inside a small opaque black garbage bag for additional privacy. Upon retrieval, study staff would ensure the stool collection kit contained the neat stool specimen and the container was tightly sealed. Tubes were labelled with the participant, study visit number, date, and time received. Labelled tubes were double-checked to ensure participant ID matched the ID number marked on the outer side of the bag. The kits were then immediately placed on ice. Neat stool specimens were transported on ice to the National Public Health Laboratory, where specimens underwent further processing and were frozen at −20 °C within 4–6 h until further analysis. Additionally, women were given the metal pot to keep and use for additional study visits where follow-up stool collection was needed.

Missing stool specimens were documented, and women were followed up by staff on the morning of the initial study visit. If a woman could not pass stool or was not available for a study visit that day, stool specimens were collected within seven days of the original study visit date. In this event, study staff called women to arrange another stool pickup, ensuring that pickup happened within 2 h of bowel movement and placed on ice, driven to the National laboratory and frozen at −20 °C within 4–6 h.

How to Collect Stool

Collect first morning stool, bring to health centre and give to study nurse on the same day

1. Put on gloves

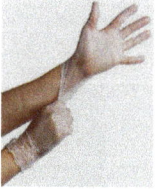

2. Sit on provided metal pot

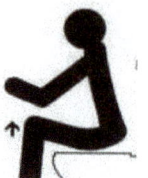

MAKE SURE POT IS CLEAN.

DO NOT ALLOW ANY WATER TO ENTER POT.

3. Poop into pot

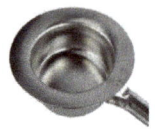

4. Open stool container tube

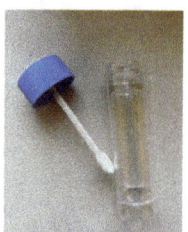

5. Use scoop to collect portion of stool from pot

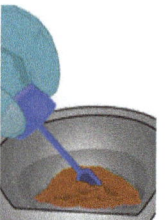

6. Place stool sample and scoop into stool collection tube and seal securely

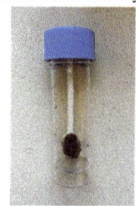

7. Place collection tube into "stool collection kit" along with fecal swab tube

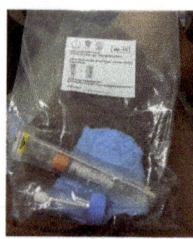

8. Throw away gloves and wash hands

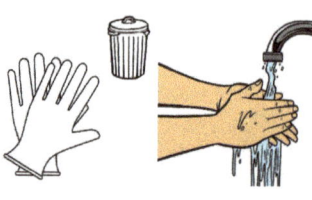

Figure 2. Participant stool collection infographic (English translation).

3. Results

During recruitment, n = 1286 women were screened for study inclusion eligibility, of which n = 577 did not meet the inclusion criteria, and n = 229 declined to participate. No women declined to participate due to the requirement of a stool specimen collection. A total of 480 women were enrolled in the study, and n = 456 (95%) women provided a stool specimen at baseline (baseline blood collection, not stool collection, was required for enrollment). A total of n = 441 (92%) women remained in the study until completion at 12 weeks, with n = 434 (90%) women providing a 12-week stool specimen, depicted in Figure 3. Women who provided a baseline stool specimen (n = 456) and those that did not give a baseline stool specimen (n = 22) differed by education level achieved (fisher's exact, p = 0.044), breastfeeding status (fisher's exact, p = 0.007), reported diarrhea (3+ loose bowel movements in 24 h) (fisher's exact, p = 0.023), pain when passing stool (fisher's exact,

$p = 0.015$), blood in stool (fisher's exact, $p = 0.028$), and if women had previously taken antibiotics (fisher's exact, $p = 0.006$) (Table 1).

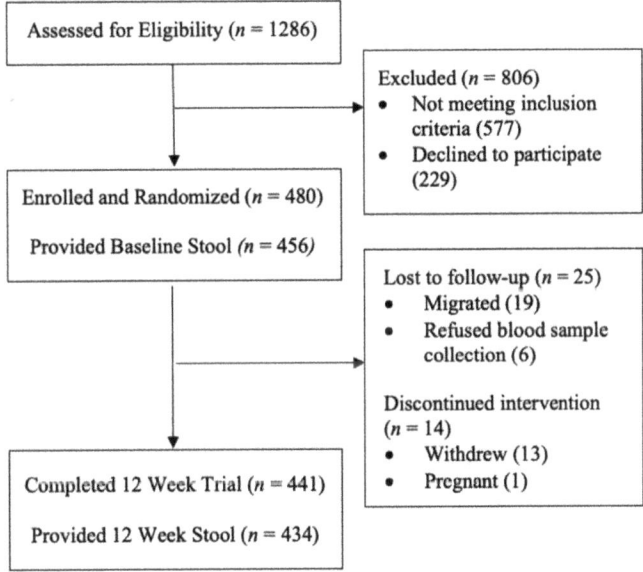

Figure 3. Participant flow chart.

Table 1. Baseline participant characteristics of enrolled Cambodian women by provision of baseline stool specimen.

	Provided Baseline Stool Specimen	No Baseline Stool Specimen	p-Value [1]
Total enrolled, n (%)	458 (95%)	22 (5%)	
Woman's age, y, median (IQR)	34.5 (28.0, 40.0)	31.5 (29.0, 36.0)	0.387
Married	397/458 (87%)	19/22 (86%)	0.624
Completed education, (%)			0.044 *
Primary	242/416 (58%)	9/22 (41%)	
Lower secondary	106/416 (26%)	12/22 (55%)	
Upper secondary	54/416 (13%)	1/22 (4%)	
Higher education/university	14/416 (3%)	0/22 (0%)	
BMI (kg/m^2)	23.5 ± 3.8	22.7 ± 3.6	0.295
Currently breastfeeding	40/141 (28%)	43/145 (30%)	0.007 *
Currently use birth control	56/161 (35%)	70/158 (44%)	0.826
Previously taken antibiotics	202/458 (44%)	11/22 (50%)	0.006 *
Experienced gastrointestinal upset			
Diarrhea	67/241 (28%)	0/13 (0%)	0.023 *
Nausea	126/241 (52%)	7/13 (54%)	1.00
Constipation	31/241 (13%)	3/13 (23%)	0.392
Pain when passing stool	71/241 (7%)	4/13 (31%)	0.015 *
Blood in Stool	11/241 (5%)	3/13 (23%)	0.028 *

Total n = 480. Values are n (%) or median (IQR). [1] Independent samples t-test (parametric) and Wilcoxon rank sum tests (non-parametric) for continuous variables and Fisher's exact tests for categorical variables. * Statistically significant at $p < 0.05$.

Throughout the study duration, research staff informally collected feedback from participants on their experience in the stool collection method. Some specific comments from research participants included: constipation made stool collection a challenge, this was their first time providing a stool specimen, and lastly, in general, participants expressed greater hesitation and fear towards blood collection than stool collection. It should be emphasized that this data was not systematically collected and may be biased by many factors, such as response bias. Research staff shared that verbal communication was more productive and helpful to participants than the written instructions (Khmer translated infographic).

DNA was extracted from a subsample ($n = 150$) of thawed neat stool using QIAamp PowerFecal Pro DNA Kit [10], and DNA yield was checked via NanoDrop spectrophotometer reading. All extracted specimens yielded DNA suitable for PCR amplification and were thus uncompromised during specimen collection, transportation, and storage.

4. Discussion

With the call and opportunity to promote inclusivity in microbiome research, an appropriate, low-cost and appropriate stool collection method is warranted for use in rural and low-resource settings [8,11]. The collection of stool specimens from a large cohort of rural-dwelling women could present challenges regarding participant recruitment, specimen collection, retention, and management of staff resources. We describe the development, assembly and use of a simple, low-cost at-home stool collection kit for rural or low-resource settings where modern toilets with seats are unavailable. Using this at-home stool collection kit was reported as easy and safe.

Other authors have reported using at-home adult stool collection tools but are also limited by the availability of a modern toilet with a toilet seat [5,6]. Further, contemporary over-the-toilet seat stool collection supplies (e.g., flushable collection paper secured to the toilet seat) cannot be procured in some countries, such as Cambodia, and instructions are not available in different languages. In rural and low-resource settings, even when improved sanitation infrastructure is built, there is still a lack of facilities allowing for straightforward and sterile stool collection. Our kit was <$5 USD, thus, it is a low-cost option for single and multiple follow-up stool specimen collections.

To our knowledge, no authors have reported on the development and use of a simple adult stool collection kit for use at an individual's home in a rural or low-resource setting. There is no consensus or guidance on an appropriate or detailed method of stool collection in rural or low-resource settings. In other reports in rural and low-resource settings, the general practice is to collect the stool specimen at the local health centre [12], which may be unfeasible for studies with large sample sizes and for women who cannot defecate 'on demand'. Our stool collection method is novel, as it allows participants to independently collect a stool specimen in the comfort and privacy of their home and when they feel the 'urge' to defecate. This approach also reduces the burden on local health facilities and research staff and is optimal for use in large-scale research.

Ensuring that specimen collection methods are culturally acceptable is essential to improve participation and minimize attrition rates in the study population. On account of our high study retention rate (92%) and stool specimen collection rate at 12 weeks (90%), we infer participants generally accepted this stool specimen collection method. However, these findings may have been affected by response bias. We should reiterate that our high study retention rate was likely due to our experienced field research staff's strong rapport with study participants. Detailed staff training resulted in the clear communication of stool collection instructions. We also recognize the limitations of this method of stool specimen collection. Although the metal pots were stored together in heavy-duty plastic bags to prevent contamination by dirt and debris, they were not stored in a sanitized environment, allowing for possible contamination during storage and transportation. As a lesson learned, we recommend that collection pots/containers be wrapped in protective sealing and stored in clean areas. Alternatively, the collection pots/containers could be sanitized prior to defecation at each specimen collection time point, if participants were provided with such materials. Secondly, our research group provided clear bags for the transportation of stool specimens to the health centre. Still, most participants opted to put the clear participant labelled bag inside in their own small black garbage bag for privacy. Therefore, we recommend supplying a discrete, non-opaque bag or container for participants to return specimens to the study staff. Lastly, it would be advantageous to conduct a standardized assessment of user acceptability of this stool specimen collection technique in future work.

5. Conclusions

In response to the growing field of human gut microbiome study, we describe the development, assembly and use of a simple, low-cost at-home stool collection kit for rural or low-resource settings where modern toilets with seats are unavailable. This method for the collection of stool specimens was feasible, generally acceptable, and has strong potential for similar or adapted stool collection procedures among adults residing in other rural or low-resource settings.

Author Contributions: Conceptualization, J.A.J.F. and C.D.K.; methodology, J.A.J.F. and C.D.K.; software, J.A.J.F.; validation, J.A.J.F.; formal analysis, J.A.J.F.; investigation, J.A.J.F.; resources, C.D.K.; data curation, J.A.J.F.; writing—original draft preparation, J.A.J.F.; writing—review and editing, C.D.K.; visualization, J.A.J.F.; supervision, C.D.K.; project administration, J.A.J.F.; funding acquisition, C.D.K. All authors have read and agreed to the published version of the manuscript.

Funding: This trial was funded by a Canadian Institutes of Health Research (CIHR) Project Grant (ID400771).

Institutional Review Board Statement: The study was conducted according to the guidelines of the Declaration of Helsinki and approved by the Clinical Research Ethics Board at the University of British Columbia in Vancouver, Canada (H18-02610), and the National Ethics Committee for Health Research in Phnom Penh, Cambodia (273-NECHR).

Informed Consent Statement: Informed consent was obtained from all subjects involved in the study.

Data Availability Statement: All relevant data are within the manuscript.

Conflicts of Interest: The authors declare no conflict of interest.

References

1. Marchesi, J.R.; Adams, D.H.; Fava, F.; Hermes, G.D.A.; Hirschfield, G.M.; Hold, G.; Quraishi, M.N.; Kinross, J.; Smidt, H.; Tuohy, K.M.; et al. The gut microbiota and host health: A new clinical frontier. *Gut* **2016**, *65*, 330–339. [CrossRef] [PubMed]
2. Hamady, M.; Knight, R. Microbial community profiling for human microbiome projects: Tools, techniques, and challenges. *Genome Res.* **2009**, *19*, 1141–1152. [CrossRef] [PubMed]
3. Allaband, C.; McDonald, D.; Vázquez-Baeza, Y.; Minich, J.J.; Tripathi, A.; Brenner, D.A.; Loomba, R.; Smarr, L.; Sandborn, W.J.; Schnabl, B.; et al. Microbiome 101: Studying, Analyzing, and Interpreting Gut Microbiome Data for Clinicians. *Clin. Gastroenterol. Hepatol.* **2019**, *17*, 218–230. [CrossRef]
4. Church, T.R.; Yeazel, M.W.; Jones, R.M.; Kochevar, L.K.; Watt, G.D.; Mongin, S.J.; Cordes, J.E.; Engelhard, D. A randomized trial of direct mailing of fecal occult blood tests to increase colorectal cancer screening. *J. Natl. Cancer Inst.* **2004**, *96*, 770–780. [CrossRef]
5. Wu, W.K.; Chen, C.C.; Panyod, S.; Chen, R.A.; Wu, M.S.; Sheen, L.Y.; Chang, S.C. Optimization of fecal sample processing for microbiome study—The journey from bathroom to bench. *J. Formos. Med. Assoc.* **2019**, *118*, 545–555. [CrossRef] [PubMed]
6. Hogue, S.R.; Gomez, M.F.; da Silva, W.V.; Pierce, C.M. A Customized At-Home Stool Collection Protocol for Use in Microbiome Studies Conducted in Cancer Patient Populations. *Microb. Ecol.* **2019**, *78*, 1030–1034. [CrossRef] [PubMed]
7. DNAgenotek. Available online: https://www.dnagenotek.com/row/products/collection-microbiome/omnigene-gut-kit/OM-200.100.html (accessed on 29 July 2021).
8. Porras, A.M.; Brito, I.L. The internationalization of human microbiome research. *Curr. Opin. Microbiol.* **2019**, *50*, 50–55. [CrossRef] [PubMed]
9. Fischer, J.A.; Pei, L.X.; Goldfarb, D.M.; Albert, A.; Elango, R.; Kroeun, H.; Karakochuk, C.D. Is untargeted iron supplementation harmful when iron deficiency is not the major cause of anaemia? Study protocol for a double-blind, randomised controlled trial among non-pregnant Cambodian women. *BMJ Open* **2020**, *10*, e037232. [CrossRef] [PubMed]
10. Qiagen. Available online: https://www.qiagen.com/us/products/discovery-and-translational-research/dna-rna-purification/dna-purification/genomic-dna/qiaamp-powerfecal-pro-dna-kit/ (accessed on 11 June 2021).
11. Andrews, K.; Gonzalez, A. Contextual risk factors impacting the colonization and development of the intestinal microbiota: Implications for children in low- and middle-income countries. *Dev. Psychobiol.* **2019**, *61*, 714–728. [CrossRef] [PubMed]
12. Bodhidatta, L.; McDaniel, P.; Sornsakrin, S.; Srijan, A.; Serichantalergs, O.; Mason, C.J. Case-control study of diarrheal disease etiology in a remote rural area in western Thailand. *Am. J. Trop. Med. Hyg.* **2010**, *83*, 1106–1109. [CrossRef] [PubMed]

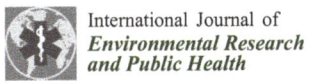

Review

Nicotinic Acetylcholine Receptor Involvement in Inflammatory Bowel Disease and Interactions with Gut Microbiota

Lola Rueda Ruzafa [1], José Luis Cedillo [2] and Arik J. Hone [3,4,*]

[1] Laboratory of Neuroscience, Biomedical Research Center (CINBIO), University of Vigo, 36310 Vigo, Spain; lolarrzg@gmail.com
[2] Department of Pharmacology and Therapeutics, Universidad Autónoma de Madrid, 28034 Madrid, Spain; jose_cedillo_mireles@hotmail.com
[3] MIRECC, George E. Whalen Veterans Affairs Medical Center, Salt Lake City, UT 84148, USA
[4] School of Biological Sciences, University of Utah, Salt Lake City, UT 84112, USA
* Correspondence: uuneurotox@yahoo.com; Tel.: +1-801-581-8370

Abstract: The gut-brain axis describes a complex interplay between the central nervous system and organs of the gastrointestinal tract. Sensory neurons of dorsal root and nodose ganglia, neurons of the autonomic nervous system, and immune cells collect and relay information about the status of the gut to the brain. A critical component in this bi-directional communication system is the vagus nerve which is essential for coordinating the immune system's response to the activities of commensal bacteria in the gut and to pathogenic strains and their toxins. Local control of gut function is provided by networks of neurons in the enteric nervous system also called the 'gut-brain'. One element common to all of these gut-brain systems is the expression of nicotinic acetylcholine receptors. These ligand-gated ion channels serve myriad roles in the gut-brain axis including mediating fast synaptic transmission between autonomic pre- and postganglionic neurons, modulation of neurotransmitter release from peripheral sensory and enteric neurons, and modulation of cytokine release from immune cells. Here we review the role of nicotinic receptors in the gut-brain axis with a focus on the interplay of these receptors with the gut microbiome and their involvement in dysregulation of gut function and inflammatory bowel diseases.

Keywords: nicotinic acetylcholine receptors; α7 and α9 nicotinic receptor subtypes; cholinergic anti-inflammatory pathway; gut-brain axis; gut microbiome; dysbiosis; inflammatory bowel disease; COVID-19

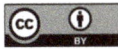

1. Nicotinic Acetylcholine Receptors

1.1. Nicotinic Acetylcholine Receptors, Composition, Subtypes, and Pharmacological Properties

Nicotinic acetylcholine receptors (nAChRs) are ligand-gated ion channels ubiquitously expressed throughout the central (CNS) and peripheral (PNS) nervous systems [1,2]. Nicotinic receptors are composed of five individual subunits that assemble in pentameric fashion to form a central ion-conducting channel [3,4]. There are 17 individual subunits, designated by Greek letters, and include α1–α10, β1–β4, δ, ε, and γ. Because of the number and diversity of subunits, numerous distinct nAChR subtypes are possible but can nevertheless be classified into two broad categories: heteromeric subtypes composed of α and β subunits and homomeric subtypes composed of α subunits only. Most heteromeric subtypes contain α and β subunits, for example α3β4, a subtype highly expressed by ganglionic neurons of the PNS [5]. However, heteromeric nAChRs composed strictly of α subunits have also been described and include α9α10 [6–8] and α7α8 subtypes [9]. Adding to the diversity of potential subtypes, more than one α or β subunit may be present in a given nAChR complex such as α3β2β4* receptors (the asterisk denotes the potential or known presence of additional subunits in native receptor complexes) which are expressed by rodent adrenal chromaffin cells [10] and neurons of superior cervical and nodose ganglia [11,12]. Homomeric receptor subtypes include α7, α8, α9, and α10 [13–15]. It should be noted that α8 subunits are not expressed in mammals and homomeric α10 nAChRs have only been reported in nonmammalian organisms [16].

Each of the various nAChR subtypes possesses different pharmacological and biophysical properties including sensitivities to the neurotransmitters acetylcholine and choline, desensitization properties, and permeabilities to cations [17–20]. Receptor subtypes that contain the β2 subunit such as α3β2, α4β2, and α6β2 have generally been found to be more sensitive to activation by acetylcholine than the closely related α3β4, α4β4, and α6β4 subtypes [21,22]. Subtypes that contain the β2 subunit are insensitive to the acetylcholine precursor and metabolite choline whereas those containing β4 subunits are weakly activated by choline [23]. By contrast, choline is a full agonist of homomeric α7 nAChRs [24] and a partial agonist of α9 and α9α10 subtypes [8,13,25]. Nicotinic receptors are so named because they are activated by the tobacco plant alkaloid nicotine, but curiously, α9 and α9α10 nAChRs are not activated by nicotine and instead are inhibited by this ligand [8,13,25].

1.2. Nicotinic Acetylcholine Receptor Expression by Sensory and Autonomic Ganglion Neurons that Innervate the Gut

Innervation of the gut by neurons of the inferior ganglion of the vagus nerve (nodose ganglion) and dorsal root ganglion (DRG) neurons provide the CNS with sensory information concerning the physiological state of the gut. Although the functional characterization of the nAChRs expressed by nodose ganglion neurons using subtype-selective ligands is lacking, immunoprecipitation assays suggest the presence of several subtypes that contain α2, α3, α4, α5, β2, or β4 subunits [12]. Pharmacological and electrophysiological assays of lumbar DRG neurons from rat suggest that these neurons mainly express α3β4*, α6β4*, and α7 nAChRs [26–28]. Innervation of mouse gut by DRG neurons is provided by ganglia located at levels T8-L1 and L6-S1 [29] and have been shown to express α4β2*, α7, and α3β4* nAChRs based on receptor sensitivities to subtype-selective antagonists [30,31]. The functional role of nAChRs in DRG neurons is poorly understood, but α3β4*, α6β4*, and α7 nAChRs have been reported to be expressed by putative nociceptors and may therefore be involved in nociception [28,32,33]. Additionally, α7 nAChRs located on DRG neuron terminals in the dorsal horn of the spinal cord modulate the release of glutamate and have been proposed to be involved in nicotine mediated analgesia [34].

The main nAChR subtypes expressed by autonomic nervous system (ANS) neurons almost certainly contain the α3 subunit as evidenced by CHRNA3 gene knockout mice that show perinatal mortality and severe ANS dysfunction [35,36]. However, sparse functional information is available concerning the exact subtypes expressed by both ANS and enteric nervous system (ENS) neurons innervating the gut. Immunohistochemical studies of ENS plexuses in mice, rats, and guinea pigs suggest neuronal expression of a heterogenous population of nAChRs that contain α3, α5, β2, β4, or α7 subunits [37–39]. Functional assays of mouse myenteric plexus neurons demonstrated the presence of at least α3β2* and α3β4* but transcripts for α7 nAChRs were also present [40]. Similar results were found for neurons of the submucosal plexus in guinea pig [41]. Lastly, immunohistochemical studies of myenteric plexuses of mouse colon revealed the expression of α3 subunits in glial cells that also express nitric oxide synthase II [42]. Stimulation of glial cells with the nicotinic agonist dimethylpiperazine increased the production of nitric oxide which functions as a signaling molecule between glia and myenteric neurons. Glial cells and neurons thus coordinate regulation of ion transport in the epithelia through stimulation of nAChRs and the production of nitric oxide. Table 1 lists the expression patterns of nAChRs in neurons that innervate gut structures.

Table 1. nAChR expression in neurons that innervate the gastrointestinal tract

Neural Structure	nAChR Subunits [a]	Functional nAChRs [b]	Target Organ in the Gastrointestinal Tract	Ref.
Nodose ganglia [c]	α2, α3, α4, α5, α6, α7, β2, β3, β4	α3β4 *	Proximal small intestine and colon	[12,43,44]
Dorsal root ganglia [c,e]	α3, α4, α5, α6, α7, β2, β4	α3β4 *, α4β2 *, α6β4 *, α7	Small and large intestines	[26,27,43,45,46]
Celiac ganglia [c]	α3, α7	α3 *,[f], α7 [f]	Distal esophagus, stomach, proximal duodenum, liver, biliary system, spleen, adrenal glands	[47,48]
Superior mesenteric ganglia [c]	α7	α7 [f]	Duodenum, jejunum, ileum, cecum, appendix, ascending colon, proximal transverse colon	[47]
Inferior mesenteric ganglia [c,d]	α3, α5, β4	α3β4 *	Distal transverse, descending, and sigmoid, colon, rectum, upper anal canal	[49]
Inferior hypogastric plexus [c,d]	α3, β4, α7	unknown	Urogential organs, pelvic viscera	[50,51]
Myenteric plexus [c,d,e]	α3, α5, α7, β2, β4	α3β2 *, α3β4 *, α7	Circular and longitudinal muscles of the gut wall, submucosa, epithelia, stomach, small and large intestines, colon	[37,39,52,53]

[a] Subunits detected by molecular biology techniques; [b] nAChR subtypes detected by functional assays; [c] rodent; [d] guinea pig; [e] human; [f] probable functional expression; * denotes the potential presence of other subunits.

Alterations in the expression patterns of α3β4 nAChRs in neurons of the ANS can result is dysregulation of gut function in humans. Several neurological conditions such as idiopathic, paraneoplastic, and diabetic autonomic neuropathies are associated with the presence of receptor binding (blocking) autoantibodies in patient serum [54]. In autoimmune ganglionopathies where autoantibodies against the α3 subunit are produced, gross ANS dysfunction occurs [55]. Similarly, patients with megacystis microcolon intestinal hypoperistalsis syndrome show significantly decreased expression of the α3 subunit [56], and patients with diverticular disease show decreased β4 subunit mRNA expression in the myenteric plexus [53]. These studies indicate an essential role of α3-containing nAChRs in the gut-brain axis.

2. The Gut-Brain Axis

2.1. Neural Communication between the Brain and the Gut

It has been well established that a bi-directional relationship exists between the CNS and the gut, and influences myriad pathological conditions from psychiatric to gastrointestinal disorders [57,58]. This 'gut-brain axis' controls a number of physiological processes via the brain, autonomic, and enteric nervous systems. Some of the principal components of this system are the vagus nerve, the hypothalamic-pituitary-adrenal axis (HPA axis), and the immune and circulatory systems. Critical to the bi-directional communication between the brain and the gut are neurons that innervate gut structures and the neurotransmitters they release for communication and autocrine/paracrine functions. Neurons of dorsal root and nodose ganglia along with intrinsic primary afferent neurons (Dogiel Type II neurons) of the ENS provide sensory functions to gut structures and relay information concerning gut homeostasis to the CNS [43,57]. Ganglionic neurons of the ANS found in the superior and inferior mesenteric ganglia, celiac, middle and inferior cervical ganglia provide direct PNS innervation to visceral organs although those that specifically innervate structures of the gut are largely found in the celiac, superior and inferior mesenteric ganglia [59] (Figure 1). Direct, local control of gut function is mediated almost entirely by the ENS or the gut-brain which is made up of neural networks or plexuses and include the submucosal and myenteric plexuses [59]. Each of these gut-brain systems is involved in maintaining gut homeostasis and responding to alterations in gut function including those that cause gastrointestinal inflammation.

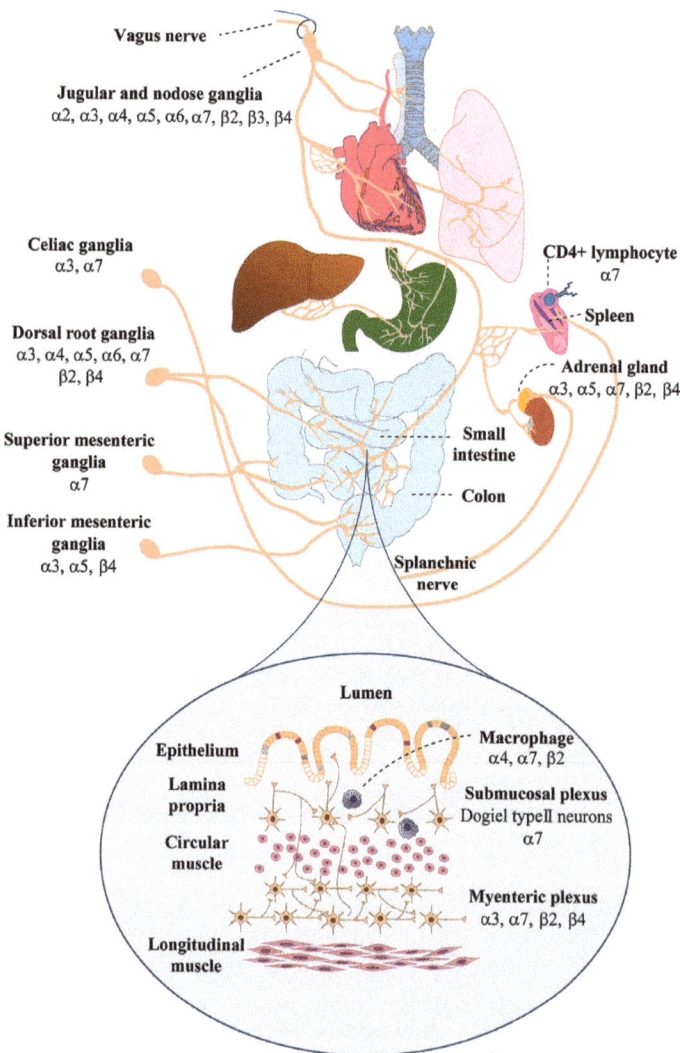

Figure 1. Cartoon representation depicting organs and structures of the gastrointestinal tract and the neurons that innervate them that express nAChR subunits. The inset in the lower part of the cartoon details the structures of the intestines; the myenteric and submucosal plexuses are shown along with select cell types.

2.2. Inflammatory Control in the Gut Involves the Vagus Nerve and α7 nAChRs

The cholinergic anti-inflammatory pathway (CAP) is referred to as the neuroinflammatory reflex in which the nervous and immune systems 'cooperate' to control excessive inflammation, and one mechanism by which this occurs is through activity of the vagus nerve. The vagus nerve is composed of 80% sensory afferent fibers and 20% motor efferent fibers [60]. Vagal nerve fibers innervate the gastrointestinal tract, lungs, heart, pancreas, adrenal glands, and liver and are responsible for the control/modulation of heart rate, digestion, intestinal movement, hormone and neurotransmitter secretion. Correct function of this nerve is essential for numerous physiological processes of the gut-brain axis [61]. Activation of vagal efferents leads to the release of acetylcholine in visceral organs with the exception of the spleen as this organ is innervated by the splenic nerve, which is adregenergic [62]. The splenic nerve releases noradrenaline and activates adrenergic receptors expressed by a specific subpopulation of resident CD4$^+$ T-cells that are capable of synthesizing and releasing acetylcholine that, in turn, activates resident macrophage expressed α7 nAChRs to inhibit the release of pro-inflammatory cytokines [63]. The anti-inflammatory effects of α7 nAChR activation have been observed through stimulation of enteric macrophages through vagal nerve activity [63–65]. This anti-inflammatory mechanism occurs via activation of α7 nAChRs, recruitment and activation of Janus kinase-2 (JAK-2), and subsequent phosphorylation of signal transducer and activator of transcription-3 (STAT-3) which dimerizes and translocates to the nucleus to inhibit pro-inflammatory cytokine gene expression including tumor necrosis factor-α (TNF-α) and interleukin-6 (IL-6) among others [66,67]. Additionally, activation of α7 nAChRs is associated with inhibition of Nf-κB nuclear translocation [68,69] and activation of the phosphoinositide 3-kinase/protein kinase B (PI3K/Akt) signaling pathways [70,71]. Inhibition of these pathways disrupts signaling through the inflammasome complex [72] and ultimately results in the suppression of TNF-α, Il-6, IL-1β and other pro-inflammatory cytokine secretion. At the systems level, vagal-nerve stimulation has been shown to reduce plasmatic TNF-α levels after lipopolysaccharide (LPS) injection in mice and α7 nAChRs were demonstrated to be a key player in this anti-inflammatory effect [73,74].

Several studies have shown that stimulation of α7 by acetylcholine, choline, nicotine, other agonists and positive allosteric modulators (PAMs) reduces the production of pro-inflammatory cytokines and improves outcomes in animal models of endotoxemic shock [74–78]. The anti-inflammatory role of this receptor is further supported by studies utilizing specific antagonists of α7 receptors, CHRNA7 knock-out mice [63,74,79,80], or overexpression of its dominant-negative duplicated form dupα7 [81] which has only been found in humans. Elevated expression levels of dupα7 in human large and small intestines are associated with inflammatory bowel disease (IBD) [82]. Control of inflammation through the CAP has been demonstrated in animal models of human disease including sepsis, IBD, arthritis, hemorrhagic shock, asthma, and pancreatitis [75,83–89]. In humans, the importance of the role α7 nAChRs play in the CAP and the regulation of exacerbated inflammation has been shown in sterile endotoxemia [90,91] and sepsis [92]. Activation of the CAP via vagal-nerve stimulation is currently used to treat depression [93], epilepsy [94], stroke [95], and migraines [96]. Vagal-nerve stimulation may also be potentially useful in treating Crohn's disease, ulcerative colitis, and other inflammatory bowel conditions [97] as has been demonstrated in rodent models of irritable bowel syndrome (IBS) [98] and postoperative ileus [99].

Inflammatory bowel disease is a highly prevalent and multifactorial disorder characterized by chronic inflammation of the gastrointestinal tract and significantly affects the quality of life of patients who suffer from it. The two main types are ulcerative colitis, which is limited to the colon, and Crohn's disease which can affect any section of the intestinal tract [100]. The vagus nerve plays a role in regulating intestinal inflammation in IBD [101], and the proposed mechanism involves ENS neurons and macrophages located in the submucosal plexus [102]. Release of acetylcholine by the vagus nerve contacting ENS neurons decreases the release of TNF-α, IL-1β, IL-6, and IL-18 by submucosal macrophages expressing α7 nAChRs. In dysbiosis and pathologies such as ulcerative colitis, lymphocytes and macrophages are recruited to the site of inflammation where adhesion molecules are over expressed [103]. In a mouse model of colitis, nicotine suppressed the expression of mucosal addressin cell-adhesion molecule-1 (MAdCAM-1) protein in the mucosal venules of the inflamed colon [104]. In the mouse dextran sodium sulfate (DSS) model of colitis, nicotine reduced lumbar DRG neuron hyperexcitability through activation of α7 nAChRs [105]. Electrical stimulation of the vagal nerve in a mouse model of endotoxemia reversed LPS-induced decreases in tight-junction proteins, via an α7-mediated mechanism, and increased intestinal permeability [106]. Furthermore, intraperitoneal injection of nicotine reduced gut permeability by maintaining localization of intestinal tight-junction proteins after burn-induced gut injury in mice [107]. These finding have led to consideration of a potential protective role of nicotine on bowel wall integrity. However, nicotine also induces significant increases in triglycerides, LDL-cholesterol, and serum glucose along with a decrease in HDL-cholesterol in animals fed a high-fat diet and increased plasmatic levels of certain cytokines raising concerns about its usefulness as an anti-inflammatory therapeutic in IBD [108]. However, other subtype-selective agonists of nAChRs have also shown beneficial effects in animal models of IBD.

Treatment with galantamine, a PAM of nAChRs, succeeded in preventing ulcers and reducing inflammatory mediators such as intracellular adhesion molecule-1 (ICAM-1) in the 2,4,6-trinitrobenzene sulfonic acid (TNBS) model of colitis in rats [109]. The effects of galantamine were abolished by the α7 nAChR antagonist methyllycaconitine. Similarly, use of the α7-selective agonist PNU-282987 improved oxidative enzyme myeloperoxidase activity and reduced IL-6 and IFN-γ levels in the mouse DSS model of colitis [110]. Subsequent treatment with methyllycaconitine reversed the beneficial effects of PNU-282987. Varenicline, a non-selective agonist of α7 nAChRs, improved colonic motility and the cholinergic response in a rat IBS model [111]. Other α7-selective agonists including encenicline and AR-R17779 have shown anti-inflammatory effects in mouse models of colitis and postoperative ileus. Encenicline reduced the infiltration of immune cells into inflamed colonic tissue in TNBS- and DSS- induced colitis [112], and AR-R17779 stimulated the CAP and reduced NF-κB transcription in peritoneal macrophages in postoperative ileus [99]. These studies indicate an important role of α7 nAChRs in IBD. Nevertheless, other studies have reported that stimulation of α7 nAChRs did not reduce intestinal inflammation although the hyperalgesia associated with colonic inflammation was reduced [113]. Overall, however, selective stimulation of α7 nAChRs has shown to be effective in reducing signs and symptoms of disease in a variety of bowel conditions characterized by excessive inflammation. Table 2 lists the effects of activation of α7 nAChRs on IBD. Other nAChR subtypes including α4β2* have been reported to be expressed by a subset of intestinal and peritoneal macrophages that do not express α7 receptors and are not directly involved in the anti-inflammatory effects of the CAP but instead serve a phagocytotic function in the gut [114].

Table 2. Effects of nAChR ligands on murine models and human patients with IBD

Ligand	Mechanism of Action	Disease-modifying Mechanisms	Effects on IBD	Ref.
Nicotine	Non-selective agonist	Suppression of MAdCAM-1; reduced regenerative spike action-potentials	Decreased signs and symptoms of DSS-induced colitis in mice Reduced colonic DRG neuron hyperexcitability in DSS-induced colitis in mice	[30,104]
Galantamine	Non-selective PAM	Reduced NF-κB, TNF-α levels, MPO, and neutrophil infiltration	Decreased signs and symptoms of TNBS-induced colitis in mice	[109]
PNU-282987	α7-selective agonist	Reduced infiltration of leucocytes Reduced infiltration of macrophages, and reduced levels of IL-6, and IFN-γ	Attenuated colonic inflammation in DSS-treated mice Decreased signs and symptoms of DSS-induced colitis in mice	[110,115]
PNU-120596	α7-selective PAM	Decreased IL-1β and TNF-α in LPS-treated mice	Decreased symptoms related to anxiety and depression in mice	[116]
GTS-21	partial α7 agonist	Decreased TNF-α in plasma	Probable decreased colonic inflammation in patients with ulcerative colitis	[117]
AR-R17779	α7 agonist	Reduced colonic infiltration of CD4$^+$ and CD8$^+$ lymphocytes; inhibition of macrophage activation	Decreased signs and symptoms of TNBS-induced colitis in mice Decreased signs and symptoms of postoperative ileus in mice	[99,114]
Encenicline	partial α7 agonist	Reduced colonic infiltration of macrophages, neutrophils, and B lymphocytes	Decreased signs and symptoms of TNBS- and DSS induced colitis in mice	[112]
RgIA	α9 antagonist	Reduced levels of colonic TNF-α	Decreased signs and symptoms of DSS-induced colitis in mice	[118]

Dextran sodium sulfate, DSS; a 2,4,6-trinitrobenzene sulfonic acid, TNBS; oxidative enzyme myeloperoxidase, MPO; mucosal vascular addressin cell adhesion molecule-1, MAdCAM-1.

2.3. Nicotinic Acetylcholine Receptor Subunits α9 and α10 are Novel Players in IBD

Although the role of the α7 nAChR in IBD has been well studied and firmly established, recently nAChRs containing α9 and α10 subunits have emerged as new targets for treating inflammation. It has been shown that inhibiting the α9α10 receptor with the selective antagonist α-conotoxin RgIA reduced the severity of inflammation in the DSS model of colitis in mice [118]. RgIA and its analogs have been shown to have disease-modifying effects in a number of neuropathic and inflammatory disease models including sciatic nerve injury, diabetic neuropathy, and neuropathies associated with the use of the anti-cancer drugs paclitaxel and oxaliplatin [119–122]. An important mechanism through which RgIA exerts the observed therapeutic effects is by inhibiting the recruitment of lymphocytes and macrophages to damaged nerve tissues, although the exact mechanisms by which this occurs are currently unknown. However, experiments with nicotine, acetylcholine, or choline in a human monocyte cell line (U937) and mouse peripheral blood mononuclear cells showed that ATP-mediated release of IL-1β, through nAChRs containing α7, α9 or α10 subunits, is inhibited by these nicotinic ligands [123,124]. Phosphocholine, a molecule structurally similar to choline, also inhibited ATP-evoked currents and IL-1β release in U937 cells through α7 and α9α10 nAChRs [123,125,126].

3. Bacterial Types in the Gastrointestinal Tract

3.1. The Gut Microbiome Plays an Important Role in Communication between the Nervous System and the Gut

A critical component of the gut-brain axis is the make-up of the microbiota found in the different compartments of the gastrointestinal tract. Among the different strains of bacteria present are *Lactobacillus* and *Streptococcus*, found in the stomach and duodenum, *Lactobacillus, Streptococcus, Bacteroides, Bifidobacterium,* and *Fusobacteria* in the jejunum and ileum, and *Bacteroides, Bifidobacterium, Streptococcus, Eubacteria, Clostridium, Vellionella, Ruminococcus, Pseudomonas,* and *Lactobacillus,* among others, in the colon [127]. These bacteria have multiple roles including protective, structural, and metabolic functions for example through the fermentation of dietary fiber into short-chain fatty acids (SCFAs) and the synthesis of B and K vitamins [128,129]. Short-chain fatty acids play an important role in regulating inflammation in the intestines through inhibition of the NF-κB pathway and reduction of macrophage-produced pro-inflammatory cytokines [130,131]. Alterations in the levels of these commensal bacteria can result in intestinal dysbiosis (an imbalance in the populations of intestinal microbiota). Table 3 lists some of the commensal bacteria found in the lower gastrointestinal tract and their roles.

Table 3. Bacterial types, location within the gastrointestinal tract, and function

Bacteria	Location in the GI Tract	Functional Role	Ref.
Lactobacillus	Stomach, duodenum, jejunum, ileum, colon	Improved digestion and absorption of nutrients; inhibition of the growth of pathogens by activating the immune system [a,b]	[132–134]
Streptococcus	Jejunum, ileum, colon	Modulation of the immune system through altered cytokine release from immune cells[c]	[135,136]
Bacteroides	Jejunum, ileum, colon	Production of SCFAs involved in energy homeostasis and regulation of intestinal inflammation[d]	[137]
Bifidobacterium	Jejunum, ileum, colon	Inhibition of the growth of pathogens by activating the immune system; amino-acid and vitamin synthesis[d]	[138,139]
Veillonella	Colon	Production of SCFAs involved in energy homeostasis[c,d]	[140]
Eubacteria	Colon	Production of SCFAs involved in energy homeostasis and regulation of intestinal inflammation[c]	[141]
Clostridia	Colon	Participation in resistance to the colonization of pathogens; production of SCFAs[c]; maintenance of gut homeostasis[c]	[142–144]
Peptostreptococcus	Colon	Maintenance of epithelial barrier and modulation of intestinal inflammation[c,d]	[145]

[a] Dog; [b] cat; [c] human; [d] rodent.

3.2. Gut Dysbiosis

Gastrointestinal dysbiosis is associated with a number of pathophysiological conditions including neurodegenerative diseases, psychiatric conditions, diabetes, obesity, autism, and IBD [146]. Alterations in the normal populations of intestinal microbiota can allow the proliferation of harmful bacterial strains and the toxins they produce. Celiac disease and IBS are associated with a decrease in intestinal microbial diversity in general, with alterations in *Firmicutes/Bacteroidetes* ratio and in members of the *Proteobacteria* phylum [147,148]. For instance, elevated levels of endotoxins in the bloodstream such as LPS, derived from the outer membrane of gram-negative bacteria, is a common alteration that can cause a severe immune system response that leads to systemic inflammation and sepsis. Peripheral blood mononuclear cells from patients with IBS show elevated levels of pro-inflammatory cytokine release when challenged with LPS from *Escherichia coli* [149]. Similarly, *Clostridium difficile*, the bacteria responsible for diarrhea associated with overuse of certain antibiotics and the etiology of pseudomembranous colitis, attacks the lining of the intestine through the release of toxins A and B. Both toxins induce damage to the intestinal epithelium, increase permeability of the mucosal barrier, and generate an inflammatory response [150,151].

3.3. Effects of nAChR Stimulation by Nicotine on Intestinal Microbiota Populations

As mentioned above, the composition of commensal intestinal microbiota is essential for proper gastrointestinal function. Alterations in the proportion of certain bacterial strains produce negative impacts that lead to the onset, progression, and/or maintenance of IBDs. In relation to nAChRs, results from several studies have shown a disruptive effect from nicotine on the composition of intestinal microbiota populations in mice [108,152]. During a 9-week smoking cessation period, an increase in *Firmicutes* and *Actinobacteria* and a decrease in *Bacteroidetes* and *Proteobacteria* was found in human fecal samples [153]. In mice, chronic oral administration of nicotine increased bacterial alpha-diversity including members of the *Lactobacillus* and *Lachnospiraceae* genera and *Firmicutes* phylum [108]. Interestingly, administration of nicotine in the drinking water of mice showed a sex-dependent effect on the bacterial composition of the intestinal microbiome [152]. The relative abundance of bacteria from the *Christensenellaceae* and *Anaeroplasmataceae* families showed significant reductions in female mice after a 13-week exposure to nicotine whereas males showed decreased *Dehalobacteriaceae* bacteria. Similarly, daily exposure to tobacco smoke increased cecal *Clostridium clostridiforme* and decreased *Lactoccoci*, *Ruminococcus albus*, *Enterobacteriaceae* and *Bifidobacterium* compared to controls in mice and rats [154,155]. In addition, SCFAs such as butyrate, propionate, and acetate were reduced by the effect of smoke exposure [154]. Activation of the free fatty acid receptor 3 (FFA3) by SCFAs has been shown to reduce colonic motility and abolish chloride secretion involving nAChRs via G protein-coupled receptors in rats [156,157]. Thus, the composition of gut microbiota is essential for maintaining the ability of the host organism to regulate intestinal inflammation and respond to pathogenic organisms that target the intestinal tract. Table 4 lists the effects of nicotine on the bacterial composition of gut microbiota.

Table 4. Effects of nicotine on gut microbiota and their function.

Bacteria	Effect on Bacterial Levels	Effects on Gut Function	Ref.
alpha-diversity	Increased in mice	Improvement of gut barrier function by production metabolites and antimicrobial substances	[108]
Lactobacillus	Increased in mice	Improvement of gut barrier function and prevent inflammation by production of SCFAs, lactate and antimicrobial substances	[108]
Lachnospiraceae	Increased in mice	Improvement of gut barrier function by production of beneficial metabolites such as SCFAs	[108]
Christensenellaceae	Decreased in female mice	Development of metabolic syndrome	[152]
Anaeroplasmataceae	Decreased in female mice	Alteration of the intestinal transit	[152]
Dehalobacteriaceae	Decreased in male mice	Development of metabolic syndrome	[152]

4. Potential Involvement of nAChRs in COVID-19 and Associated Dysbiosis

The Pathophysiology of COVID-19 May Involve α7 nAChRs and Inhibition of the CAP

In late December of 2019, a novel strain of coronavirus was reported in Hubei province, China in patients with viral pneumonia and was determined to be similar to other coronaviruses that causes severe acute respiratory syndrome (SARS) [158]. The sequence of this virus, SARS-CoV-2, was quickly determined and showed high similarity to other members of the coronavirus family including SARS-CoV-1 and RaTG13 but with one notable difference [158]. Unlike SARS-CoV-1 and RaTG13, SARS-CoV-2 contains additional residues (681-PRRA-684) between the S1 and S2 domains of the spike protein [159,160]. These residues serve as a cleavage site for the furin enzyme and have been proposed to impart increased infectiousness of SARS-CoV-2 relative to other members of the SARS-CoV family. This hypothesis is controversial, however, and requires further investigation [161,162].

Researchers at the Pasteur Institute and the Sorbonne in Paris, France observed that the sequence of the furin cleavage site along with seven residues (674-YQTQTNS-680) upstream and one arginine-685 residue downstream were similar to a motif found in neurotoxins from *Elapidea* serpents [163] (Figure 2). This motif allows serpent neurotoxins to bind to and inhibit nAChRs, most notably α7 nAChRs, which led Changeux and his colleagues to hypothesize that inhibition of α7 receptors by the SARS-CoV-2 spike protein may contribute to the pathophysiology of COVID-19 and specifically to elevated levels of cytokines. Computational modeling experiments later suggested that the spike protein may potentially interact with receptors that contain α7 subunits and/or α9-containing subtypes [164]. Given the possibility that the spike protein interacts with α7 nAChRs, inhibition of this receptor has been proposed as a contributor to the so-called 'cytokine storm' through inhibition the CAP [163–165].

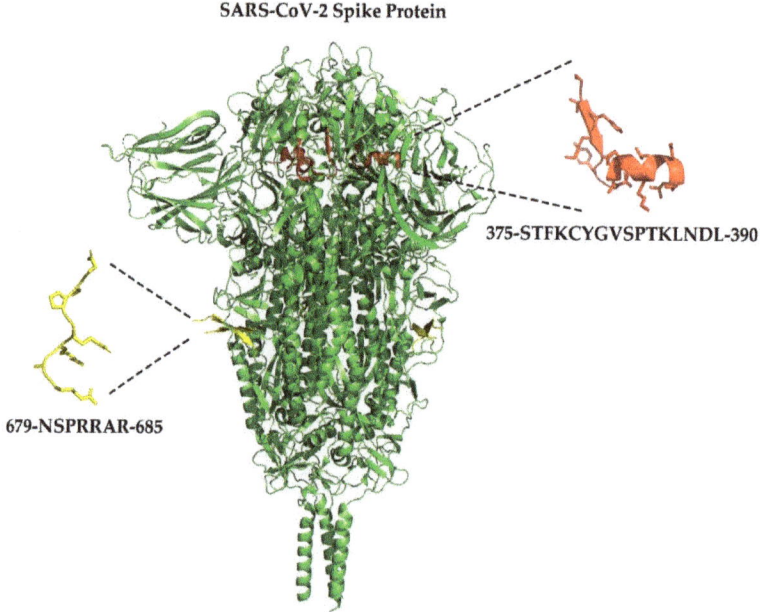

Figure 2. Cartoon representation of the SARS-CoV-2 spike protein trimer (green) showing the proposed domains that interact with α7 and α9α10 nAChRs. Note that residues 675-QTNSPRRARSVA-686 are unresolved in this structure. Residues highlighted in yellow are those that show homology with sequences of the three-finger neurotoxins from *Elapidea* serpents including α-bungarotoxin from *Bungurus multicintus* and α-cobratoxin from *Naja naja* species [163]. Residues highlighted in red have also been proposed to interact with α7 and α9α10 nAChRs [164]. Rendition of the spike protein was accomplished using PyMOL [166] and adapted from Cai et al., 2020 (PDB:6XR8) [167]; rendition of the NSPRRAR sequence was adapted from Daly et al., 2020 (PDB: 7JJC) [168].

SARS-CoV-2 not only produces acute respiratory distress but has shown a propensity for inducing severe dysfunction of neurological, pulmonary, cardiovascular, and gastrointestinal systems. Some patients develop acute gastrointestinal distress including diarrhea and vomiting which initially led to the assumption that patients with IBD would experience more severe gastrointestinal symptoms than those without due to the presence of significant angiotensin-converting enzyme-2 receptor expression in the ileum and colon as suggested by analysis of transcriptomics data [169]. In addition, immunosuppressive therapies are often first-line treatments for IBD. However, analysis of clinical data has, in fact, suggested the contrary leading to speculation that immunotherapies with biologics and other immune system modulators may actually reduce COVID-19-related symptoms by suppressing the cytokine storm [170–173]. Similarly, pharmacological stimulation of α7 receptors and the CAP has been proposed as a mechanism to 'calm the storm' [174]. As discussed above, α7 is highly involved in inflammatory conditions of the gastrointestinal tract and low expression levels of α7 receptors are associated with worse outcomes in Crohn's, other IBDs, and sepsis [82,92]. The systemic presence of an antagonist of α7 receptors would almost certainly worsen the gastrointestinal symptoms associated with COVID-19 by inhibiting the anti-inflammatory actions of the CAP. Therefore, treatment with an agonist such as nicotine might be beneficial and do two things: (1) bind to the ligand-binding site of α7 receptors and compete with or inhibit spike protein binding while simultaneously activating the receptor, and (2) stimulate the CAP to inhibit the cytokine storm. Indeed, such a treatment has been proposed by several authors [165,175,176].

The gastrointestinal symptoms associated with COVID-19, as experienced by some patients, including increased prevalence of diarrhea and vomiting may cause alterations in the gut microbiome and influence the severity of the disease [177,178]. COVID-19 has been shown to be associated with reduced bacterial diversity in the gut and increased prevalence of harmful strains of bacteria [179]. Analysis of fecal samples from patients with COVID-19 found differences in the gut microbiome in those with high fecal levels of SARS-CoV-2 mRNA compared to those with low levels of mRNA [180]. Specifically, patients with high levels of viral mRNA showed increased prevalence, relative to those with low or no fecal viral mRNA, of *Collinsella aerofaciens* and *Morganella morganii*, bacteria that are associated with opportunistic infections in humans. By contrast, patients with low (or no) detectable levels of viral mRNA showed higher levels of bacteria known to produce SCFAs including members of *Parabacteroides*, *Bacteroides*, and *Lachnospiraceae* families. Therefore, alterations in the gut microbiome in patients with COVID-19 may influence the course and severity of the disease. Treatment of COVID-19 with probiotics to combat such alterations has been suggested as a way to ameliorate COVID-19 symptoms [178,181].

5. Conclusions

The aim of this Review was to evaluate the involvement of nAChRs in the gut-brain axis by examining their role in different physiological and pathophysiological processes of the gastrointestinal tract. The extensive expression of nAChRs by neurons that innervate gastrointestinal organs influences numerous physiological processes including gut motility, sensory detection of signaling molecules released by other neurons, immune cells, and bacteria. Importantly, control of gut inflammation through α7 and α9 nAChRs, the vagus nerve, and the CAP is essential. We note that there is a surprising lack on information concerning several important areas of nAChR research on the gut-brain axis. First, sparse information is available detailing the functional nAChR subtypes expressed by ENS neurons and glial cells. Research on the role of glial cells in general in gut function is also lacking. Determining the subtype composition of these receptors is important in the context of designing pharmacotherapeutics that treat IBD. Gene knock-out of CHRNA3 in mice produces gross ANS dysfunction, and certain human diseases of the gut involve production of antibodies against α3 and β4 subunits. It is highly likely that ENS neurons express the α3β4* subtype, but it is possible that multiple different subtypes containing α3 and β4 subunits are present, for example α3β2β4*, α3β4α5* and α3β2*, which are highly expressed by other PNS neurons. Each of these nAChRs subtypes may show different sensitivities to ligands. Nevertheless, it is critical that potential drugs used to treat IBD be devoid of activity on α3β4 subtypes to avoid secondary side effects associated with excessive activation or inhibition of α3β4 receptors. Additionally, sparse information is available concerning the expression of the α7 subtype in the ENS and essentially nothing is known about the expression of subtypes containing α9 subunits. Secondly, information about the interaction of commensal bacteria and enterotoxins, produced by pathogenic strains, with nAChRs is lacking. It is known that bacteria from *Firmicutes* species and from *Bacteroides* and *Eubacteria* genera and other commensal bacteria produce SCFAs. These fatty-acid molecules reach millimolar concentrations in the intestines and are involved in the esterification of choline. Choline and its various derivatives have been shown to modulate the release of cytokines from murine macrophages and human monocytes through α7- and/or α9-containing nAChRs as well as decrease chloride secretion from intestinal epithelia. Alterations in SCFA-producing populations of bacteria may therefore affect activities of nAChRs expressed by sensory neurons innervating the gut, ENS neurons, and immune cells and ultimately affect regulation of gut homeostasis. Lastly, although numerous studies detailing the effects of nicotine on gut microbiota have been reported, little information is available concerning the effects of other nAChR compounds including those listed in Table 2. In the context of pharmacotherapy of IBD with nAChR compounds, it is important to determine the potential effects these compounds might have on commensal bacterial populations. Clearly, more research is needed to elucidate the nAChR subtypes expressed in the gut-brain axis, their interactions with bacteria, and the effects of experimental nicotinic IBD therapeutics on commensal bacteria.

Author Contributions: Writing—original draft preparation, L.R.R., J.L.C., A.J.H.; writing—review and editing, L.R.R., J.L.C., A.J.H.; visualization, L.R.R., J.L.C., A.J.H.; project administration, A.J.H. All authors have read and agreed to the published version of the manuscript.

Funding: This research received no external funding.

Institutional Review Board Statement: Not applicable.

Informed Consent Statement: Not applicable.

Data Availability Statement: Published data for the x-ray crystallography structures of the SARS-CoV-2 spike protein and its peptide fragment are archived in the Protein Data Bank (PDB:6XR8 and PDB:7JJC) at rcsb.org.

Conflicts of Interest: The authors declare no conflict of interest.

References

1. Gotti, C.; Zoli, M.; Clementi, F. Brain nicotinic acetylcholine receptors: Native subtypes and their relevance. *Trends Pharmacol. Sci.* **2006**, *27*, 482–491. [CrossRef]
2. Skok, V.I. Nicotinic acetylcholine receptors in autonomic ganglia. *Auton. Neurosci.* **2002**, *97*, 1–11. [CrossRef]
3. Albuquerque, E.X.; Pereira, E.F.R.; Alkondon, M.; Rogers, S.W. Mammalian Nicotinic Acetylcholine Receptors: From Structure to Function. *Physiol. Rev.* **2009**, *89*, 73–120. [CrossRef]
4. Dani, J.A. Neuronal Nicotinic Acetylcholine Receptor Structure and Function and Response to Nicotine. *Int. Rev. Neurobiol.* **2015**, *124*, 3–19. [CrossRef] [PubMed]
5. De Biasi, M. Nicotinic mechanisms in the autonomic control of organ systems. *J. Neurobiol.* **2002**, *53*, 568–579. [CrossRef] [PubMed]
6. Elgoyhen, A.B.; Vetter, D.E.; Katz, E.; Rothlin, C.V.; Heinemann, S.F.; Boulter, J. 10: A determinant of nicotinic cholinergic receptor function in mammalian vestibular and cochlear mechanosensory hair cells. *Proc. Natl. Acad. Sci. USA* **2001**, *98*, 3501–3506. [CrossRef] [PubMed]
7. Lustig, L.R.; Peng, H.; Hiel, H.; Yamamoto, T.; Fuchs, P.A. Molecular Cloning and Mapping of the Human Nicotinic Acetylcholine Receptor α10 (CHRNA10). *Genomics* **2001**, *73*, 272–283. [CrossRef]
8. Sgard, F.; Charpantier, E.; Bertrand, S.; Walker, N.; Caput, D.; Graham, D.; Bertrand, D.; Besnard, F. A Novel Human Nicotinic Receptor Subunit, α10, That Confers Functionality to the α9-Subunit. *Mol. Pharmacol.* **2002**, *61*, 150–159. [CrossRef]
9. Keyser, K.; Britto, L.; Schoepfer, R.; Whiting, P.; Cooper, J.; Conroy, W.; Prechtl, A.B.-; Karten, H.; Lindstrom, J. Three subtypes of alpha-bungarotoxin-sensitive nicotinic acetylcholine receptors are expressed in chick retina. *J. Neurosci.* **1993**, *13*, 442–454. [CrossRef]
10. Hone, A.J.; Rueda-Ruzafa, L.; Gordon, T.J.; Gajewiak, J.; Christensen, S.; Dyhring, T.; Albillos, A.; McIntosh, J.M. Expression of α3β2β4 nicotinic acetylcholine receptors by rat adrenal chromaffin cells determined using novel conopeptide antagonists. *J. Neurochem.* **2020**, *154*, 158–176. [CrossRef] [PubMed]
11. David, R.; Ciuraszkiewicz, A.; Simeone, X.; Orr-Urtreger, A.; Papke, R.L.; McIntosh, J.M.; Huck, S.; Scholze, P. Biochemical and functional properties of distinct nicotinic acetylcholine receptors in the superior cervical ganglion of mice with targeted deletions of nAChR subunit genes. *Eur. J. Neurosci.* **2010**, *31*, 978–993. [CrossRef] [PubMed]
12. Mao, D.; Yasuda, R.P.; Fan, H.; Wolfe, B.B.; Kellar, K.J. Heterogeneity of Nicotinic Cholinergic Receptors in Rat Superior Cervical and Nodose Ganglia. *Mol. Pharmacol.* **2006**, *70*, 1693–1699. [CrossRef] [PubMed]
13. Elgoyhen, A.B.; Johnson, D.S.; Boulter, J.; Vetter, D.E.; Heinemann, S. α9: An acetylcholine receptor with novel pharmacological properties expressed in rat cochlear hair cells. *Cell* **1994**, *79*, 705–715. [CrossRef]

14. Seguela, P.; Wadiche, J.; Dineley-Miller, K.; Dani, J.; Patrick, J.W. Molecular cloning, functional properties, and distribution of rat brain alpha 7: A nicotinic cation channel highly permeable to calcium. *J. Neurosci.* **1993**, *13*, 596–604. [CrossRef] [PubMed]
15. Gerzanich, V.; Anand, R.; Lindstrom, J. Homomers of alpha 8 and alpha 7 subunits of nicotinic receptors exhibit similar channel but contrasting binding site properties. *Mol. Pharmacol.* **1994**, *45*, 212–220. [PubMed]
16. Marcovich, I.; Moglie, M.J.; Freixas, A.E.C.; Trigila, A.P.; Franchini, L.F.; Plazas, P.V.; Lipovsek, M.; Elgoyhen, A.B. Distinct Evolutionary Trajectories of Neuronal and Hair Cell Nicotinic Acetylcholine Receptors. *Mol. Biol. Evol.* **2020**, *37*, 1070–1089. [CrossRef]
17. Corringer, P.-J.; Bertrand, S.; Bohler, S.; Edelstein, S.J.; Changeux, J.-P.; Bertrand, D. Critical Elements Determining Diversity in Agonist Binding and Desensitization of Neuronal Nicotinic Acetylcholine Receptors. *J. Neurosci.* **1998**, *18*, 648–657. [CrossRef]
18. Ragozzino, D.; Barabino, B.; Fucile, S.; Eusebi, F. Ca2+permeability of mouse and chick nicotinic acetylcholine receptors expressed in transiently transfected human cells. *J. Physiol.* **1998**, *507*, 749–758. [CrossRef]
19. Fucile, S.; Sucapane, A.; Eusebi, F. Ca2+ permeability through rat cloned α9-containing nicotinic acetylcholine receptors. *Cell Calcium* **2006**, *39*, 349–355. [CrossRef]
20. Ciuraszkiewicz, A.; Schreibmayer, W.; Platzer, D.; Orr-Urtreger, A.; Scholze, P.; Huck, S. Single-channel properties of α3β4, α3β4α5 and α3β4β2 nicotinic acetylcholine receptors in mice lacking specific nicotinic acetylcholine receptor subunits. *J. Physiol.* **2013**, *591*, 3271–3288. [CrossRef]
21. Parker, M.J.; Beck, A.; Luetje, C.W. Neuronal nicotinic receptor beta2 and beta4 subunits confer large differences in agonist binding affinity. *Mol. Pharmacol.* **1998**, *54*, 1132–1139. [CrossRef] [PubMed]
22. Kuryatov, A.; Olale, F.; Cooper, J.; Choi, C.; Lindstrom, J. Human α6 AChR subtypes: Subunit composition, assembly, and pharmacological responses. *Neuropharmacology* **2000**, *39*, 2570–2590. [CrossRef]
23. Alkondon, M.; Pereira, E.F.R.; Cartes, W.S.; Maelicke, A.; Albuquerque, E.X. Choline is a Selective Agonist of α7 Nicotinic Acetylcholine Receptors in the Rat Brain Neurons. *Eur. J. Neurosci.* **1997**, *9*, 2734–2742. [CrossRef] [PubMed]
24. Papke, R.L.; McCormack, T.J.; Jack, B.A.; Wang, D.; Bugaj-Gaweda, B.; Schiff, H.C.; Buhr, J.D.; Waber, A.J.; Stokes, C. Rhesus monkey α7 nicotinic acetylcholine receptors: Comparisons to human α7 receptors expressed in Xenopus oocytes. *Eur. J. Pharmacol.* **2005**, *524*, 11–18. [CrossRef]
25. Christensen, S.B.; Hone, A.J.; Roux, I.; Kniazeff, J.; Pin, J.-P.; Upert, G.; Servent, D.; Glowatzki, E.; McIntosh, J.M. RgIA4 Potently Blocks Mouse α9α10 nAChRs and Provides Long Lasting Protection against Oxaliplatin-Induced Cold Allodynia. *Front. Cell. Neurosci.* **2017**, *11*, 219. [CrossRef]
26. Hone, A.J.; Meyer, E.L.; McIntyre, M.; McIntosh, J.M. Nicotinic acetylcholine receptors in dorsal root ganglion neurons include the α6β4 subtype. *FASEB J.* **2011**, *26*, 917–926. [CrossRef]
27. Genzen, J.R.; Van Cleve, W.; McGehee, D.S. Dorsal Root Ganglion Neurons Express Multiple Nicotinic Acetylcholine Receptor Subtypes. *J. Neurophysiol.* **2001**, *86*, 1773–1782. [CrossRef]
28. Rau, K.K.; Johnson, R.D.; Cooper, B.Y. Nicotinic AChR in Subclassified Capsaicin-Sensitive and -Insensitive Nociceptors of the Rat DRG. *J. Neurophysiol.* **2005**, *93*, 1358–1371. [CrossRef]
29. Robinson, D.R.; McNaughton, P.A.; Evans, M.L.; Hicks, G.A. Characterization of the primary spinal afferent innervation of the mouse colon using retrograde labelling. *Neurogastroenterol. Motil.* **2004**, *16*, 113–124. [CrossRef]
30. Abdrakhmanova, G.R.; AlSharari, S.; Kang, M.; Damaj, M.I.; Akbarali, H.I. α7-nAChR-mediated suppression of hyperexcitability of colonic dorsal root ganglia neurons in experimental colitis. *Am. J. Physiol. Liver Physiol.* **2010**, *299*, G761–G768. [CrossRef]
31. Smith, N.J.; Hone, A.J.; Memon, T.; Bossi, S.; Smith, T.E.; McIntosh, J.M.; Olivera, B.M.; Teichert, R.W. Comparative functional expression of nAChR subtypes in rodent DRG neurons. *Front. Cell. Neurosci.* **2013**, *7*, 225. [CrossRef] [PubMed]
32. Wieskopf, J.S.; Mathur, J.; Limapichat, W.; Post, M.R.; Al-Qazzaz, M.; Sorge, R.E.; Martin, L.J.; Zaykin, D.V.; Smith, S.B.; Freitas, K.; et al. The nicotinic α6 subunit gene determines variability in chronic pain sensitivity via cross-inhibition of P2X2/3 receptors. *Sci. Transl. Med.* **2015**, *7*, 225. [CrossRef] [PubMed]
33. Spies, M.; Lips, K.S.; Kurzen, H.; Kummer, W.; Haberberger, R.V. Nicotinic Acetylcholine Receptors Containing Subunits α3 and α5 in Rat Nociceptive Dorsal Root Ganglion Neurons. *J. Mol. Neurosci.* **2006**, *30*, 55–56. [CrossRef]
34. Genzen, J.R.; McGehee, D.S. Short- and long-term enhancement of excitatory transmission in the spinal cord dorsal horn by nicotinic acetylcholine receptors. *Proc. Natl. Acad. Sci. USA* **2003**, *100*, 6807–6812. [CrossRef] [PubMed]
35. De Biasi, M.; Nigro, F.; Xu, W. Nicotinic acetylcholine receptors in the autonomic control of bladder function. *Eur. J. Pharmacol.* **2000**, *393*, 137–140. [CrossRef]
36. Xu, W.; Orr-Urtreger, A.; Nigro, F.; Gelber, S.; Sutcliffe, C.B.; Armstrong, D.; Patrick, J.W.; Role, L.W.; Beaudet, A.L.; De Biasi, M. Multiorgan autonomic dysfunction in mice lacking the beta2 and the beta4 subunits of neuronal nicotinic acetylcholine receptors. *J. Neurosci.* **1999**, *19*, 9298–9305. [CrossRef]
37. Zhou, X.; Ren, J.; Brown, E.; Schneider, D.A.; Caraballo-Lopez, Y.; Galligan, J.J. Pharmacological Properties of Nicotinic Acetylcholine Receptors Expressed by Guinea Pig Small Intestinal Myenteric Neurons. *J. Pharmacol. Exp. Ther.* **2002**, *302*, 889–897. [CrossRef]
38. Garza, A.; Huang, L.Z.; Son, J.-H.; Winzer-Serhan, U.H. Expression of nicotinic acetylcholine receptors and subunit messenger RNAs in the enteric nervous system of the neonatal rat. *Neuroscience* **2009**, *158*, 1521–1529. [CrossRef]
39. Obaid, A.; Nelson, M.E.; Lindström, J.; Salzberg, B.M. Optical studies of nicotinic acetylcholine receptor subtypes in the guinea-pig enteric nervous system. *J. Exp. Biol.* **2005**, *208*, 2981–3001. [CrossRef]

40. Foong, J.P.P.; Hirst, C.S.; Hao, M.M.; McKeown, S.J.; Boesmans, W.; Young, H.M.; Bornstein, J.C.; Berghe, P.V. Changes in Nicotinic Neurotransmission during Enteric Nervous System Development. *J. Neurosci.* **2015**, *35*, 7106–7115. [CrossRef]
41. Glushakov, A.V.; Voytenko, L.P.; Skok, M.V.; Skok, V. Distribution of neuronal nicotinic acetylcholine receptors containing different alpha-subunits in the submucosal plexus of the guinea-pig. *Auton. Neurosci.* **2004**, *110*, 19–26. [CrossRef] [PubMed]
42. MacEachern, S.J.; Patel, B.A.; McKay, D.M.; Sharkey, K. Nitric oxide regulation of colonic epithelial ion transport: A novel role for enteric glia in the myenteric plexus. *J. Physiol.* **2011**, *589*, 3333–3348. [CrossRef] [PubMed]
43. Lai, N.Y.; Mills, K.; Chiu, I.M. Sensory neuron regulation of gastrointestinal inflammation and bacterial host defence. *J. Intern. Med.* **2017**, *282*, 5–23. [CrossRef] [PubMed]
44. Keiger, C.H.; Walker, J.C. Individual variation in the expression profiles of nicotinic receptors in the olfactory bulb and trigeminal ganglion and identification of α2, α6, α9, and β3 transcripts. *Biochem. Pharmacol.* **2000**, *59*, 233–240. [CrossRef]
45. Zhang, X.; Hartung, J.E.; Friedman, R.L.; Koerber, H.R.; Belfer, I.; Gold, M.S. Nicotine Evoked Currents in Human Primary Sensory Neurons. *J. Pain* **2019**, *20*, 810–818. [CrossRef] [PubMed]
46. Ray, P.R.; Torck, A.; Quigley, L.; Wangzhou, A.; Neiman, M.; Rao, C.; Lam, T.; Kim, J.-Y.; Kim, T.H.; Zhang, M.Q.; et al. Comparative transcriptome profiling of the human and mouse dorsal root ganglia. *Pain* **2018**, *159*, 1325–1345. [CrossRef]
47. Downs, A.; Bond, C.; Hoover, D.B. Localization of α7 nicotinic acetylcholine receptor mRNA and protein within the cholinergic anti-inflammatory pathway. *Neuroscience* **2014**, *266*, 178–185. [CrossRef]
48. Mundinger, T.O.; Mei, Q.; Taborsky, G.J., Jr. Impaired activation of celiac ganglion neurons in vivo after damage to their sympathetic nerve terminals. *J. Neurosci. Res.* **2008**, *86*, 1981–1993. [CrossRef]
49. Koval, O.M.; Voitenko, L.P.; Skok, M.V.; Lykhmus, E.Y.; Tsetlin, V.; Zhmak, M.N.; Skok, V. The β-subunit composition of nicotinic acetylcholine receptors in the neurons of the guinea pig inferior mesenteric ganglion. *Neurosci. Lett.* **2004**, *365*, 143–146. [CrossRef]
50. Bentley, G.A. Pharmacological studies on the hypogastric ganglion of the rat and guinea-pig. *Br. J. Pharmacol.* **1972**, *44*, 492–509. [CrossRef]
51. Girard, B.M.; Merriam, L.A.; Tompkins, J.D.; Vizzard, M.A.; Parsons, R.L. Decrease in neuronal nicotinic acetylcholine receptor subunit and PSD-93 transcript levels in the male mouse MPG after cavernous nerve injury or explant culture. *Am. J. Physiol. Physiol.* **2013**, *305*, F1504–F1512. [CrossRef] [PubMed]
52. Kirchgessner, A.L.; Liu, M.T. Immunohistochemical localization of nicotinic acetylcholine receptors in the guinea pig bowel and pancreas. *J. Comp. Neurol.* **1998**, *390*, 497–514. [CrossRef]
53. Barrenschee, M.; Cossais, F.; Böttner, M.; Egberts, J.-H.; Becker, T.; Wedel, T. Impaired Expression of Neuregulin 1 and Nicotinic Acetylcholine Receptor β4 Subunit in Diverticular Disease. *Front. Cell. Neurosci.* **2019**, *13*, 563. [CrossRef] [PubMed]
54. Vernino, S.; Low, P.A.; Fealey, R.D.; Stewart, J.D.; Farrugia, G.; Lennon, V.A. Autoantibodies to Ganglionic Acetylcholine Receptors in Autoimmune Autonomic Neuropathies. *N. Engl. J. Med.* **2000**, *343*, 847–855. [CrossRef]
55. Vernino, S.; Hopkins, S.; Wang, Z. Autonomic ganglia, acetylcholine receptor antibodies, and autoimmune ganglionopathy. *Auton. Neurosci.* **2009**, *146*, 3–7. [CrossRef]
56. Richardson, C.E.; Morgan, J.M.; Jasani, B.; Green, J.T.; Rhodes, J.; Williams, G.T.; Lindstrom, J.; Wonnacott, S.; Thomas, G.A.; Smith, V. Megacystis-microcolon-intestinal hypoperistalsis syndrome and the absence of the α3 nicotinic acetylcholine receptor subunit. *Gastroenterology* **2001**, *121*, 350–357. [CrossRef]
57. Abdullah, N.; Defaye, M.; Altier, C. Neural control of gut homeostasis. *Am. J. Physiol. Liver Physiol.* **2020**, *319*, G718–G732. [CrossRef]
58. Breit, S.; Kupferberg, A.; Rogler, G.; Hasler, G. Vagus Nerve as Modulator of the Brain–Gut Axis in Psychiatric and Inflammatory Disorders. *Front. Psychiatry* **2018**, *9*, 44. [CrossRef]
59. Kruepunga, N.; Hikspoors, J.P.J.M.; Hülsman, C.J.M.; Mommen, G.M.C.; Köhler, S.E.; Lamers, W.H. Development of extrinsic innervation in the abdominal intestines of human embryos. *J. Anat.* **2020**, *237*, 655–671. [CrossRef]
60. Berthoud, H.-R.; Neuhuber, W.L. Functional and chemical anatomy of the afferent vagal system. *Auton. Neurosci.* **2000**, *85*, 1–17. [CrossRef]
61. Tracey, K.J. The inflammatory reflex. *Nature* **2002**, *420*, 853–859. [CrossRef] [PubMed]
62. Rosas-Ballina, M.; Ochani, M.; Parrish, W.R.; Ochani, K.; Harris, Y.T.; Huston, J.M.; Chavan, S.; Tracey, K.J. Splenic nerve is required for cholinergic antiinflammatory pathway control of TNF in endotoxemia. *Proc. Natl. Acad. Sci. USA* **2008**, *105*, 11008–11013. [CrossRef] [PubMed]
63. Rosas-Ballina, M.; Olofsson, P.S.; Ochani, M.; Valdés-Ferrer, S.I.; Levine, Y.A.; Reardon, C.; Tusche, M.W.; Pavlov, V.A.; Andersson, U.; Chavan, S.; et al. Acetylcholine-Synthesizing T Cells Relay Neural Signals in a Vagus Nerve Circuit. *Science* **2011**, *334*, 98–101. [CrossRef] [PubMed]
64. Nezami, B.G.; Srinivasan, S. Enteric Nervous System in the Small Intestine: Pathophysiology and Clinical Implications. *Curr. Gastroenterol. Rep.* **2010**, *12*, 358–365. [CrossRef]
65. Metz, C.N.; Pavlov, V.A. Vagus nerve cholinergic circuitry to the liver and the gastrointestinal tract in the neuroimmune communicatome. *Am. J. Physiol. Liver Physiol.* **2018**, *315*, G651–G658. [CrossRef]
66. Arredondo, J.; Chernyavsky, A.I.; Jolkovsky, D.L.; Pinkerton, K.E.; Grando, S.A. Receptor-mediated tobacco toxicity: Cooperation of the Ras/Raf-1/MEK1/ERK and JAK-2/STAT-3 pathways downstream of α7 nicotinic receptor in oral keratinocytes. *FASEB J.* **2006**, *20*, 2093–2101. [CrossRef]

67. De Jonge, W.J.; Van Der Zanden, E.P.; The, F.O.; Bijlsma, M.F.; Van Westerloo, D.J.; Bennink, R.J.; Berthoud, H.-R.; Uematsu, S.; Akira, S.; Wijngaard, R.M.V.D.; et al. Stimulation of the vagus nerve attenuates macrophage activation by activating the Jak2-STAT3 signaling pathway. *Nat. Immunol.* **2005**, *6*, 844–851. [CrossRef]
68. Hoentjen, F.; Sartor, R.B.; Ozaki, M.; Jobin, C. STAT3 regulates NF-κB recruitment to the IL-12p40 promoter in dendritic cells. *Blood* **2005**, *105*, 689–696. [CrossRef]
69. Yoshida, Y.; Kumar, A.; Koyama, Y.; Peng, H.; Arman, A.; Boch, J.A.; Auron, P.E. Interleukin 1 Activates STAT3/Nuclear Factor-κB Cross-talk via a Unique TRAF6- and p65-dependent Mechanism. *J. Biol. Chem.* **2004**, *279*, 1768–1776. [CrossRef]
70. Tyagi, E.; Agrawal, R.; Nath, C.; Shukla, R. Cholinergic protection via α7 nicotinic acetylcholine receptors and PI3K-Akt pathway in LPS-induced neuroinflammation. *Neurochem. Int.* **2010**, *56*, 135–142. [CrossRef]
71. Kim, T.-H.; Kim, S.-J.; Lee, S.-M. Stimulation of the α7 Nicotinic Acetylcholine Receptor Protects against Sepsis by Inhibiting Toll-like Receptor via Phosphoinositide 3-Kinase Activation. *J. Infect. Dis.* **2013**, *209*, 1668–1677. [CrossRef] [PubMed]
72. Lu, B.; Kwan, K.; Levine, Y.A.; Olofsson, P.S.; Yang, H.; Li, J.; Joshi, S.; Wang, H.; Andersson, U.; Chavan, S.S.; et al. α7 Nicotinic Acetylcholine Receptor Signaling Inhibits Inflammasome Activation by Preventing Mitochondrial DNA Release. *Mol. Med.* **2014**, *20*, 350–358. [CrossRef] [PubMed]
73. Borovikova, L.V.; Ivanova, S.; Zhang, M.; Yang, H.; Botchkina, G.I.; Watkins, L.R.; Wang, H.; Abumrad, N.N.; Eaton, J.W.; Tracey, K.J. Vagus nerve stimulation attenuates the systemic inflammatory response to endotoxin. *Nat. Cell Biol.* **2000**, *405*, 458–462. [CrossRef] [PubMed]
74. Wang, H.; Yu, M.; Ochani, M.; Amella, C.A.; Tanovic, M.; Susarla, S.; Li, J.H.; Wang, H.; Yang, H.; Ulloa, L.; et al. Nicotinic acetylcholine receptor α7 subunit is an essential regulator of inflammation. *Nat. Cell Biol.* **2002**, *421*, 384–388. [CrossRef]
75. Parrish, W.R.; Czura, C.J.; Tracey, K.J.; Puerta, M. Experimental Therapeutic Strategies for Severe Sepsis. *Ann. N. Y. Acad. Sci.* **2008**, *1144*, 210–236. [CrossRef]
76. Pavlov, V.A.; Ochani, M.; Yang, L.-H.; Gallowitsch-Puerta, M.; Ochani, K.; Lin, X.; Levi, J.; Parrish, W.R.; Rosas-Ballina, M.; Czura, C.J.; et al. Selective α7-nicotinic acetylcholine receptor agonist GTS-21 improves survival in murine endotoxemia and severe sepsis. *Crit. Care Med.* **2007**, *35*, 1139–1144. [CrossRef]
77. Wang, H.; Liao, H.; Ochani, M.; Justiniani, M.; Lin, X.; Yang, L.; Al-Abed, Y.; Wang, H.; Metz, C.N.; Miller, E.J.; et al. Cholinergic agonists inhibit HMGB1 release and improve survival in experimental sepsis. *Nat. Med.* **2004**, *10*, 1216–1221. [CrossRef]
78. Tsoyi, K.; Jang, H.J.; Kim, J.W.; Chang, H.K.; Lee, Y.S.; Pae, H.-O.; Kim, H.J.; Seo, H.G.; Lee, J.H.; Chung, H.-T.; et al. Stimulation of Alpha7 Nicotinic Acetylcholine Receptor by Nicotine Attenuates Inflammatory Response in Macrophages and Improves Survival in Experimental Model of Sepsis Through Heme Oxygenase-1 Induction. *Antioxid. Redox Signal.* **2011**, *14*, 2057–2070. [CrossRef]
79. Olofsson, P.S.; Rosas-Ballina, M.; Levine, Y.A.; Tracey, K.J. Rethinking inflammation: Neural circuits in the regulation of immunity. *Immunol. Rev.* **2012**, *248*, 188–204. [CrossRef]
80. Zhao, Y.X.; He, W.; Jing, X.H.; Liu, J.L.; Rong, P.J.; Ben, H.; Liu, K.; Zhu, B. Transcutaneous Auricular Vagus Nerve Stimulation Protects Endotoxemic Rat from Lipopolysaccharide-Induced Inflammation. *Evid. Based Complement. Altern. Med.* **2012**, *2012*, 1–10. [CrossRef]
81. Maldifassi, M.C.; Martín-Sánchez, C.; Atienza, G.; Cedillo, J.L.; Arnalich, F.; Bordas, A.; Zafra, F.; Giménez, C.; Extremera, M.; Renart, J.; et al. Interaction of the α7-nicotinic subunit with its human-specific duplicated dupα7 isoform in mammalian cells: Relevance in human inflammatory responses. *J. Biol. Chem.* **2018**, *293*, 13874–13888. [CrossRef] [PubMed]
82. Baird, A.; Coimbra, R.; Dang, X.; Eliceiri, B.P.; Costantini, T.W. Up-regulation of the human-specific CHRFAM7A gene in inflammatory bowel disease. *BBA Clin.* **2016**, *5*, 66–71. [CrossRef] [PubMed]
83. Kessler, W.; Diedrich, S.; Menges, P.; Ebker, T.; Nielson, M.; Partecke, L.I.; Traeger, T.; Cziupka, K.; Van Der Linde, J.; Puls, R.; et al. The Role of the Vagus Nerve: Modulation of the Inflammatory Reaction in Murine Polymicrobial Sepsis. *Mediat. Inflamm.* **2012**, *2012*, 1–9. [CrossRef] [PubMed]
84. Levy, G.; Fishman, J.; Xu, D.; Chandler, B.T.J.; Feketova, E.; Dong, W.; Qin, Y.; Alli, V.; Ulloa, L.; Deitch, E.A. Parasympathetic Stimulation Via the Vagus Nerve Prevents Systemic Organ Dysfunction by Abrogating Gut Injury and Lymph Toxicity in Trauma and Hemorrhagic Shock. *Shock* **2013**, *39*, 39–44. [CrossRef]
85. Li, T.; Zuo, X.; Zhou, Y.; Wang, Y.; Zhuang, H.; Zhang, L.; Zhang, H.; Xiao, X. The Vagus Nerve and Nicotinic Receptors Involve Inhibition of HMGB1 Release and Early Pro-inflammatory Cytokines Function in Collagen-Induced Arthritis. *J. Clin. Immunol.* **2009**, *30*, 213–220. [CrossRef]
86. Meregnani, J.; Clarencon, D.; Vivier, M.; Peinnequin, A.; Mouret, C.; Sinniger, V.; Picq, C.; Job, A.; Canini, F.; Jacquier-Sarlin, M.; et al. Anti-inflammatory effect of vagus nerve stimulation in a rat model of inflammatory bowel disease. *Auton. Neurosci.* **2011**, *160*, 82–89. [CrossRef]
87. Van Westerloo, D.J.; Giebelen, I.A.; Florquin, S.; Bruno, M.J.; LaRosa, G.J.; Ulloa, L.; Tracey, K.J.; Van Der Poll, T. The Vagus Nerve and Nicotinic Receptors Modulate Experimental Pancreatitis Severity in Mice. *Gastroenterology* **2006**, *130*, 1822–1830. [CrossRef]
88. Schneider, L.; Jabrailova, B.; Soliman, H.; Hofer, S.; Strobel, O.; Hackert, T.; Büchler, M.W.; Werner, J. Pharmacological Cholinergic Stimulation as a Therapeutic Tool in Experimental Necrotizing Pancreatitis. *Pancreas* **2014**, *43*, 41–46. [CrossRef]
89. Feng, X.; Li, L.; Feng, J.; He, W.; Li, N.; Shi, T.; Jie, Z.; Su, X. Vagal-α7nAChR signaling attenuates allergic asthma responses and facilitates asthma tolerance by regulating inflammatory group 2 innate lymphoid cells. *Immunol. Cell Biol.* **2020**. [CrossRef]
90. Kox, M.; Pompe, J.C.; De Gouberville, M.C.G.; Van Der Hoeven, J.G.; Hoedemaekers, C.W.E.; Pickkers, P. Effects of the α7 Nicotinic Acetylcholine Receptor Agonist Gts-21 on the Innate Immune Response in Humans. *Shock* **2011**, *36*, 5–11. [CrossRef]

91. Wittebole, X.; Hahm, S.; Coyle, S.M.; Kumar, A.; Calvano, S.E.; Lowry, S.F. Nicotine exposure alters in vivo human responses to endotoxin. *Clin. Exp. Immunol.* **2006**, *147*, 28–34. [CrossRef] [PubMed]
92. Cedillo, J.L.; Arnalich, F.; Martín-Sánchez, C.; Quesada, A.; Rios, J.J.; Maldifassi, M.C.; Atienza, G.; Renart, J.; Fernández, F.A.; García-Rio, F.; et al. Usefulness of α7 Nicotinic Receptor Messenger RNA Levels in Peripheral Blood Mononuclear Cells as a Marker for Cholinergic Antiinflammatory Pathway Activity in Septic Patients: Results of a Pilot Study. *J. Infect. Dis.* **2014**, *211*, 146–155. [CrossRef] [PubMed]
93. Nicholson, W.; Kempf, M.-C.; Moneyham, L.; Vance, D.E. The potential role of vagus-nerve stimulation in the treatment of HIV-associated depression: A review of literature. *Neuropsychiatr. Dis. Treat.* **2017**, *13*, 1677–1689. [CrossRef] [PubMed]
94. Toffa, D.H.; Touma, L.; El Meskine, T.; Bouthillier, A.; Nguyen, D.K. Learnings from 30 years of reported efficacy and safety of vagus nerve stimulation (VNS) for epilepsy treatment: A critical review. *Seizure* **2020**, *83*, 104–123. [CrossRef]
95. Jiang, W.-; Zhang, C.; Wang, J.-X.; Sun, F.-H.; Xie, Y.-J.; Ou, X.; Yang, S.-B. The effect of VNS on the rehabilitation of stroke: A meta-analysis of randomized controlled studies. *J. Clin. Neurosci.* **2020**, *81*, 421–425. [CrossRef]
96. Lendvai, I.S.; Maier, A.; Scheele, D.; Hurlemann, R.; Kinfe, T.M. Spotlight on cervical vagus nerve stimulation for the treatment of primary headache disorders: A review. *J. Pain Res.* **2018**, *11*, 1613–1625. [CrossRef]
97. Bonaz, B.; Sinniger, V.; Hoffmann, D.; Clarençon, D.; Mathieu, N.; Dantzer, C.; Vercueil, L.; Picq, C.; Trocmé, C.; Faure, P.; et al. Chronic vagus nerve stimulation in Crohn's disease: A 6-month follow-up pilot study. *Neurogastroenterol. Motil.* **2016**, *28*, 948–953. [CrossRef]
98. Ghia, J.E.; Blennerhassett, P.; Kumar–Ondiveeran, H.; Verdu, E.F.; Collins, S.M. The Vagus Nerve: A Tonic Inhibitory Influence Associated With Inflammatory Bowel Disease in a Murine Model. *Gastroenterology* **2006**, *131*, 1122–1130. [CrossRef]
99. The, F.O.; Boeckxstaens, G.E.; Snoek, S.A.; Cash, J.L.; Bennink, R.; LaRosa, G.J.; Wijngaard, R.M.V.D.; Greaves, D.R.; De Jonge, W.J. Activation of the Cholinergic Anti-Inflammatory Pathway Ameliorates Postoperative Ileus in Mice. *Gastroenterology* **2007**, *133*, 1219–1228. [CrossRef]
100. Yu, Y.R.; Rodriguez, J.R. Clinical presentation of Crohn's, ulcerative colitis, and indeterminate colitis: Symptoms, extraintestinal manifestations, and disease phenotypes. *Semin. Pediatr. Surg.* **2017**, *26*, 349–355. [CrossRef]
101. Matteoli, G.; Boeckxstaens, G.E. The vagal innervation of the gut and immune homeostasis. *Gut* **2012**, *62*, 1214–1222. [CrossRef] [PubMed]
102. Cailotto, C.; Gomez-Pinilla, P.J.; Costes, L.M.; Van Der Vliet, J.; Di Giovangiulio, M.; Nemethova, A.; Matteoli, G.; Boeckxstaens, G.E. Neuro-Anatomical Evidence Indicating Indirect Modulation of Macrophages by Vagal Efferents in the Intestine but Not in the Spleen. *PLoS ONE* **2014**, *9*, e87785. [CrossRef] [PubMed]
103. Ahluwalia, B.; Moraes, L.; Magnusson, M.K.; Öhman, L. Immunopathogenesis of inflammatory bowel disease and mechanisms of biological therapies. *Scand. J. Gastroenterol.* **2018**, *53*, 379–389. [CrossRef] [PubMed]
104. Maruta, K.; Watanabe, C.; Hozumi, H.; Kurihara, C.; Furuhashi, H.; Takajo, T.; Okada, Y.; Shirakabe, K.; Higashiyama, M.; Komoto, S.; et al. Nicotine treatment ameliorates DSS-induced colitis by suppressing MAdCAM-1 expression and leukocyte recruitment. *J. Leukoc. Biol.* **2018**, *104*, 1013–1022. [CrossRef] [PubMed]
105. Abdrakhmanova, G.R.; Kang, M.; Damaj, M.I.; Akbarali, H.I. Nicotine suppresses hyperexcitability of colonic sensory neurons and visceral hypersensivity in mouse model of colonic inflammation. *Am. J. Physiol. Liver Physiol.* **2012**, *302*, G740–G747. [CrossRef] [PubMed]
106. Zhou, H.; Liang, H.; Li, Z.-F.; Xiang, H.; Liu, W.; Li, J.-G. Vagus Nerve Stimulation Attenuates Intestinal Epithelial Tight Junctions Disruption in Endotoxemic Mice Through α7 Nicotinic Acetylcholine Receptors. *Shock* **2013**, *40*, 144–151. [CrossRef]
107. Costantini, T.W.; Krzyzaniak, M.; Cheadle, G.A.; Putnam, J.G.; Hageny, A.-M.; Lopez, N.; Eliceiri, B.P.; Bansal, V.; Coimbra, R. Targeting α-7 Nicotinic Acetylcholine Receptor in the Enteric Nervous System. *Am. J. Pathol.* **2012**, *181*, 478–486. [CrossRef]
108. Wang, R.; Li, S.; Jin, L.; Zhang, W.; Liu, N.; Wang, H.; Wang, Z.; Wei, P.; Li, F.; Yu, J.; et al. Four-week administration of nicotine moderately impacts blood metabolic profile and gut microbiota in a diet-dependent manner. *Biomed. Pharmacother.* **2019**, *115*, 108945. [CrossRef]
109. Wazea, S.A.; Wadie, W.; Bahgat, A.K.; El-Abhar, H.S. Galantamine anti-colitic effect: Role of alpha-7 nicotinic acetylcholine receptor in modulating Jak/STAT3, NF-κB/HMGB1/RAGE and p-AKT/Bcl-2 pathways. *Sci. Rep.* **2018**, *8*, 5110. [CrossRef]
110. Tasaka, Y.; Yasunaga, D.; Kiyoi, T.; Tanaka, M.; Tanaka, A.; Suemaru, K.; Araki, H. Involvement of stimulation of α7 nicotinic acetylcholine receptors in the suppressive effect of tropisetron on dextran sulfate sodium-induced colitis in mice. *J. Pharmacol. Sci.* **2015**, *127*, 275–283. [CrossRef]
111. Regmi, B.; Shah, M.K. Possible implications of animal models for the assessment of visceral pain. *Anim. Model. Exp. Med.* **2020**, *3*, 215–228. [CrossRef] [PubMed]
112. Salaga, M.; Blomster, L.V.; Czyk, A.P.-P.; Zielinska, M.; Jacenik, D.; Cygankiewicz, A.; Krajewska, W.M.; Mikkelsen, J.D.; Fichna, J.; Piechota-Polanczyk, A. Encenicline, a 7 nicotinic acetylcholine receptor partial agonist, reduces immune cell infiltration in the colon and improves experimental colitis in mice. *J. Pharmacol. Exp. Ther.* **2015**, *356*, 157–169. [CrossRef] [PubMed]
113. Da Costa, R.; Motta, E.M.; Manjavachi, M.N.; Cola, M.; Calixto, J.B. Activation of the alpha-7 nicotinic acetylcholine receptor (α7 nAchR) reverses referred mechanical hyperalgesia induced by colonic inflammation in mice. *Neuropharmacology* **2012**, *63*, 798–805. [CrossRef] [PubMed]

114. Van Der Zanden, E.P.; Snoek, S.A.; Heinsbroek, S.E.; Stanisor, O.I.; Verseijden, C.; Boeckxstaens, G.E.; Peppelenbosch, M.P.; Greaves, D.R.; Gordon, S.; De Jonge, W.J. Vagus Nerve Activity Augments Intestinal Macrophage Phagocytosis via Nicotinic Acetylcholine Receptor α4β2. *Gastroenterology* **2009**, *137*, 1029–1039.e4. [CrossRef] [PubMed]
115. Xiao, J.; Zhang, G.; Gao, S.; Shen, J.; Feng, H.; He, Z.; Xu, C. Combined administration of SHP2 inhibitor SHP099 and the α7nAChR agonist PNU282987 protect mice against DSS-induced colitis. *Mol. Med. Rep.* **2020**, *22*, 2235–2244. [CrossRef] [PubMed]
116. AlZarea, S.; Rahman, S. Alpha-7 nicotinic receptor allosteric modulator PNU120596 prevents lipopolysaccharide-induced anxiety, cognitive deficit and depression-like behaviors in mice. *Behav. Brain Res.* **2019**, *366*, 19–28. [CrossRef]
117. Engler, H.; Elsenbruch, S.; Rebernik, L.; Köcke, J.; Cramer, H.; Schöls, M.; Langhorst, J. Stress burden and neuroendocrine regulation of cytokine production in patients with ulcerative colitis in remission. *Psychoneuroendocrinology* **2018**, *98*, 101–107. [CrossRef]
118. AlSharari, S.D.; Toma, W.; Mahmood, H.M.; McIntosh, J.M.; Damaj, M.I. The α9α10 nicotinic acetylcholine receptors antagonist α-conotoxin RgIA reverses colitis signs in murine dextran sodium sulfate model. *Eur. J. Pharmacol.* **2020**, *883*, 173320. [CrossRef]
119. Romero, H.K.; Christensen, S.B.; Mannelli, L.D.C.; Gajewiak, J.; Ramachandra, R.; Elmslie, K.S.; Vetter, D.E.; Ghelardini, C.; Iadonato, S.P.; Mercado, J.L.; et al. Inhibition of α9α10 nicotinic acetylcholine receptors prevents chemotherapy-induced neuropathic pain. *Proc. Natl. Acad. Sci. USA* **2017**, *114*, E1825–E1832. [CrossRef]
120. Mannelli, L.D.C.; Cinci, L.; Micheli, L.; Zanardelli, M.; Pacini, A.; McIntosh, M.J.; Ghelardini, C. α-Conotoxin RgIA protects against the development of nerve injury-induced chronic pain and prevents both neuronal and glial derangement. *Pain* **2014**, *155*, 1986–1995. [CrossRef]
121. Huynh, P.N.; Giuvelis, D.; Christensen, S.B.; Tucker, K.L.; McIntosh, J.M. RgIA4 Accelerates Recovery from Paclitaxel-Induced Neuropathic Pain in Rats. *Mar. Drugs* **2019**, *18*, 12. [CrossRef] [PubMed]
122. Pacini, A.; Micheli, L.; Maresca, M.; Branca, J.J.V.; McIntosh, J.M.; Ghelardini, C.; Mannelli, L.D.C. The α9α10 nicotinic receptor antagonist α-conotoxin RgIA prevents neuropathic pain induced by oxaliplatin treatment. *Exp. Neurol.* **2016**, *282*, 37–48. [CrossRef] [PubMed]
123. Zakrzewicz, A.; Richter, K.; Agné, A.; Wilker, S.; Siebers, K.; Fink, B.; Krasteva-Christ, G.; Althaus, M.; Padberg, W.; Hone, A.J.; et al. Canonical and Novel Non-Canonical Cholinergic Agonists Inhibit ATP-Induced Release of Monocytic Interleukin-1β via Different Combinations of Nicotinic Acetylcholine Receptor Subunits α7, α9 and α10. *Front. Cell. Neurosci.* **2017**, *11*, 189. [CrossRef] [PubMed]
124. Richter, K.; Mathes, V.; Fronius, M.; Althaus, M.; Hecker, A.; Krasteva-Christ, G.; Padberg, W.; Hone, A.J.; McIntosh, J.M.; Zakrzewicz, A.; et al. Phosphocholine—An agonist of metabotropic but not of ionotropic functions of α9-containing nicotinic acetylcholine receptors. *Sci. Rep.* **2016**, *6*, 28660. [CrossRef] [PubMed]
125. Hecker, A.; Küllmar, M.; Wilker, S.; Richter, K.; Zakrzewicz, A.; Atanasova, S.; Mathes, V.; Timm, T.; Lerner, S.; Klein, J.; et al. Phosphocholine-Modified Macromolecules and Canonical Nicotinic Agonists Inhibit ATP-Induced IL-1β Release. *J. Immunol.* **2015**, *195*, 2325–2334. [CrossRef]
126. Richter, K.; Ogiemwonyi-Schaefer, R.; Wilker, S.; Chaveiro, A.I.; Agné, A.; Hecker, M.; Reichert, M.; Amati, A.-L.; Schlüter, K.-D.; Manzini, I.; et al. Amyloid Beta Peptide (Aβ$_{1-42}$) Reverses the Cholinergic Control of Monocytic IL-1β Release. *J. Clin. Med.* **2020**, *9*, 2887. [CrossRef] [PubMed]
127. Cresci, A.M.G.; Izzo, C. Chapter 4—Gut Microbiome. In *Adult Short Bowel Syndrome*; Elsevier: Amsterdam, The Netherlands, 2019; pp. 45–54.
128. Uebanso, T.; Shimohata, T.; Mawatari, K.; Takahashi, A. Functional Roles of B-Vitamins in the Gut and Gut Microbiome. *Mol. Nutr. Food Res.* **2020**, *64*, 2000426. [CrossRef]
129. Gordon, C.; Behan, J.; Costello, M. Newly identified vitamin K-producing bacteria isolated from the neonatal faecal flora. *Microb. Ecol. Health Dis.* **2006**, *18*, 133–138.
130. Tan, J.; McKenzie, C.; Potamitis, M.; Thorburn, A.N.; Mackay, C.R.; Macia, L. The Role of Short-Chain Fatty Acids in Health and Disease. *Adv. Immunol.* **2014**, *121*, 91–119. [CrossRef]
131. Park, J.-S.; Lee, E.-J.; Lee, J.-C.; Kim, W.-K.; Kim, H.-S. Anti-inflammatory effects of short chain fatty acids in IFN-γ-stimulated RAW 264.7 murine macrophage cells: Involvement of NF-κB and ERK signaling pathways. *Int. Immunopharmacol.* **2007**, *7*, 70–77. [CrossRef]
132. Rastall, R.A. Bacteria in the Gut: Friends and Foes and How to Alter the Balance. *J. Nutr.* **2004**, *134*, 2022S–2026S. [CrossRef] [PubMed]
133. Marshall-Jones, Z.V.; Baillon, M.-L.A.; Croft, J.M.; Butterwick, R.F. Effects of Lactobacillus acidophilus DSM13241 as a probiotic in healthy adult cats. *Am. J. Veter. Res.* **2006**, *67*, 1005–1012. [CrossRef] [PubMed]
134. Baillon, M.-L.A.; Marshall-Jones, Z.V.; Butterwick, R.F. Effects of probiotic Lactobacillus acidophilus strain DSM13241 in healthy adult dogs. *Am. J. Veter. Res.* **2004**, *65*, 338–343. [CrossRef]
135. Ménard, S.; Laharie, D.; Asensio, C.; Vidal-Martinez, T.; Candalh, C.; Rullier, A.; Zerbib, F.; Mégraud, F.; Matysiak-Budnik, T.; Heyman, M. Bifidobacterium breve and Streptococcus thermophilus Secretion Products Enhance T Helper 1 Immune Response and Intestinal Barrier in Mice. *Exp. Biol. Med.* **2005**, *230*, 749–756. [CrossRef]
136. Dargahi, N.; Johnson, J.; Apostolopoulos, V. Streptococcus thermophilus alters the expression of genes associated with innate and adaptive immunity in human peripheral blood mononuclear cells. *PLoS ONE* **2020**, *15*, e0228531. [CrossRef] [PubMed]

137. Wrzosek, L.; Miquel, S.; Noordine, M.-L.; Bouet, S.; Chevalier-Curt, M.J.; Robert, V.; Philippe, C.; Bridonneau, C.; Cherbuy, C.; Robbe-Masselot, C.; et al. Bacteroides thetaiotaomicron and Faecalibacterium prausnitzii influence the production of mucus glycans and the development of goblet cells in the colonic epithelium of a gnotobiotic model rodent. *BMC Biol.* **2013**, *11*, 61. [CrossRef]
138. Tanner, S.A.; Chassard, C.; Rigozzi, E.; Lacroix, C.; Stevens, M.J.A. Bifidobacterium thermophilum RBL67 impacts on growth and virulence gene expression of Salmonella enterica subsp. enterica serovar Typhimurium. *BMC Microbiol.* **2016**, *16*, 1–16. [CrossRef]
139. Lee, J.-H.; O'Sullivan, D.J. Genomic Insights into Bifidobacteria. *Microbiol. Mol. Biol. Rev.* **2010**, *74*, 378–416. [CrossRef] [PubMed]
140. Scheiman, J.; Luber, J.M.; Chavkin, T.A.; Macdonald, T.; Tung, A.; Pham, L.-D.; Wibowo, M.C.; Wurth, R.C.; Punthambaker, S.; Tierney, B.T.; et al. Meta-omics analysis of elite athletes identifies a performance-enhancing microbe that functions via lactate metabolism. *Nat. Med.* **2019**, *25*, 1104–1109. [CrossRef]
141. Bunesova, V.; Lacroix, C.; Schwab, C. Mucin Cross-Feeding of Infant Bifidobacteria and Eubacterium hallii. *Microb. Ecol.* **2018**, *75*, 228–238. [CrossRef]
142. Lopetuso, L.R.; Scaldaferri, F.; Petito, V.; Gasbarrini, A. Commensal clostridia: Leading players in the maintenance of gut homeostasis. *Gut Pathog.* **2013**, *5*, 1–23. [CrossRef] [PubMed]
143. Drago, L.; Toscano, M.; Rodighiero, V.; De Vecchi, E.; Mogna, G. Cultivable and Pyrosequenced Fecal Microflora in Centenarians and Young Subjects. *J. Clin. Gastroenterol.* **2012**, *46*, S81–S84. [CrossRef] [PubMed]
144. Pryde, S.E.; Duncan, S.H.; Hold, G.L.; Stewart, C.S.; Flint, H.J. The microbiology of butyrate formation in the human colon. *FEMS Microbiol. Lett.* **2002**, *217*, 133–139. [CrossRef]
145. Wlodarska, M.; Luo, C.; Kolde, R.; D'Hennezel, E.; Annand, J.W.; Heim, C.E.; Krastel, P.; Schmitt, E.K.; Omar, A.S.; Creasey, E.A.; et al. Indoleacrylic Acid Produced by Commensal Peptostreptococcus Species Suppresses Inflammation. *Cell Host Microbe* **2017**, *22*, 25–37.e6. [CrossRef] [PubMed]
146. Kho, Z.Y.; Lal, S.K. The Human Gut Microbiome—A Potential Controller of Wellness and Disease. *Front. Microbiol.* **2018**, *9*, 1835. [CrossRef] [PubMed]
147. Jeffery, I.B.; O'Toole, P.W.; Öhman, L.; Claesson, M.J.; Deane, J.; Quigley, E.M.M.; Simrén, M. An irritable bowel syndrome subtype defined by species-specific alterations in faecal microbiota. *Gut* **2011**, *61*, 997–1006. [CrossRef]
148. Sánchez, E.; Donat, E.; Ribes-Koninckx, C.; Fernández-Murga, M.L.; Sanz, Y. Duodenal-Mucosal Bacteria Associated with Celiac Disease in Children. *Appl. Environ. Microbiol.* **2013**, *79*, 5472–5479. [CrossRef]
149. Liebregts, T.; Adam, B.; Bredack, C.; Röth, A.; Heinzel, S.; Lester, S.; Downie–Doyle, S.; Smith, E.; Drew, P.; Talley, N.J.; et al. Immune Activation in Patients with Irritable Bowel Syndrome. *Gastroenterology* **2007**, *132*, 913–920. [CrossRef]
150. Kuehne, S.A.; Cartman, S.T.; Heap, J.T.; Kelly, M.L.; Cockayne, A.; Minton, N.P. The role of toxin A and toxin B in Clostridium difficile infection. *Nature* **2010**, *467*, 711–713. [CrossRef]
151. Savidge, T.C.; Pan, W.-H.; Newman, P.; O'Brien, M.J.; Anton, P.M.; Pothoulakis, C. Clostridium difficile toxin B is an inflammatory enterotoxin in human intestine. *Gastroenterology* **2003**, *125*, 413–420. [CrossRef]
152. Chi, L.; Mahbub, R.; Gao, B.; Bian, X.; Tu, P.; Ru, H.; Lu, K. Nicotine Alters the Gut Microbiome and Metabolites of Gut–Brain Interactions in a Sex-Specific Manner. *Chem. Res. Toxicol.* **2017**, *30*, 2110–2119. [CrossRef] [PubMed]
153. Biedermann, L.; Zeitz, J.; Mwinyi, J.; Sutter-Minder, E.; Rehman, A.; Ott, S.J.; Steurer-Stey, C.; Frei, A.; Frei, P.; Scharl, M.; et al. Smoking Cessation Induces Profound Changes in the Composition of the Intestinal Microbiota in Humans. *PLoS ONE* **2013**, *8*, e59260. [CrossRef] [PubMed]
154. Tomoda, K.; Kubo, K.; Asahara, T.; Andoh, A.; Nomoto, K.; Nishii, Y.; Yamamoto, Y.; Yoshikawa, M.; Kimura, H. Cigarette smoke decreases organic acids levels and population of bifidobacterium in the caecum of rats. *J. Toxicol. Sci.* **2011**, *36*, 261–266. [CrossRef] [PubMed]
155. Wang, H. Side-stream smoking reduces intestinal inflammation and increases expression of tight junction proteins. *World J. Gastroenterol.* **2012**, *18*, 2180–2187. [CrossRef]
156. Kaji, I.; Akiba, Y.; Konno, K.; Watanabe, M.; Kimura, S.; Iwanaga, T.; Kuri, A.; Iwamoto, K.-I.; Kuwahara, A.; Kaunitz, J.D. Neural FFA3 activation inversely regulates anion secretion evoked by nicotinic ACh receptor activation in rat proximal colon. *J. Physiol.* **2016**, *594*, 3339–3352. [CrossRef]
157. Kaji, I.; Akiba, Y.; Furuyama, T.; Adelson, D.W.; Iwamoto, K.; Watanabe, M.; Kuwahara, A.; Kaunitz, J.D. Free fatty acid receptor 3 activation suppresses neurogenic motility in rat proximal colon. *Neurogastroenterol. Motil.* **2017**, *30*, e13157. [CrossRef]
158. Zhu, N.; Zhang, D.; Wang, W.; Li, X.; Yang, B.; Song, J.; Zhao, X.; Huang, B.; Shi, W.; Lu, R.; et al. A Novel Coronavirus from Patients with Pneumonia in China, 2019. *N. Engl. J. Med.* **2020**, *382*, 727–733. [CrossRef]
159. Zhou, P.; Yang, X.-L.; Wang, X.-G.; Hu, B.; Zhang, L.; Zhang, W.; Si, H.-R.; Zhu, Y.; Li, B.; Huang, C.-L.; et al. A pneumonia outbreak associated with a new coronavirus of probable bat origin. *Nature* **2020**, *579*, 270–273. [CrossRef]
160. Walls, A.C.; Park, Y.-J.; Tortorici, M.A.; Wall, A.; McGuire, A.T.; Veesler, D. Structure, Function, and Antigenicity of the SARS-CoV-2 Spike Glycoprotein. *Cell* **2020**, *181*, 281–292.e6. [CrossRef]
161. Xia, S.; Lan, Q.; Su, S.; Wang, X.; Xu, W.; Liu, Z.; Zhu, Y.; Wang, Q.; Lu, L.; Jiang, S. The role of furin cleavage site in SARS-CoV-2 spike protein-mediated membrane fusion in the presence or absence of trypsin. *Signal Transduct. Target. Ther.* **2020**, *5*, 1–3. [CrossRef]

162. Coutard, B.; Valle, C.; De Lamballerie, X.; Canard, B.; Seidah, N.; Decroly, E. The spike glycoprotein of the new coronavirus 2019-nCoV contains a furin-like cleavage site absent in CoV of the same clade. *Antivir. Res.* **2020**, *176*, 104742. [CrossRef] [PubMed]
163. Changeux, J.-P.; Amoura, Z.; Rey, F.A.; Miyara, M. A nicotinic hypothesis for Covid-19 with preventive and therapeutic implications. *Comptes Rendus. Biol.* **2020**, *343*, 33–39. [CrossRef] [PubMed]
164. Farsalinos, K.; Eliopoulos, E.; Leonidas, D.D.; Papadopoulos, G.E.; Tzartos, S.J.; Poulas, K. Nicotinic Cholinergic System and COVID-19: In Silico Identification of an Interaction between SARS-CoV-2 and Nicotinic Receptors with Potential Therapeutic Targeting Implications. *Int. J. Mol. Sci.* **2020**, *21*, 5807. [CrossRef]
165. Farsalinos, K.; Niaura, R.; Le Houezec, J.; Barbouni, A.; Tsatsakis, A.; Kouretas, D.; Vantarakis, A.; Poulas, K. Editorial: Nicotine and SARS-CoV-2: COVID-19 may be a disease of the nicotinic cholinergic system. *Toxicol. Rep.* **2020**, *7*, 658–663. [CrossRef] [PubMed]
166. Schrödinger. *PyMOL Molecular Graphics System Version 2.3*; Schrödinger: New York, NY, USA, 2019.
167. Cai, Y.; Zhang, J.; Xiao, T.; Peng, H.; Sterling, S.M.; Jr, R.M.W.; Rawson, S.; Rits-Volloch, S.; Chen, B. Distinct conformational states of SARS-CoV-2 spike protein. *Science* **2020**, *369*, eabd4251. [CrossRef]
168. Daly, J.L.; Simonetti, B.; Klein, K.; Chen, K.-E.; Williamson, M.K.; Antón-Plágaro, C.; Shoemark, D.K.; Simón-Gracia, L.; Bauer, M.; Hollandi, R.; et al. Neuropilin-1 is a host factor for SARS-CoV-2 infection. *Science* **2020**, *370*, 861–865. [CrossRef]
169. Zhang, H.; Kang, Z.; Gong, H.; Xu, D.; Wang, J.; Li, Z.; Li, Z.; Cui, X.; Xiao, J.; Zhan, J.; et al. Digestive system is a potential route of COVID-19: An analysis of single-cell coexpression pattern of key proteins in viral entry process. *Gut* **2020**, *69*, 1010–1018. [CrossRef]
170. Mao, R.; Qiu, Y.; He, J.-S.; Tan, J.-Y.; Li, X.-H.; Liang, J.; Shen, J.; Zhu, L.-R.; Chen, Y.; Iacucci, M.; et al. Manifestations and prognosis of gastrointestinal and liver involvement in patients with COVID-19: A systematic review and meta-analysis. *Lancet Gastroenterol. Hepatol.* **2020**, *5*, 667–678. [CrossRef]
171. Guerra, I.; Algaba, A.; Jimenez, L.; Mar Aller, M.; Garza, D.; Bonillo, D.; Molina Esteban, L.M.; Bermejo, F. Incidence, Clinical Characteristics, and Evolution of SARS-CoV-2 Infection in Patients with Inflammatory Bowel Disease: A Single-Center Study in Madrid, Spain. *Inflamm. Bowel Dis.* **2020**, *27*, 25–33. [CrossRef]
172. Rodríguez-Lago, I.; De La Piscina, P.R.; Elorza, A.; Merino, O.; De Zárate, J.O.; Cabriada, J.L. Characteristics and Prognosis of Patients With Inflammatory Bowel Disease During the SARS-CoV-2 Pandemic in the Basque Country (Spain). *Gastroenterology* **2020**, *159*, 781–783. [CrossRef]
173. D'Amico, F.; Danese, S.; Peyrin-Biroulet, L. Systematic Review on Inflammatory Bowel Disease Patients With Coronavirus Disease 2019: It Is Time to Take Stock. *Clin. Gastroenterol. Hepatol.* **2020**, *18*, 2689–2700. [CrossRef] [PubMed]
174. Gonzalez-Rubio, J.; Navarro-Lopez, C.; Lopez-Najera, E.; Lopez-Najera, A.; Najera, A.; Navarro-Lopez, J.D.; Najera, A. Cytokine Release Syndrome (CRS) and Nicotine in COVID-19 Patients: Trying to Calm the Storm. *Front. Immunol.* **2020**, *11*, 1359. [CrossRef] [PubMed]
175. Bonaz, B.; Sinniger, V.; Pellissier, S. Targeting the cholinergic anti-inflammatory pathway with vagus nerve stimulation in patients with Covid-19? *Bioelectron. Med.* **2020**, *6*, 1–7. [CrossRef] [PubMed]
176. Ahmad, F. COVID-19 induced ARDS, and the use of galantamine to activate the cholinergic anti-inflammatory pathway. *Med Hypotheses* **2020**, *145*, 110331. [CrossRef]
177. Segal, J.P.; Mak, J.W.Y.; Mullish, B.H.; Alexander, J.L.; Ng, S.C.; Marchesi, J.R. The gut microbiome: An under-recognised contributor to the COVID-19 pandemic? *Ther. Adv. Gastroenterol.* **2020**, *13*, 1756284820974914. [CrossRef]
178. Din, A.U.; Mazhar, M.; Waseem, M.; Ahmad, W.; Bibi, A.; Hassan, A.; Ali, N.; Gang, W.; Qian, G.; Ullah, R.; et al. SARS-CoV-2 microbiome dysbiosis linked disorders and possible probiotics role. *Biomed. Pharmacother.* **2021**, *133*, 110947. [CrossRef]
179. Gu, S.; Chen, Y.; Wu, Z.; Chen, Y.; Gao, H.; Lv, L.; Guo, F.; Zhang, X.; Luo, R.; Huang, C.; et al. Alterations of the Gut Microbiota in Patients with COVID-19 or H1N1 Influenza. *Clin. Infect. Dis.* **2020**, *71*, 2669–2678. [CrossRef]
180. Zuo, T.; Liu, Q.; Zhang, F.; Lui, G.C.; Tso, E.Y.; Yeoh, Y.K.; Chen, Z.; Boon, S.S.; Chan, F.K.; Chan, P.K.; et al. Depicting SARS-CoV-2 faecal viral activity in association with gut microbiota composition in patients with COVID-19. *Gut* **2020**, *70*, 276–284. [CrossRef]
181. Conte, L.; Toraldo, D.M. Targeting the gut–lung microbiota axis by means of a high-fibre diet and probiotics may have anti-inflammatory effects in COVID-19 infection. *Ther. Adv. Respir. Dis.* **2020**, *14*, 1753466620937170. [CrossRef]

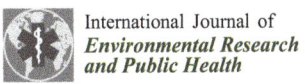

Review

The Microbiota-Bone-Allergy Interplay

Maria Maddalena Sirufo [1,2], Francesca De Pietro [1,2], Alessandra Catalogna [1,2], Lia Ginaldi [1,2] and Massimo De Martinis [1,2,*]

[1] Department of Life, Health and Environmental Sciences, University of L'Aquila, Piazzale Salvatore Tommasi n. 1, 67100 L'Aquila, Italy; maddalena.sirufo@gmail.com (M.M.S.); fra722@hotmail.it (F.D.P.); alessandra.cat4@gmail.com (A.C.); lia.ginaldi@cc.univaq.it (L.G.)

[2] Allergy and Clinical Immunology Unit, Center for the Diagnosis and Treatment of Osteoporosis, AUSL 04, 64100 Teramo, Italy

* Correspondence: demartinis@cc.univaq.it; Tel.: +39-0861-429548

Abstract: Emerging knowledge suggests an increasing importance of gut microbiota in health and disease. Allergy and bone metabolism are closely interconnected, and the possible negative effects of common therapies are not the only aspects of this relationship. The immune system is influenced by the microbiota-host interactions, and several pieces of evidence suggest the existence of an interplay between microbiota, bone metabolism, and allergies. Understanding these inter-relationships is essential for the development of new potential strategies of treatment and prevention targeting microbiota. A wide range of substances and germs, prebiotics and probiotics, are capable of influencing and modifying the microbiota. Prebiotics and probiotics have been shown in several studies to have different actions based on various factors such as sex, hormonal status, and age. In this review, we summarize the latest knowledge on the topic, and we discuss practical implications and the need for further studies.

Keywords: microbiota; gut microbiota; allergy; osteoporosis; bone metabolism; food allergy; skeletal health; inflammation; osteoimmunology

1. Introduction

The term microbiota defines the whole of microorganisms, not only bacteria but also fungi, protozoa, and viruses present in our organism. In particular, the human gastrointestinal tract is colonized by about 10^{13}–10^{14} microorganisms, of which 15,000 different bacterial strains are located mainly in the colon in a symbiotic relationship with the host [1]. In normal conditions, the microbiota is characterized by the predominance of obligate anaerobic members of *Firmicutes* and *Bacteroidetes phyla*, which guarantee intestinal and general health, while the loss of homeostasis, known as dysbiosis, is linked to the proliferation of some bacterial populations such as the Enterobacteriaceae or the absence of important commensal bacteria helps to create a more favorable environment for the growth of pathogens, predisposing the organism to pathological conditions [2,3] (Figure 1). According to what was recently reported in a study by the Human Microbiome Project and the European consortium Meta HIT, the human intestinal bacterial flora, despite being composed of a very high number of different species, can be divided into three most represented genus: *Bacteroides* and *Prevotella*, belonging to the phylum *Bacteroidetes*, and *Ruminococcus* belonging to the phylum *Firmicutes* [4]. In the time from birth to adulthood, the microbiota undergoes numerous changes; in fact, the neonatal microbiota is precociously formed by *Escherichia coli* of the birth canal followed by *Bacteroides*, *Bifidobacteria*, and *Clostridium* in the first week of life and reaches stabilization already appearing similar to that of adults only around 2–3 years old [5]. The intestinal microbiota has many important functions for maintaining the health of the host, such as the formation and maintenance of the intestinal barrier, through the production of short-chain fatty acids (SCFAs) resulting from the fermentation of undigested nutrients, immunostimulation, and immunotolerance, synthesis

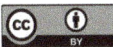

of substances, metabolic-trophic function, metabolism of drugs and toxins [6]. The balance between the intestinal microbiota and the host is maintained through various mechanisms, including the secretion of gastric acid, mucus, bile salts, and mucous Ig, mucosal pH, intestinal motility, local and systemic immunity, and interactions between different microbial species. An alteration in the microbiota-host relationship could potentially cause the onset of gastrointestinal or extra-intestinal diseases, defined as "intestinal microbiota related diseases". Among the most known, we remember allergic diseases, inflammatory bowel diseases, obesity, metabolic syndrome, type 1 and 2 diabetes, cardiovascular disease and even osteoporosis (OP) [1].

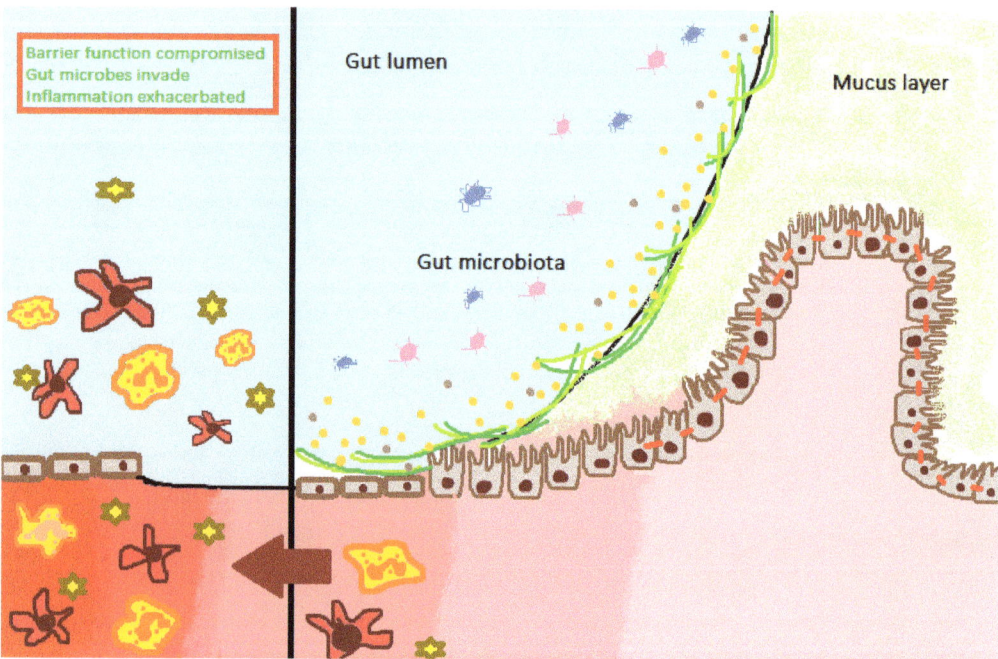

Figure 1. The human gastrointestinal tract is colonized by about 10^{13}–10^{14} microorganisms, of which 15,000 different bacterial strains are located mainly in the colon in a symbiotic relationship with the host. In normal conditions, the microbiota is characterized by the predominance of obligate anaerobic members of Firmicutes and Bacteriodetes phyla, which guarantee intestinal and general health, while the loss of homeostasis, dysbiosis, linked to the proliferation of some bacterial populations such as the Enterobacteriaceae or the absence of important commensal bacteria helps to create a more favorable environment for the growth of pathogens, predisposing the organism to pathological conditions.

2. Osteoporosis

OP is defined as a systemic and metabolic bone disease characterized by a decreased bone mass per unit of volume and a deterioration of the microstructure of the bone tissue, thus increasing the risk of fracture caused by bone fragility. OP is a female-dominated disease more common in postmenopausal women, with a male/female ratio of 1:6 [7,8]. In physiological conditions, there is a balance between osteogenesis, promoted by osteoblasts, and bone resorption by osteoclasts, regulated by a complex molecular mechanism in which estrogens, parathyroid hormone, vitamin D, and inflammatory cytokines are important factors [9–12]. Osteoblasts secrete the nuclear factor receptor activator ligand κB (RANKL), which interacts with the RANK receptor, a member of the tumor necrosis factor family expressed by osteoclasts and their precursors. The RANK/RANKL interaction, which promotes the differentiation and survival of osteoclasts, is controlled by the soluble decoy receptor Osteoprotegerin (OPG), a natural inhibitor of RANKL. The alteration of these mechanisms, therefore, leads to the prevalence of the RANK /RANKL interaction and to increased bone resorption with consequent OP [13–16]. It has been observed that the loss of estrogens, a condition typical of the postmenopausal state, increases the expression of proinflammatory cytokines, namely interleukin (IL)-1, IL-6, IL-7, IL-17 TNFα, Macrophage colony-stimulating factor (MCSF), and RANKL by osteoblasts, T cells and B cells. Among these cells, T helper lymphocytes (Th)17 are thought to play a particularly critical role in bone loss associated with estrogen deficiency while, regulatory T cells (Tregs) are capable of producing different cytokines, including Transforming Growth Factor (TGF) beta 1, IL-4 and IL-10, inhibiting bone resorption, and reducing the production of effector cytokines [17–22].

3. Microbiota and Osteoporosis

The microbiota can, through the regulation of mineral absorption of calcium, phosphorous, and magnesium and the production of incretins, serotonin, and gut-derived factors, influence the health of bone. Many studies have already shown that the intestinal microbiome is closely related to bone metabolism, the absorption of bone minerals in physiological conditions, and to the pathogenesis of OP [8,23–25].

In the studies carried out by Collins et al., it was observed that bone mass was higher in germ-free (GF) mice than in conventional mice; GF mice also had a reduced number of osteoclasts per bone surface and a reduced frequency of CD4+ T cells and osteoclast precursors in their bone marrow [23]. These results varied following colonization of the germ-free gut with a conventional microbiota, suggesting the beneficial action of probiotics in the prevention of OP [26].

Uchida et al. found that, comparing the primary osteoblasts isolated from alveolar bones and scalps of the GF mice and the osteoblasts isolated from the specific pathogen-free (SPF) mice, the last expressed substantially more osteocalcin, alkaline phosphatase (ALP), and insulin-like growth factor-I/II (IGF-I/IGF-II), with a decreased ratio of OPG/RANKL. In the end, the bone density of SPF mice was lower than GF mice, indicating that the gut microbiome has a greater regulatory impact on osteoclasts and bone density [27].

Another important study conducted by Jing-Jing Ni et al. about the valuation of the causal relationship between gut microbiota to bone mineral density (BMD) discovered that an increase in the *Clostridiales* class and in the *Lachnospiraceae* family was negatively correlated to BMD, demonstrating the causal relationship between microbiota and bone development [28].

Significant changes in the intestinal microbiota were observed in patients with OP. In fact, while in healthy controls, the composition of the intestinal microbiota was given by the maximum presence of *Bacteroides, Faecalibacterium,* and *Prevotella,* in OP patients, it was possible to observe a variation of the bacterial composition with an increase in the proportion of *Firmicutes* and a decrease in the proportion of *Bacteroidetes* than in healthy people [29].

The diet is therefore essential for the absorption of nutrients and for the composition of the microbiota; high consumption of fats is associated with a reduction in the Bacteriodetes/Firmicutes ratio and metabolic imbalances for the host, as found in patients with OP. On the contrary, a low-calorie diet removes harmful substances, leading to beneficial effects for the host [30,31]. An important role concerning the composition of the intestinal microbiota is played, also, by the use of antibiotics. Prolonged therapy can change the normal composition of the bacterial flora, altering its biological metabolism. This leads to impaired intestinal absorption, especially a deficiency of minerals important for bone health, thus contributing to the development of OP [32].

The link between the microbiota and BMD is now established; in particular, bacterial overgrowth has been associated with malabsorption and the consequent alteration in the metabolism of calcium, carbohydrates, vitamins B and K, essential elements for bone metabolism. Furthermore, a high concentration of probiotics *Lactobacillus reuteri* and *Bifidobacterium longum* facilitate the absorption of calcium, magnesium, and phosphorus, increasing BMD. Some species of Lactobacilli, intervening in the degradation of proteins present in milk, are the main ones responsible for the beneficial effects of milk found in bone health [33–35].

Alterations of the microbiota are able to lead to a dysfunction of the intestinal barrier with an increase in serum lipopolysaccharide (LPS) and consequent increase in intestinal permeability and osteoclasts survival [36,37].

Moreover, the intestinal microbiota is able to influence bone metabolism both directly, through the production of SCFAs, above all butyrate, and through the influence on metabolic hormones such as serotonin, an important factor in the development and maintenance of bone.

SCFAs play a very important role in bone formation and mineralization, acting on the osteoprotegerin pathway, suppressing the RANKL pathway, and influencing the glucagon-like peptide 1, involved in osteoblast-adipocyte differentiation of bone mesenchymal stem cells [38–43] (Figure 2).

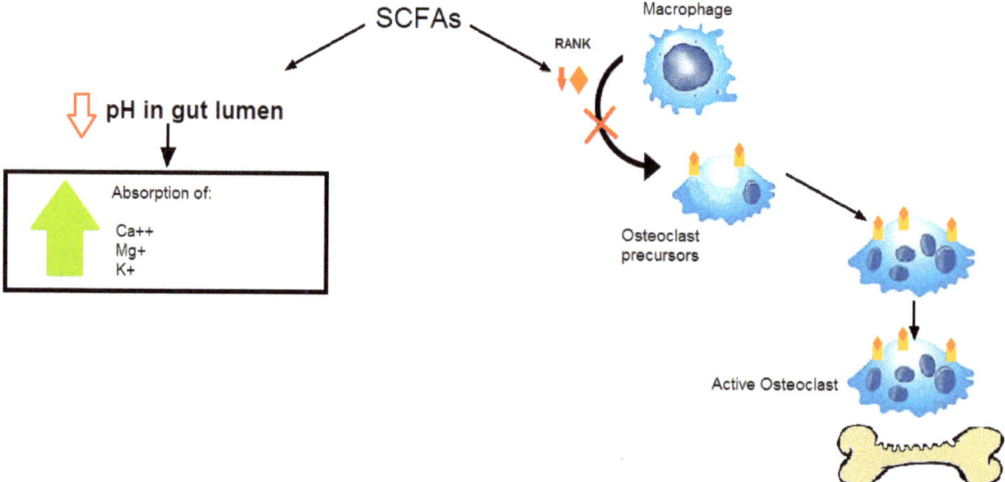

Figure 2. SCFAs play a very important role in bone formation and mineralization by acting on the osteoprotegerin pathway, reducing osteoclastogenesis by suppressing the RANKL pathway, and reducing the pH of the intestinal tract by subsequently increasing the absorption of minerals.

A mechanism underlying the changes in the gut microbiota in patients with OP has been hypothesized to involve the immune-inflammatory axis as a key bridge linking the intestinal microbiota to bone metabolism [44–48].

In particular, the microbiota can increase TNF-α, one of the activators of the RANK-RANKL pathway, which leads to increased bone resorption by altering bone homeostasis in mice [23].

Finally, the microbiota also appears to influence flavonoids and diethylstilbestrol, estrogens of intestinal origin, whose alteration influences bone homeostasis, being the estrogen deficiency directly involved in the risk of postmenopausal OP [49,50].

It is possible to hypothesize the modulation of the microbiota as a therapy limiting the progress of the OP in addition to conventional therapies. One of the strategies that can be used is the administration of probiotics, live microorganisms that restore intestinal permeability, improve the immune barrier function of the intestine, promote the production of IgA, and inhibit the release of proinflammatory cytokines. Several studies were conducted to evaluate the beneficial action of probiotics on the prevention of primary OP, highlighting complex bone protection mechanisms.

Particularly in vitro studies, *Lactobacillus reuteri* was able to inhibit the differentiation of osteoclasts from monocytic macrophages, releasing an anti-osteoclastogenic factor capable of modulating osteoclastogenesis [51]. Furthermore, a secreted component of *Lactobacillus reuteri* was sufficient to inhibit TNFα-induced suppression on pre-osteoblastic cells [52]. It has also been shown that *Lactobacillus reuteri* secretes histamine, capable of suppressing the production of TNFα by human monocytoid cells [53]. *Lactobacillus helveticus* and *Lactobacillus casei* have a direct effect on bone cells [54]. In particular, the addition of *Lactobacillus helveticus* fermented milk products to primary bone marrow cultures showed an increased calcium accumulation in osteoblast cultures, suggesting its role as an enhancer in osteoblast differentiation [55]. Both *Lactobacillus rhamnosus GG* (LGG) and the commercially available probiotic supplement reduce expression of TNFα, IL-17, and RANKL in cells isolated from the small intestine and bone marrow in mice who underwent ovariectomy [56].

The mechanisms by which probiotics act in human cells are very complex and not fully explored. The direct action of probiotics on osteoclasts must be considered limited in humans, while probably a key role is played in the intestine. Bacteria have been shown to be essential for the synthesis of numerous vitamins and enzymes required for matrix formation and bone growth, including Vitamin D, K, C, and folate. Furthermore, bacteria of the genus *Bifidobacteria* are capable of producing SCFA, which can reduce the pH of the intestinal tract by subsequently increasing the absorption of minerals. Some studies demonstrate that *Lactobacillus reuteri* is able to suppress the gene expression of proinflammatory and pro-osteoclastogenic cytokines, both in the intestine and in the bone marrow. Probiotic bacteria can directly increase calcium transport across the intestinal barrier by reducing intestinal inflammation [25,51,57–61].

The results showed that probiotic preparations prevent increased intestinal permeability caused by the depletion of sex steroids, thus limiting the production of osteoclasts. This serves as a proof of concept that the gut microbiome and probiotic preparations are involved in trabecular bone loss caused by sex steroid deficiency [8].

4. Allergy

Food allergy (FA) is an unexpected reaction resulting from an immunological alteration, in which a specific and reproducible immune response is triggered by the ingestion of food antigens normally tolerated by the population [62].

Although the prevalence rate of FA is variable in relation to age and geographical location, about 10% of the population is affected by FA, with a prevalence in childhood and in developing countries [63–65]. All foods can cause FA, but the most commonly involved are peanuts, cow's milk, hen's egg, tree nuts, fish, shellfish, wheat, seeds, and soy [66]. The essential process for avoiding the development of FA is oral tolerance. It derives from oral exposure to food antigens and is mediated by dendritic cells (DCs), able to stimulate the differentiation of naive T cells into positive forkhead box P3 (Foxp3) T cells that produce IL-10, leading to the inhibition of sensitization to specific food allergens. Proinflammatory cytokines produced by intestinal epithelial cells in association with pathogen-associated molecular patterns (PAMPs) or damage-associated molecular patterns (DAMPs) lead to the production of inflammatory cytokines that switch antigen-presenting cells into a proinflammatory phenotype, increasing Th2 cells, that drive the allergic response through the production of IL-4, the expansion of eosinophils and mast cells and the isotypic switch of B cells towards the production of IgE. The onset of FA is linked to the breakdown of oral tolerance. The first phase of sensitization, at the first contact with the antigen, leads to the production of specific IgEs, which are anchored to specific receptors on mast cells and basophils. At the second contact with the allergen, the cells are activated by the binding of the antigen to the IgEs, releasing various mediators including histamine, TNF-α, platelet activation factor (PAF), leukotrienes, IL-4, IL-5, IL-9, IL-13, IL-31, and IL-33, which lead to a range of symptoms from the skin to life-threatening one [67,68].

Increasing evidence suggests that the gut microbiome contributes to the pathophysiology of such inflammatory disorders [69–72]. In particular, dysbiosis is associated with the pathogenesis of food allergies (Table 1) [73–84].

Table 1. Association between the most frequent food allergy and microbiota.

Food Allergy	Associated Bacteria
Cow's milk	↓Clostridia, Firmicutes
Cow's milk, egg, peanut	↑Enterobacteriaceae ↓Bacteroidaceae
Peanut	↓Clostridiales ↑Bacteroidales
Egg white, cow's milk, wheat, peanut, soy bean	↓Bacteroidetes ↑Firmicutes

Bacteroidetes and Firmicutes makeup 90% of the microbiota and are involved in the pathogenesis of FA. The association with FA has been identified especially for *Clostridia* species, able to increase the production of Treg, with resulting inhibition of allergic inflammation and promotion of oral tolerance. *Bacteroides fragilis*, a species of Bacteroidetes, was also capable of producing polysaccharide A (PSA), which increased the suppressive capacity of Treg cells and the production of IL-10 by Foxp3 + T cells in a murine study. Several studies identify a lower abundance of bacterial class Clostridia, phylum Firmicutes, in children with food allergy compared to healthy children [3].

Fazlollahi M. et al. studied 141 children with egg allergy compared with healthy controls, highlighting a preponderance of Lachnospiraceae, Streptococcaceae, and Leuconostocaceae in the early gut microbiome of children with egg allergy. The association found between the presence of the families of *Lachnospiraceae* and *Ruminococcaceae* and egg sensitization has, therefore, led the authors to identify the early diversity of the microbiota in egg-sensitized children as a target for preventive or therapeutic interventions [81].

Intestinal microorganisms such as *Clostridium leptum*, *Eubacterium rectal*, and *Faecalibacterium prausnitzii*, are able to produce SCFA, whose fermentation produces butyrate, propionate, acetate, and valerate with a higher concentration in the colon. SCFAs have direct immune-modulatory effects and are a key factor in promoting immunological tolerance towards harmless antigens and preventing inflammation (Figure 3).

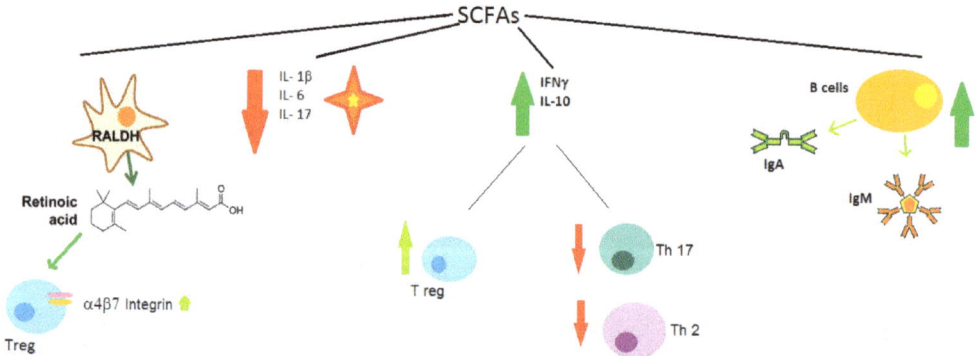

Figure 3. SCFAs effects in immunological tolerance: induce gut dendritic cells (DC) to express retinal aldehyde dehydrogenase (RALDH), with result in the production of retinoic acid that upregulates expression of the gut-homing integrins α4β7 on peripheral regulatory T cells (Treg); promote immune tolerance, regulate the antibody response through the production of IgA and IgM; stimulate the production of anti-inflammatory mediators such as IFNγ and IL-10, which induce the expansion of Treg cells and the suppression of proinflammatory T helper 17 (Th17) and Th2 cells; reduce the production of proinflammatory cytokines including IL-1β, IL-6, and IL-17.

In addition to the production of SCFA, intestinal bacteria also produce polyamines (PA) (spermidine, spermine, putrescine, cadaverine) essential for maintaining the intestinal barrier function through upregulation of junctional proteins.

The rise of food allergy in modern society has led to the postulation of the hygiene hypothesis, according to which lack of early childhood exposure to infectious agents suppresses the development of the immune system with the rise of atopic diseases. Recent work has revisited the hygiene hypothesis model to include mode of delivery, antibiotic intake, diet, and synthetic chemicals as factors in altering gut microbiota [3]. After the introduction of the complementary diet, the composition of the microbiota varies according to the diet applied with evident compositional differences between a diet rich in fiber, characterized by *Alistipes*, *Bilophila*, and *Bacteroides*, and higher abundance of *Roseburia*, *Ruminococcus*, and *Eubacterium*, and diet rich in fat. In general, *Lactobacillus*, *Clostridium*, *Ruminococcus*, *Peptostreptococcus*, and *Bacteroides* are species that, through the catabolization of tryptophan, are able to regulate the immune response and the proliferation of T lymphocytes with consequent induction of the expression of the IL-10 receptor-1 (IL-10R1) and inhibition of proinflammatory cytokines [85]. In this context, it is clear that a diet that is higher in fat but low in fiber, like the Western one, maybe the cause of the increased prevalence of FA in Western countries [86].

About that, Mckenzie et al. have described the "nutrition-gut microbiome-physiology axis", an essential link between diet, gut microbiota, and allergic diseases. It was also shown that food diversity was associated with greater expression of Foxp3, suggesting a protective effect of a diversified diet against the development of FA. On the contrary, reduced Foxp3 expression was present in children with a less diversified diet [1].

Data supporting the ability of the microbiota to influence allergic sensitization was found in mice treated with antibiotics and GF, which developed greater allergic sensitization than controls. In particular, Jiménez-Saiz R et al. demonstrated that eosinophil-deficient GF mice had intestinal fibrosis and were less prone to allergic sensitization than GF controls, establishing the role of the microbiota in regulating the frequency and activation of eosinophils in the intestinal mucosa [87].

More commonly, Clostridiales and Lactobacillales appear to have beneficial effects on food tolerance, while Bacteroidales and Enterobacteriales have ambivalent effects. In particular, children with AD and FA had a microbiota more colonized by *Escherichia coli* and *Bifidobacterium pseudocatenulatum* and less by *Bifidobacterium adolescentis*, *Akkermansia muciniphila*, *Bifidobacterium breve*, and *Faecalibacterium prausnitzii* compared to children with AD without FA. The authors, therefore, established an association, also in this case, between early colonization with potentially more pathogenic bacteria, such as *Clostridium difficile* or *Stafilococcus aureus*, and the development of FA, and *vice-versa* colonization with more beneficial bacteria such as *Bifidobacteria* and food tolerance [1]. In particular, studies in the literature have revealed the desensitizing effects of *Lactobacillus rhamnosus* GG in cow's milk and in peanut allergy [3,88,89].

The World Allergy Organization (WAO), regarding probiotic supplementation, concluded that there was weak evidence to support their action in reducing the risk of developing allergic disorders in pediatric patients but that nevertheless, a small reduction in risk could be connected [90].

5. Discussion

The alteration of the microbiota appears to be a common ground for both OP and FA. In particular, an altered intestinal barrier can be considered common damage to both diseases. The intestinal barrier is defined as a functional unit that constantly balances the antigenic charge of the intestinal lumen with a complex immunological and non-immunological organization of the intestinal mucosa. It performs two fundamental functions for the survival of the individual: allow the absorption of nutrients and defend the body from the penetration of harmful macromolecules mediated by the tight junctions of the apical epithelial cells. It has recently been observed that tight junctions are regulated in their functioning by cytokines produced in the intestine and can be altered by various factors, including alcohol consumption, dietary imbalances, and the action of bacterial toxins [91]. Alteration of the intestinal barrier and the gut microbiota cause the development of an important inflammatory substrate in the intestine, which leads to FA and the loss of estrogen typical of primary OP. A study by Li et al. found that depletion of hormones increases inflammation in the intestine through a greater antigenic load that crosses the intestinal barrier [22]. Estrogens seem to have an ambivalent role in promoting the development of allergic diseases and the degranulation of mast cells in association with exposure to allergens. Andrè et al. also found involvement of the use of oral contraceptives in the etiology of urticaria and chronic angioneurotic edema [91].

The intestinal microbiota is also able to influence the estrogens circulating level through the secretion of β-glucuronidase, an enzyme that activates them. The integrity of the intestinal barrier, normally preserved by the presence of four phyla, Bacteriodetes, Firmicutes, Actinobacteria, and Proteobacteria, is altered by dysbiosis, in which the reduction in cell-cell junctions increases intestinal permeability, resulting in bacterial translocation inducing a systemic inflammatory state at the basis of various pathological processes. Furthermore, it is important to underline that dysbiosis leads to a reduced deconjugation of estrogens with a reduction in their circulation, leading to the activation of CD4 + T cells. CD4 + T cells produce RANKL, OPG, and TNF-α, promoting osteoclast activation and bone absorption through the OPG- RANK-RANKL signal transduction pathway.

There is evidence that the inflammatory process is at the basis of both OP and FA. Several proinflammatory and anti-inflammatory mediators are involved in the immunopathogenesis of FA, in which allergens can stimulate Th1, Th2, and Th17 cytokines in a heterogeneous way. Kara et al. [92] have hypothesized the monitoring of cytokines such as TNF-α and IL-6 in the follow-up of patients with FA, while Nadelkopoulou et al. [93] have investigated the role of IL-10 in the treatment of FA. TNF-a and IL-1 are also the main cytokines involved in bone metabolism and bone loss related to estrogen deficiency. The role of IL-33 is being debated [94], its activity contributing to the development of various allergological conditions through its action on mast cells, eosinophils, Th2 cells, Tregs, natural killers, basophils, dendritic cells, and activated macrophages, but at the same time appears to have a protective role on bone by inhibiting RANKL-dependent osteoclastogenesis [91–99].

Bone health is highly dependent on diet and nutritional style that determines the type of microbiota in host organisms. The intestinal microbiome, in fact, contributes to the production of proteins and enzymes related to digestion and energy metabolism since it ferments undigested nutrients transforming them into SCFA, leading to a decrease in intestinal permeability and greater absorption of minerals such as calcium. There are several factors linked to the microbiota that unite OP and FA; in particular, a key role is played by SCAF with immunomodulatory and anti-inflammatory effects, exercised through the promotion of immune tolerance, the production of IgA and IgM, the reduction in the production of proinflammatory cytokines including IL-1β, IL-6, and IL-17 [41], and the production of anti-inflammatory IFNγ and IL-10 with consequent expansion of Treg cells and suppression of proinflammatory Th17 and Th2 cells.

The strong influence of the diet on the microbiota and consequently on the OP and allergic manifestations has led to evaluate the fundamental role of nutrition. In fact, a diet rich in fat can reduce the absorption of essential elements for bone health, including vitamin D, K, C, and folate. Moreover, the high-fat diet of Western countries is one of the factors that can contribute to the increased prevalence of allergies in Western countries [100].

Diet-induced obesity has been demonstrated to be a factor of increased susceptibility for FA, and in particular, the microbiota associated with the high-fat diet was found to be able to increase the propensity for FA as evidence of the connection between diet-microbiota and FA [101]. It has been reported that heat-killed lactic acid bacteria (LAB) increased the percentage of peripheral CD4 + CD25 + Foxp3 + Treg cells and relieve symptoms in the pollen season when administered to patients with mild Japanese cedar pollinosis. Although not through the microbiota, LAB is thought to act directly on the immune system. In particular, increased Treg, along with SCFA, is considered a promising target for improving both allergies and bone metabolic balance [102]. Roduit et al. analyzed the levels of SCFA in fecal samples of 301 children at the age of 1, reporting that children with the highest levels of butyrate and propionate were less likely to suffer from asthma by the age of 3 and 6 years and showed significantly lower allergic sensitization with a decrease in food allergy risks and allergic rhinitis diagnosis. More recently, Cait et al. examined the role of bacterial butyrate production in the gut during early childhood in the development of atopic disease and concluded that the lack of genes encoding key enzymes for both the breakdown of carbohydrates and the production of butyrate was the basis of allergic sensitization [1].

Although OP and allergies are two conditions with a high prevalence in the general population and the relationship between fracture risk and allergic diseases such as asthma, atopic dermatitis, urticaria, FA is now well established, to date, we do not yet have adequate epidemiological studies on the prevalence of allergies in patients with OP [103–109]. This probably partially depends on the recent recognition of their interrelationship other than the difficulty in including all together so many "allergic" pathologies with such different peculiarities. The currently available data in the literature refer to single pathologies and limited series. Furthermore, the available studies evaluate the presence of OP in allergic diseases and not the prevalence of allergies in patients with OP. Even in recent studies conducted to evaluate the prevalence of comorbidities in subjects with OP, no data relating to allergies emerge [110], probably because there is still not enough awareness of the influence of allergic disease on bone health. Furthermore, the retrospective analysis conducted in Italy on 64.852 subjects at high risk for fracture collected between 2016 and 2020, through the DeFRAcalc79, does not take into account allergic diseases among the variables for calculating the risk of OP [111].

Vitamin D plays an important role in the pathogenesis of OP and also in the regulation of intestinal tight junctions, leading to the hypothesis that its deficiency may compromise the integrity of the barrier or induce alterations in the composition of the intestinal microbiota, increasing the risk of FA and of OP. Vitamin D, in fact, is important in the maintenance of bone health through the regulation of serum calcium homeostasis. The lack of vitamin D increases bone resorption in order to maintain the right serum calcium levels, making up for the lack of calcium reabsorbed by the gut induced by vitamin D deficiency [112].

Sardecka-Milewska et al. found that children with cow's milk allergy have lower serum concentrations of vitamin D than healthy children [113]. The role of vitamin D in the development of FA is further confirmed by Koplin et al., who documented an attenuated association between low serum levels of vitamin D and food allergy only in subjects with polymorphisms associated with lower levels of vitamin D-binding protein. This involvement of vitamin D in FA could be linked to the ability of vitamin D to induce the expression of IL-10 by Treg cells, leading to oral tolerance and its maintenance [114,115].

Finally, it is also essential to remember the relationships between microbiota and microRNA (miRNA). The latter are small non-coding RNAs capable of regulating gene expression. The importance of the role of miRNAs in many pathological conditions [116–118], including allergies [119] and OP [120,121], is emerging. Being able to fully understand the relationship between miRNA and microbiota could allow to have new disease markers and pave the way for new targeted and personalized therapeutic strategies [122].

The importance of the unaltered microbiota is underlined by the fact that the growing tendency to use antibiotics leads to impaired intestinal absorption with a deficiency of minerals important for bone health, thus contributing to the development of OP, on the other hand, the use of antibiotics compromises the development of oral tolerance mechanisms leading to increased development of FA.

On this basis is founded the use of prebiotics and probiotics for beneficial modulation of the intestinal microbiota both in OP and in allergological pathologies. For example, it has been shown that LGG is able to reduce the expression of TNFα, IL-17, and RANKL in cells isolated from the small intestine and bone marrow of mice, decreasing bone resorption, and also have desensitizing effects in cow's milk and peanut allergy [45,88]. The data in this review based on the current literature highlight how the microbiota and some bacterial species can influence the propensity to develop diseases, including allergies and OP. In particular, the supplementation of beneficial bacteria and diet corrections seems to improve the outcome and prevent the onset of these diseases.

6. Conclusions

Although further studies are needed on the topic, current evidence shows the driving role of the microbiota and its modulation on both bone remodeling and allergic sensitization processes. The full understanding of the existing interplay between microbiota, bone metabolism, and allergies can design new pathophysiological scenarios and open new and stimulating horizons for preventive and therapeutic strategies.

Author Contributions: All authors contributed equally to this work. All authors have read and agreed to the published version of the manuscript.

Funding: This research received no external funding.

Institutional Review Board Statement: Not applicable.

Informed Consent Statement: Not applicable.

Data Availability Statement: Not applicable.

Conflicts of Interest: The authors declare no conflict of interest.

References

1. Nance, C.L.; Deniskin, R.; Diaz, V.C.; Paul, M.; Anvari, S.; Anagnostou, A. The Role of the Microbiome in Food Allergy: A Review. *Children* **2020**, *7*, 50. [CrossRef]
2. Yoo, J.Y.; Groer, M.; Dutra, S.V.O.; Sarkar, A.; McSkimming, D.I. Gut Microbiota and Immune System Interactions. *Microorganisms* **2020**, *8*, 1587. [CrossRef] [PubMed]
3. Lee, K.H.; Song, Y.; Wu, W.; Yu, K.; Zhang, G. The gut microbiota, environmental factors, and links to the development of food allergy. *Clin. Mol. Allergy* **2020**, *18*, 5. [CrossRef] [PubMed]
4. Kim, S.; Jazwinski, S.M. The Gut Microbiota and Healthy Aging: A Mini-Review. *Gerontology* **2018**, *64*, 513–520. [CrossRef] [PubMed]
5. Miqdady, M.; Al Mistarihi, J.; Azaz, A.; Rawat, D. Prebiotics in the Infant Microbiome: The Past, Present, and Future. *Pediatr. Gastroenterol. Hepatol. Nutr.* **2020**, *23*, 1–14. [CrossRef] [PubMed]
6. Kreft, L.; Hoffmann, C.; Ohnmacht, C. Therapeutic Potential of the Intestinal Microbiota for Immunomodulation of Food Allergies. *Front. Immunol.* **2020**, *11*, 1853. [CrossRef] [PubMed]
7. Watts, N.B.; Bilezikian, J.P.; Camacho, P.M.; Greenspan, S.L.; Harris, S.T.; Hodgson, S.F.; Kleerekoper, M.; Luckey, M.M.; McClung, M.R.; Pollack, R.P.; et al. American Association of Clinical Endocrinologists Medical Guidelines for Clinical Practice for the diagnosis and treatment of postmenopausal osteoporosis. *Endocr. Pract.* **2010**, *16*, 1–37. [CrossRef] [PubMed]
8. Li, S.; Mao, Y.; Zhou, F.; Yang, H.; Shi, Q.; Meng, B. Gut microbiome and osteoporosis: A review. *Bone Jt. Res.* **2020**, *9*, 524–530. [CrossRef] [PubMed]
9. Irelli, A.; Sirufo, M.M.; Scipioni, T.; De Pietro, F.; Pancotti, A.; Ginaldi, L.; De Martinis, M. mTOR Links Tumor Immunity and Bone Metabolism: What are the Clinical Implications? *Int. J. Mol. Sci.* **2019**, *20*, 5841. [CrossRef]
10. De Martinis, M.; Sirufo, M.M.; Ginaldi, L. Osteoporosis: Current and Emerging Therapies Targeted to Immunological Checkpoints. *Curr. Med. Chem.* **2020**, *27*, 6356–6372. [CrossRef]
11. De Martinis, M.; Sirufo, M.M.; Polsinelli, M.; Placidi, G.; Di Silvestre, D.; Ginaldi, L. Gender Differences in Osteoporosis: A Single-Center Observational Study. *World J. Men's Health* **2021**, *39*, 750–759. [CrossRef] [PubMed]
12. Sirufo, M.M.; Ginaldi, L.; De Martinis, M. Bone Health Risks Associated with Finasteride and Dutasteride Long-Term Use. *World J. Men's Health* **2021**, *39*, 389–390. [CrossRef] [PubMed]
13. Hofbauer, L.C.; Khosla, S.; Dunstan, C.R.; Lacey, D.L.; Boyle, W.J.; Riggs, B.L. The roles of osteoprotegerin and osteoprotegerin ligand in the paracrine regulation of bone resorption. *J. Bone Miner. Res.* **2000**, *15*, 2–12. [CrossRef]
14. Hofbauer, L.C.; Khosla, S.; Dunstan, C.R.; Lacey, D.L.; Spelsberg, T.C.; Riggs, B.L. Estrogen stimulates gene expression and protein production of osteoprotegerin in human osteoblastic cells. *Endocrinology* **1999**, *140*, 4367–4370. [CrossRef]
15. Lochlin, R.M.; Khosla, S.; Turner, R.T.; Riggs, B.L. Mediators of the bisphasic responses of bone to intermittent and continuously administered parathyroid hormone. *J. Cell. Biochem.* **2003**, *89*, 180–190. [CrossRef] [PubMed]
16. Hofbauer, L.C.; Gori, F.; Riggs, B.L.; Lacey, D.L.; Dunstan, C.R.; Spelsberg, T.C.; Khosla, S. Stimulation of osteoprotegerin ligand and inhibition of osteoprotegerin production by glucocorticoids in human osteoblastic lineage cells. *Endocrinology* **1999**, *140*, 4382–4389. [CrossRef]
17. Pfeilschifter, J.; Köditz, R.; Pfohl, M.; Schatz, H. Changes in proinflammatory cytokine activity after menopause. *Endocr. Rev.* **2002**, *23*, 90–119. [CrossRef]

18. Bismar, H.; Diel, I.; Ziegler, R.; Pfeilschifter, J. Increased cytokine secretion by human bone marrow cells after menopause or discontinuation of estrogen replacement. *J. Clin. Endocrinol. Metab.* **1995**, *80*, 3351–3355.
19. D'Amelio, P.; Grimaldi, A.; Di Bella, S.; Brianza, S.Z.M.; Cristofaro, M.A.; Tamone, C.; Giribaldi, G.; Ulliers, D.; Pescarmona, G.P.; Isaia, G. Estrogen deficiency increases osteoclastogenesis up-regulating T cells activity: A key mechanism in osteoporosis. *Bone* **2008**, *43*, 92–100. [CrossRef]
20. Weitzmann, M.N.; Roggia, C.; Toraldo, G.; Weitzmann, L.; Pacifici, R. Increased production of IL-7 uncouples bone formation from bone resorption during estrogen deficiency. *J. Clin. Investig.* **2002**, *110*, 1643–1650. [CrossRef]
21. Eghbali-Fatourechi, G.; Khosla, S.; Sanyal, A.; Boyle, W.J.; Lacey, D.L.; Riggs, B.L. Role of RANK ligand in mediating increased bone resorption in early postmenopausal women. *J. Clin. Investig.* **2003**, *111*, 1221–1230. [CrossRef] [PubMed]
22. Li, J.Y.; Tawfeek, H.; Bedi, B.; Yang, X.; Adams, J.; Gao, K.Y.; Zayzafoon, M.; Weitzmann, M.N.; Pacifici, R. Ovariectomy disregulates osteoblast and osteoclast formation through the T-cell receptor CD40 ligand. *Proc. Natl. Acad. Sci. USA* **2011**, *108*, 768–773. [CrossRef]
23. Sjögren, K.; Engdahl, C.; Henning, P.; Lerner, U.H.; Tremaroli, V.; Lagerquist, M.K.; Bäckhed, F.; Ohlsson, C. The gut microbiota regulates bone mass in mice. *J. Bone Miner. Res.* **2012**, *27*, 1357–1367. [CrossRef] [PubMed]
24. Li, J.Y.; Chassaing, B.; Tyagi, A.M.; Vaccaro, C.; Luo, T.; Adams, J.; Darby, T.M.; Weitzmann, M.N.; Mulle, J.G.; Gewirtz, A.T.; et al. Sex steroid deficiency-associated bone loss is microbiota dependent and prevented by probiotics. *J. Clin. Investig.* **2016**, *126*, 2049–2063. [CrossRef] [PubMed]
25. Hernandez, C.J.; Moeller, A.H. The microbiome: A heritable contributor to bone morphology? *Semin. Cell Dev. Biol.* **2021**. [CrossRef]
26. Collins, F.L.; Rios-Arce, N.D.; Schepper, J.D.; Parameswaran, N.; McCabe, L.R. The Potential of Probiotics as a Therapy for Osteoporosis. *Microbiol. Spectr.* **2017**, *5*. [CrossRef]
27. Uchida, Y.; Irie, K.; Fukuhara, D.; Kataoka, K.; Hattori, T.; Ono, M.; Ekuni, D.; Kubota, S.; Morita, M. Commensal Microbiota Enhance Both Osteoclast and Osteoblast Activities. *Molecules* **2018**, *23*, 1517. [CrossRef]
28. Ni, J.; Yang, X.; Zhang, H.; Xu, Q.; Wei, X.; Feng, G.; Zhao, M.; Pei, Y.; Zhang, L. Assessing causal relationship from gut microbiota to heel bone mineral density. *Bone* **2020**, *143*, 115652. [CrossRef]
29. Wang, J.; Wang, Y.; Gao, W.; Wang, B.; Zhao, H.; Zeng, Y.; Ji, Y.; Hao, D. Diversity analysis of gut microbiota in osteoporosis and osteopenia patients. *PeerJ* **2017**, *5*, e3450. [CrossRef]
30. Vaughn, A.C.; Cooper, E.M.; DiLorenzo, P.M.; O'Loughlin, L.J.; Konkel, M.E.; Peters, J.H.; Hajnal, A.; Sen, T.; Lee, S.H.; de La Serre, C.B.; et al. Energy-dense diet triggers changes in gut microbiota, reorganization of gut brain vagal communication and increases body fat accumulation. *Acta Neurobiol. Exp.* **2017**, *77*, 18–30. [CrossRef]
31. Rowland, I.; Gibson, G.; Heinken, A.; Scott, K.; Swann, J.; Thiele, I.; Tuohy, K. Gut microbiota functions: Metabolism of nutrients and other food components. *Eur. J. Nutr.* **2018**, *57*, 1–24. [CrossRef] [PubMed]
32. Cox, L.M.; Yamanishi, S.; Sohn, J.; Alekseyenko, A.V.; Leung, J.M.; Cho, I.; Kim, S.G.; Li, H.; Gao, Z.; Mahana, D.; et al. Altering the intestinal microbiota during a critical developmental window has lasting metabolic consequences. *Cell* **2014**, *158*, 705–721. [CrossRef] [PubMed]
33. Saltzman, J.R.; Russell, R.M. The aging gut: Nutritional issues. *Gastroenterol. Clin. N. Am.* **1998**, *27*, 309–324. [CrossRef]
34. Quigley, E.M. Gut bacteria in health and disease. *Gastroenterol. Hepatol.* **2013**, *9*, 560–569.
35. Mohanty, D.P.; Mohapatra, S.; Misra, S.; Sahu, P.S. Milk derived bioactive peptides and their impact on human health: A review. *Saudi J. Biol. Sci.* **2016**, *23*, 577–583. [CrossRef]
36. Hou, G.Q.; Guo, C.; Song, G.H.; Fang, N.; Fan, W.J.; Chen, X.D.; Yuan, L.; Wang, Z.Q. Lipopolysaccharide (LPS) promotes osteoclast differentiation and activation by enhancing the MAPK pathway and COX-2 expression in RAW264.7 cells. *Int. J. Mol. Med.* **2013**, *32*, 503–510. [CrossRef]
37. Itoh, K.; Udagawa, N.; Kobayashi, K.; Suda, K.; Li, X.; Takami, M.; Okahashi, N.; Nishihara, T.; Takahashi, N. Lipopolysaccharide promotes the survival of osteoclasts via Toll-like receptor 4, but cytokine production of osteoclasts in response to lipopolysaccharide is different from that of macrophages. *J. Immunol.* **2003**, *170*, 3688–3695. [CrossRef]
38. Weaver, C.M.; Diet, W.C.M. Diet, gut microbiome, and bone health. *Curr. Osteoporos. Rep.* **2015**, *13*, 125–130. [CrossRef]
39. Abrams, S.A.; Griffin, I.J.; Hawthorne, K.M.; Liang, L.; Gunn, S.K.; Darlington, G.; Ellis, K.J. A combination of prebiotic short- and long-chain inulin-type fructans enhances calcium absorption and bone mineralization in young adolescents. *Am. J. Clin. Nutr.* **2005**, *82*, 471–476. [CrossRef]
40. Yadav, V.K.; Balaji, S.; Suresh, P.S.; Liu, X.S.; Lu, X.; Li, Z.; Guo, X.E.; Mann, J.J.; Balapure, A.K.; Gershon, M.D.; et al. Pharmacological inhibition of gut-derived serotonin synthesis is a potential bone anabolic treatment for osteoporosis. *Nat. Med.* **2010**, *16*, 308–312. [CrossRef]
41. Lee, H.W.; Suh, J.H.; Kim, A.Y.; Lee, Y.S.; Park, S.Y.; Kim, J.B. Histone deacetylase 1-mediated histone modification regulates osteoblast differentiation. *Mol. Endocrinol.* **2006**, *20*, 2432–2443. [CrossRef]
42. Katono, T.; Kawato, T.; Tanabe, N.; Suzuki, N.; Iida, T.; Morozumi, A.; Ochiai, K.; Maeno, M. Sodium butyrate stimulates mineralized nodule formation and osteoprotegerin expression by human osteoblasts. *Arch. Oral Biol.* **2008**, *53*, 903–909. [CrossRef] [PubMed]

43. Rahman, M.M.; Kukita, A.; Kukita, T.; Shobuike, T.; Nakamura, T.; Kohashi, O. Two histone deacetylase inhibitors, trichostatin A and sodium butyrate, suppress differentiation into osteoclasts but not into macrophages. *Blood* **2003**, *101*, 3451–3459. [CrossRef] [PubMed]
44. Bindels, L.B.; Delzenne, N.M.; Cani, P.D.; Walter, J. Towards a more comprehensive concept for prebiotics. *Nat. Rev. Gastroenterol. Hepatol.* **2015**, *12*, 303–310. [CrossRef] [PubMed]
45. Lu, Y.C.; Lin, Y.C.; Lin, Y.K.; Liu, Y.J.; Chang, K.H.; Chieng, P.U.; Chan, W.P. Prevalence of osteoporosis and low bone mass in older chinese population based on bone mineral density at multiple skeletal sites. *Sci. Rep.* **2016**, *6*, 25206. [CrossRef]
46. Scholz-Ahrens, K.E.; Ade, P.; Marten, B.; Weber, P.; Timm, W.; Acil, Y.; Gluer, C.C.; Schrezenmeir, J. Prebiotics, probiotics, and synbiotics affect mineral absorption, bone mineral content, and bone structure. *J. Nutr.* **2007**, *137*, 838s–846s. [CrossRef]
47. Ohlsson, C.; Engdahl, C.; Fak, F.; Andersson, A.; Windahl, S.H.; Farman, H.H.; Moverare-Skrtic, S.; Islander, U.; Sjogren, K. Probiotics protect mice from ovariectomy-induced cortical bone loss. *PLoS ONE* **2014**, *9*, e92368. [CrossRef]
48. Yan, J.; Herzog, J.W.; Tsang, K.; Brennan, C.A.; Bower, M.A.; Garrett, W.S.; Sartor, B.R.; Aliprantis, A.O.; Charles, J.F. Gut microbiota induce IGF-1 and promote bone formation and growth. *Proc. Natl. Acad. Sci. USA* **2016**, *113*, E7554–E7563. [CrossRef]
49. Chiang, S.S.; Pan, T.M. Beneficial effects of phytoestrogens and their metabolites produced by intestinal microflora on bone health. *Appl. Microbiol. Biotechnol.* **2013**, *97*, 1489–1500. [CrossRef]
50. Flores, R.; Shi, J.; Fuhrman, B.; Xu, X.; Veenstra, T.D.; Gail, M.H.; Gajer, P.; Ravel, J.; Goedert, J.J. Fecal microbial determinants of fecal and systemic estrogens and estrogen metabolites: A cross-sectional study. *J. Transl. Med.* **2012**, *10*, 253. [CrossRef]
51. Britton, R.A.; Irwin, R.; Quach, D.; Schaefer, L.; Zhang, J.; Lee, T.; Parameswaran, N.; McCabe, L.R. Probiotic *L. reuteri* treatment prevents bone loss in a menopausal ovariectomized mouse model. *J. Cell. Physiol.* **2014**, *229*, 1822–1830. [CrossRef] [PubMed]
52. Zhang, J.; Motyl, K.J.; Irwin, R.; MacDougald, O.A.; Britton, R.A.; McCabe, L.R. Loss of bone and Wnt10b expression in male type 1 diabetic mice is blocked by the probiotic *L. reuteri*. *Endocrinology* **2015**, *156*, 3169–3182. [CrossRef] [PubMed]
53. Thomas, C.M.; Hong, T.; Van Pijkeren, J.P.; Hemarajata, P.; Trinh, D.V.; Hu, W.; Britton, R.A.; Kalkum, M.; Versalovic, J. Histamine derived from probiotic Lactobacillus reuteri suppresses TNF via modulation of PKA and ERK signaling. *PLoS ONE* **2012**, *7*, e31951. [CrossRef] [PubMed]
54. Kim, J.G.; Lee, E.; Kim, S.H.; Whang, K.Y.; Oh, S.; Imm, J.Y. Effects of a *Lactobacillus casei* 393 fermented milk product on bone metabolism in ovariectomised rats. *Int. Dairy J.* **2009**, *19*, 690–695. [CrossRef]
55. Narva, M.; Halleen, J.; Väänänen, K.; Korpela, R. Effects of *Lactobacillus helveticus* fermented milk on bone cells in vitro. *Life Sci.* **2004**, *75*, 1727–1734. [CrossRef]
56. Caballero-Franco, C.; Keller, K.; Simone, C.; Chadee, K. The VSL # 3 probiotic formula induces mucin gene expression and secretion in colonic epithelial cells. *Am. J. Physiol. Gastrointest. Liver Physiol.* **2007**, *292*, 315–322.
57. Crittenden, R.G.; Martinez, N.R.; Playne, M.J. Synthesis and utilisation of folate by yoghurt starter cultures and probiotic bacteria. *Int. J. Food Microbiol.* **2003**, *80*, 217–222. [CrossRef]
58. Arunachalam, K.D. Role of bifidobacteria in nutrition, medicine and technology. *Nutr. Res.* **1999**, *19*, 1559–1597. [CrossRef]
59. Campbell, J.M.; Fahey, G.C.; Wolf, B.W. Selected indigestible oligosaccharides affect large bowel mass, cecal and fecal short-chain fatty acids, pH and microflora in rats. *J. Nutr.* **1997**, *127*, 130–136. [CrossRef]
60. McCabe, L.R.; Irwin, R.; Schaefer, L.; Britton, R.A. Probiotic use decreases intestinal inflammation and increases bone density in healthy male but not female mice. *J. Cell. Physiol.* **2013**, *228*, 1793–1798. [CrossRef]
61. Collins, F.L.; Irwin, R.; Bierhalter, H.; Schepper, J.; Britton, R.A.; Parameswaran, N.; McCabe, L.R. *Lactobacillus reuteri* 6475 Increases Bone Density in Intact Females Only under an Inflammatory Setting. *PLoS ONE* **2016**, *11*, e0153180. [CrossRef]
62. Bernstein, J.A.; Bernstein, I.L.; Bucchini, L.; Goldman, L.R.; Hamilton, R.G.; Lehrer, S.; Rubin, C.; Sampson, H.A. Clinical and laboratory investigation of allergy to genetically modified foods. *Environ. Health Perspect.* **2003**, *111*, 1114–1121. [CrossRef] [PubMed]
63. De Martinis, M.; Sirufo, M.M.; Viscido, A.; Ginaldi, L. Food Allergies and Ageing. *Int. J. Mol. Sci.* **2019**, *20*, 5580. [CrossRef] [PubMed]
64. De Martinis, M.; Sirufo, M.M.; Viscido, A.; Ginaldi, L. Food Allergy Insights: A Changing Landscape. *Arch. Immunol. Ther. Exp.* **2020**, *68*, 8. [CrossRef] [PubMed]
65. De Martinis, M.; Sirufo, M.M.; Ginaldi, L. Allergy and Aging: An Old/New Emerging Health Issue. *Aging Dis.* **2017**, *8*, 162–175. [CrossRef] [PubMed]
66. Sicherer, S.H.; Sampson, H.A. Food allergy: Epidemiology, pathogenesis, diagnosis, and treatment. *J. Allergy Clin. Immunol.* **2014**, *133*, 291–307. [CrossRef] [PubMed]
67. De Martinis, M.; Sirufo, M.M.; Suppa, M.; Ginaldi, L. New Perspectives in Food Allergy. *Int. J. Mol. Sci.* **2020**, *21*, 1474. [CrossRef] [PubMed]
68. Sirufo, M.M.; De Pietro, F.; Bassino, E.M.; Ginaldi, L.; De Martinis, M. Osteoporosis in Skin Diseases. *Int. J. Mol. Sci.* **2020**, *21*, 4749. [CrossRef] [PubMed]
69. Muir, A.B.; Benitez, A.J.; Dods, K.; Spergel, J.M.; Fillon, S.A. Microbiome and its impact on gastrointestinal atopy. *Allergy* **2016**, *71*, 1256–1263. [CrossRef] [PubMed]
70. Aitoro, R.; Paparo, L.; Amoroso, A.; Di Costanzo, M.; Cosenza, L.; Granata, V.; Di Scala, C.; Nocerino, R.; Trinchese, G.; Montella, M.; et al. Gut microbiota as a target for preventive and therapeutic intervention against food allergy. *Nutrients* **2017**, *9*, 672. [CrossRef]

71. West, C.E.; Renz, H.; Jenmalm, M.C.; Kozyrskyj, A.L.; Allen, K.; Vuillermin, P.; Prescott, S.L.; MacKay, C.; Salminen, S.; Wong, G.; et al. The gut microbiota and inflammatory noncommunicable diseases: Associations and potentials for gut microbiota therapies. *J. Allergy Clin. Immunol.* **2015**, *135*, 3–13. [CrossRef]
72. Kalliomäki, M.; Kirjavainen, P.; Eerola, E.; Kero, P.; Salminen, S.; Isolauri, E. Distinct patterns of neonatal gut microflora in infants in whom atopy was and was not developing. *J. Allergy Clin. Immunol.* **2001**, *107*, 129–134. [CrossRef]
73. Bunyavanich, S.; Shen, N.; Grishin, A.; Wood, R.; Burks, W.; Dawson, P.; Jones, S.M.; Leung, D.Y.M.; Sampson, H.; Sicherer, S.; et al. Early-life gut microbiome composition and milk allergy resolution. *J. Allergy Clin. Immunol.* **2016**, *138*, 1122–1130. [CrossRef] [PubMed]
74. Rachid, R.A.; Gerber, G.; Li, N.; Umetsu, D.T.; Bry, L.; Chatila, T.A. Food allergy in infancy is associated with dysbiosis of the intestinal microbiota. *J. Allergy Clin. Immunol.* **2016**, *137*, 235. [CrossRef]
75. Savage, J.H.; Lee-Sarwar, K.A.; Sordillo, J.; Bunyavanich, S.; Zhou, Y.; O'Connor, G.; Sandel, M.; Bacharier, L.B.; Zeiger, R.; Sodergren, E.; et al. A prospective microbiome-wide association study of food sensitization and food allergy in early childhood. *Allergy* **2018**, *73*, 145–152. [CrossRef]
76. Azad, M.B.; Konya, T.; Guttman, D.S.; Field, C.J.; Sears, M.R.; HayGlass, K.T.; Mandhane, P.J.; Turvey, S.E.; Subbarao, P.; Becker, A.B.; et al. Infant gut microbiota and food sensitization: Associations in the frst year of life. *Clin. Exp. Allergy* **2015**, *45*, 632–643. [CrossRef] [PubMed]
77. Hua, X.; Goedert, J.J.; Pu, A.; Yu, G.; Shi, J. Allergy associations with the adult fecal microbiota: Analysis of the American Gut Project. *EBioMedicine* **2016**, *3*, 172–179. [CrossRef]
78. Inoue, R.; Sawai, T.; Sawai, C.; Nakatani, M.; Romero-Perez, G.A.; Ozeki, M.; Nonomura, K.; Tsukahara, T. A preliminary study of gut dysbiosis in children with food allergy. *Biosci. Biotechnol. Biochem.* **2017**, *81*, 2396–2399. [CrossRef]
79. Ling, Z.; Li, Z.; Liu, X.; Cheng, Y.; Luo, Y.; Tong, X.; Yuan, L.; Wang, Y.; Sun, J.; Li, L.; et al. Altered fecal microbiota composition associated with food allergy in infants. *Appl. Environ. Microbiol.* **2014**, *80*, 2546–2554. [CrossRef]
80. Chen, C.-C.; Chen, K.-J.; Kong, M.-S.; Chang, H.-J.; Huang, J.-L. Alterations in the gut microbiotas of children with food sensitization in early life. *Pediatr. Allergy Immunol.* **2016**, *27*, 254–262. [CrossRef]
81. Fazlollahi, M.; Chun, Y.; Grishin, A.; Wood, R.A.; Burks, A.W.; Dawson, P.; Jones, S.M.; Leung, D.Y.M.; Sampson, H.A.; Sicherer, S.H.; et al. Early-life gut microbiome and egg allergy. *Allergy* **2018**, *73*, 1515–1524. [CrossRef]
82. Diaz, M.; Guadamuro, L.; Espinosa-Martos, I.; Mancabelli, L.; Jimenez, S.; Molinos-Norniella, C.; Perez-Solis, D.; Milani, C.; Rodriguez, J.M.; Ventura, M.; et al. Microbiota and derived parameters in fecal samples of infants with non-IgE cow's milk protein allergy under a restricted diet. *Nutrients* **2018**, *10*, 1481. [CrossRef]
83. Berni Canani, R.; De Filippis, F.; Nocerino, R.; Paparo, L.; Di Scala, C.; Cosenza, L.; Della Gatta, G.; Calignano, A.; De Caro, C.; Laiola, M.; et al. Gut microbiota composition and butyrate production in children afected by non-IgE-mediated cow's milk allergy. *Sci. Rep.* **2018**, *8*, 12500. [CrossRef] [PubMed]
84. Kourosh, A.; Luna, R.A.; Balderas, M.; Nance, C.; Anagnostou, A.; Devaraj, S.; Davis, C.M. Fecal microbiome signatures are diferent in food-allergic children compared to siblings and healthy children. *Pediatr. Allergy Immunol.* **2018**, *29*, 545–554. [CrossRef]
85. Lanis, J.M.; Alexeev, E.E.; Curtis, V.F.; Kitzenberg, D.A.; Kao, D.J.; Battista, K.D.; Gerich, M.E.; Glover, L.E.; Kominsky, D.J.; Colgan, S.P. Tryptophan metabolite activation of the aryl hydrocarbon receptor regulates IL-10 receptor expression on intestinal epithelia. *Mucosal. Immunol.* **2017**, *10*, 1133–1144. [CrossRef] [PubMed]
86. Tan, J.; McKenzie, C.; Vuillermin, P.J.; Goverse, G.; Vinuesa, C.G.; Mebius, R.E.; Macia, L.; Mackay, C.R. Dietary fiber and bacterial SCFA enhance oral tolerance and protect against food allergy through diverse cellular pathways. *Cell Rep.* **2016**, *15*, 2809–2824. [CrossRef] [PubMed]
87. Jiménez-Saiz, R.; Anipindi, V.C.; Galipeau, H.; Ellenbogen, Y.; Chaudhary, R.; Koenig, J.F.; Gordon, M.E.; Walker, T.D.; Mandur, T.S.; Abed, S.; et al. Microbial Regulation of Enteric Eosinophils and Its Impact on Tissue Remodeling and Th2 Immunity. *Front Immunol.* **2020**, *11*, 155. [CrossRef]
88. Berni Canani, R.; Sangwan, N.; Stefka, A.T.; Nocerino, R.; Paparo, L.; Aitoro, R.; Calignano, A.; Khan, A.A.; Gilbert, J.A.; Nagler, C.R. *Lactobacillus rhamnosus* GG-supplemented formula expands butyrate-producing bacterial strains in food allergic infants. *ISME J.* **2016**, *10*, 742–750. [CrossRef]
89. Tang, M.L.; Ponsonby, A.L.; Orsini, F.; Tey, D.; Robinson, M.; Su, E.L.; Licciardi, P.; Burks, W.; Donath, S. Administration of a probiotic with peanut oral immunotherapy: A randomized trial. *J. Allergy Clin. Immunol.* **2015**, *135*, 737–744. [CrossRef]
90. Cuello-Garcia, C.A.; Brozek, J.L.; Fiocchi, A.; Pawankar, R.; Yepes-Nuñez, J.J.; Terracciano, L.; Gandhi, S.; Agarwal, A.; Zhang, Y.; Schünemann, H.J. Probiotics for the prevention of allergy: A systematic review and meta-analysis of randomized controlled trials. *J. Allergy Clin. Immunol.* **2015**, *136*, 952–961. [CrossRef]
91. André, F.; Veysseyre-Balter, C.; Rousset, H.; Descos, L.; André, C. Exogenous oestrogen as an alternative to food allergy in the aetiology of angioneurotic oedema. *Toxicology* **2003**, *185*, 155–160. [CrossRef]
92. Kara, M.; Beser, O.F.; Konukoglu, D.; Cokugras, H.; Erkan, T.; Kutlu, T.; Cokugras, F.C. The utility of TNF-α, IL-6 and IL-10 in the diagnosis and/or follow-up food allergy. *Allergol. Immunopathol.* **2020**, *48*, 48–55. [CrossRef]
93. Nedelkopoulou, N.; Taparkou, A.; Agakidis, C.; Mavroudi, A.; Xinias, I.; Farmaki, E. IL-10 receptor expression on lymphocytes and monocytes in children with food allergy. *Pediatr. Allergy Immunol.* **2021**, *32*, 1108–1111. [CrossRef] [PubMed]
94. De Martinis, M.; Ginaldi, L.; Sirufo, M.M.; Pioggia, G.; Calapai, G.; Gangemi, S.; Mannucci, C. Alarmins in Osteoporosis, RAGE, IL-1, and IL-33 Pathways: A Literature Review. *Medicina* **2020**, *56*, 138. [CrossRef] [PubMed]

95. Sirufo, M.M.; Suppa, M.; Ginaldi, L.; De Martinis, M. Does Allergy Break Bones? Osteoporosis and Its Connection to Allergy. *Int. J. Mol. Sci.* **2020**, *21*, 712. [CrossRef]
96. De Martinis, M.; Sirufo, M.M.; Suppa, M.; Ginaldi, L. IL-33/IL-31 Axis in Osteoporosis. *Int. J. Mol. Sci.* **2020**, *21*, 1239. [CrossRef]
97. Ginaldi, L.; De Martinis, M.; Saitta, S.; Sirufo, M.M.; Mannucci, C.; Casciaro, M.; Ciccarelli, F.; Gangemi, S. Interleukin-33 serum levels in postmenopausal women with osteoporosis. *Sci. Rep.* **2019**, *9*, 3786. [CrossRef]
98. Narita, S.; Goldblum, R.M.; Watson, C.S.; Brooks, E.G.; Estes, D.M.; Curran, E.M.; Midoro-Horiuti, T. Environmental estrogens induce mast cell degranulation and enhance IgE-mediated release of allergic mediators. *Environ. Health Perspect.* **2007**, *115*, 48–52. [CrossRef]
99. Baker, J.M.; Al-Nakkash, L.; Herbst-Kralovetz, M.M. Estrogen–gut microbiome axis: Physiological and clinical implications. *Maturitas* **2017**, *103*, 45–53. [CrossRef]
100. De Martinis, M.; Sirufo, M.M.; Nocelli, C.; Fontanella, L.; Ginaldi, L. Hyperhomocysteinemia is Associated with Inflammation, Bone Resorption, Vitamin B12 and Folate Deficiency and MTHFR C677T Polymorphism in Postmenopausal Women with Decreased Bone Mineral Density. *Int. J. Environ. Res. Public Health* **2020**, *17*, 4260. [CrossRef]
101. Hussain, M.; Bonilla-Rosso, G.; Kwong Chung, C.K.C.; Bäriswyl, L.; Rodriguez, M.P.; Kim, B.S.; Engel, P.; Noti, M. High dietary fat intake induces a microbiota signature that promotes food allergy. *J. Allergy Clin. Immunol.* **2019**, *144*, 157–170.e8. [CrossRef]
102. Suzuki, S.; Kubota, N.; Kakiyama, S.; Miyazaki, K.; Sato, K.; Harima-Mizusawa, N. Effect of Lactobacillus plantarum YIT 0132 on Japanese cedar pollinosis and regulatory T cells in adults. *Allergy* **2020**, *75*, 453–456. [CrossRef] [PubMed]
103. Lowe, K.E.; Mansfield, K.E.; Delmestri, A.; Smeeth, L.; Roberts, A.; Abuabara, K.; Prieto-Alhambra, D.; Langan, S.M. Atopic eczema and fracture risk in adults: A population-based cohort study. *J. Allergy Clin. Immunol.* **2019**, *145*, 563–571. [CrossRef]
104. Garg, N.; Silverberg, J.I. Association between eczema and increased fracture and bone or joint injury in adults a us population-based study. *JAMA Dermatol.* **2015**, *151*, 33–41. [CrossRef] [PubMed]
105. Chen, Y.W.; Ramsook, A.H.; Coxson, H.O.; Bon, J.; Reid, W.D. Prevalence and Risk Factors for Osteoporosis in Individuals with COPD: A Systematic Review and Meta-analysis. *Chest* **2019**, *156*, 1092–1110. [CrossRef] [PubMed]
106. Ciccarelli, F.; De Martinis, M.; Ginaldi, L. Glucocorticoids in Patients with Rheumatic Diseases: Friends or Enemies of Bone? *Curr. Med. Chem.* **2015**, *22*, 596–603. [CrossRef]
107. Al Anouti, F.; Taha, Z.; Shamim, S.; Khalaf, K.; Al Kaabi, L.; Alsafar, H. An insight into the paradigms of osteoporosis: From genetics to biomechanics. *Bone Rep.* **2019**, *11*, 100216. [CrossRef] [PubMed]
108. Pucci, S.; Incorvaia, C. Allergy as an organ and a systemic disease. *Clin. Exp. Immunol.* **2008**, *153*, 1–2. [CrossRef]
109. Barrick, B.J.; Jalan, S.; Tollefson, M.M.; Milbrandt, T.A.; Larson, A.N.; Rank, M.A.; Lohse, C.M.; Davis, D.M.R. Associations of self-reported allergic diseases and musculoskeletal problems in children: A US population-based study. *Ann. Allergy Asthma Immunol.* **2017**, *119*, 170–176. [CrossRef]
110. Puth, M.T.; Klaschik, M.; Schmid, M.; Weckbecker, K.; Münster, E. Prevalence and comorbidity of osteoporosis- a cross-sectional analysis on 10,660 adults aged 50 years and older in Germany. *BMC Musculoskelet. Disord.* **2018**, *19*, 144. [CrossRef]
111. Adami, G.; Gatti, D.; Rossini, M.; Giollo, A.; Bertoldo, E.; Viapiana, O.; Olivi, P.; Fassio, A. Factors associated with referral for osteoporosis care in men: A real-life study of a nationwide dataset. *Arch. Osteoporos.* **2021**, *16*, 56. [CrossRef]
112. De Martinis, M.; Ginaldi, L.; Sirufo, M.M.; Bassino, E.M.; De Pietro, F.; Pioggia, G.; Gangemi, S. IL-33/Vitamin D Crosstalk in Psoriasis-Associated Osteoporosis. *Front. Immunol.* **2021**, *11*, 604055. [CrossRef]
113. Sardecka-Milewska, I.; Łoś-Rycharska, E.; Gawryjołek, J.; Toporowska-Kowalska, E.; Krogulska, A. Role of FOXP3 Expression and Serum Vitamin D and C Concentrations When Predicting Acquisition of Tolerance in Infants With Cow's Milk Allergy. *J. Investig. Allergol. Clin. Immunol.* **2020**, *30*, 182–190. [CrossRef] [PubMed]
114. Koplin, J.J.; Suaini, N.H.; Vuillermin, P.; Ellis, J.A.; Panjari, M.; Ponsonby, A.L.; Peters, R.L.; Matheson, M.C.; Martino, D.; Dang, T.; et al. Polymorphisms affecting vitamin D-binding protein modify the relationship between serum vitamin D (25[OH]D$_3$) and food allergy. *J. Allergy Clin. Immunol.* **2016**, *137*, 500–506.e4. [CrossRef] [PubMed]
115. Vuillermin, P.J.; Ponsonby, A.L.; Kemp, A.S.; Allen, K.J. Potential links between the emerging risk factors for food allergy and vitamin D status. *Clin. Exp. Allergy* **2013**, *43*, 599–607. [CrossRef]
116. Sirufo, M.M.; Ginaldi, L.; De Martinis, M. Gut microbiota-microRNA interactions in osteoarthritis. *Gene* **2021**, *803*, 145887. [CrossRef]
117. Sirufo, M.M.; Ginaldi, L.; De Martinis, M. Microbiota-miRNA interactions: Opportunities in ankylosing spondylitis. *Autoimmun. Rev.* **2021**, *20*, 102905. [CrossRef]
118. Sirufo, M.; Ginaldi, L.; De Martinis, M. Noncoding RNAs, Osteoarthritis, and the Microbiome: New Therapeutic Targets? *Arthritis Rheumatol.* **2021**, *73*, 2146, Comment on the Article by Wei et al. [CrossRef]
119. Lu, T.X.; Rothenberg, M.E. MicroRNA. *J. Allergy Clin. Immunol.* **2018**, *141*, 1202–1207. [CrossRef]
120. Sirufo, M.M.; Ginaldi, L.; De Martinis, M. MicroRNAs, bone and microbiota. *Bone* **2021**, *144*, 115824. [CrossRef] [PubMed]
121. De Martinis, M.; Ginaldi, L.; Allegra, A.; Sirufo, M.M.; Pioggia, G.; Tonacci, A.; Gangemi, S. The Osteoporosis/Microbiota Linkage: The Role of miRNA. *Int. J. Mol. Sci.* **2020**, *21*, 8887. [CrossRef] [PubMed]
122. Davoodvandi, A.; Marzban, H.; Goleij, P.; Sahebkar, A.; Morshedi, K.; Rezaei, S.; Mahjoubin-Tehran, M.; Tarrahimofrad, H.; Hamblin, M.R.; Mirzaei, H. Effects of therapeutic probiotics on modulation of microRNAs. *Cell Commun. Signal.* **2021**, *19*, 4. [CrossRef] [PubMed]

MDPI
St. Alban-Anlage 66
4052 Basel
Switzerland
Tel. +41 61 683 77 34
Fax +41 61 302 89 18
www.mdpi.com

International Journal of Environmental Research and Public Health Editorial Office
E-mail: ijerph@mdpi.com
www.mdpi.com/journal/ijerph

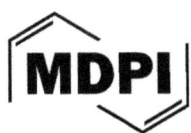

www.ingramcontent.com/pod-product-compliance
Lightning Source LLC
LaVergne TN
LVHW070718100526
838202LV00013B/1117

MDPI
St. Alban-Anlage 66
4052 Basel
Switzerland
Tel. +41 61 683 77 34
Fax +41 61 302 89 18
www.mdpi.com

International Journal of Environmental Research and Public Health Editorial Office
E-mail: ijerph@mdpi.com
www.mdpi.com/journal/ijerph

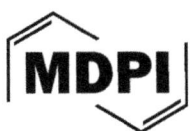